Safe and Effective Gynecological Endoscopic and Minimal Access Surgery

Safe and Effective Gynecological Endoscopic and Minimal Access Surgery

Editor

Prakash H Trivedi MD DGO DNB FCPS
Diploma in Pelvic Surgery, Germany
Advanced Hysteroscopic Surgery, France
Fellowship in ART, Australia
Director of National Institute of Laser and Endoscopic Surgery and Aakar IVF Center
Mumbai, Maharashtra, India
Professor and Head
Department of Obstetrics and Gynecology
Rajawadi Municipal Hospital
Mumbai, Maharashtra, India
Gynecological Endoscopist and Urogynecologist and Advanced Infertility Consultant
Jaslok and Bhabha Atomic Research Centre (BARC) Hospital
Mumbai, Maharashtra, India

Forewords
Mahendra Parikh
PK Shah

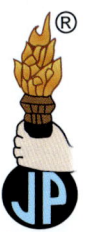

JAYPEE BROTHERS MEDICAL PUBLISHERS (P) LTD
New Delhi • Panama City • London

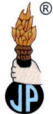 **Jaypee Brothers Medical Publishers (P) Ltd**

Headquarter

Jaypee Brothers Medical Publishers (P) Ltd
4838/24, Ansari Road, Daryaganj
New Delhi 110 002, India
Phone: +91-11-43574357
Fax: +91-11-43574314
Email: jaypee@jaypeebrothers.com

Overseas Offices

J.P. Medical Ltd.
83 Victoria Street, London
SW1H 0HW (UK)
Phone: +44-2031708910
Fax: +02-03-0086180
Email: info@jpmedpub.com

Jaypee-Highlights medical publishers Inc.
City of Knowledge, Bld. 237, Clayton
Panama City, Panama
Phone: +507-301-0496
Fax: +507-301-0499
Email: cservice@jphmedical.com

Website: www.jaypeebrothers.com
Website: www.jaypeedigital.com

© 2012, Jaypee Brothers Medical Publishers

All rights reserved. No part of this book may be reproduced in any form or by any means without the prior permission of the publisher.

Inquiries for bulk sales may be solicited at: jaypee@jaypeebrothers.com

This book has been published in good faith that the contents provided by the contributors contained herein are original, and is intended for educational purposes only. While every effort is made to ensure accuracy of information, the publisher and the editor specifically disclaim any damage, liability, or loss incurred, directly or indirectly, from the use or application of any of the contents of this work. If not specifically stated, all figures and tables are courtesy of the editor. Where appropriate, the readers should consult with a specialist or contact the manufacturer of the drug or device.

Safe and Effective Gynecological Endoscopic and Minimal Access Surgery

First Edition: **2012**

ISBN 978-93-5025-583-4

Printed at Replika Press Pvt. Ltd.

Dedicated to

All those learners, who irrespective of age or status, from small or big place, who have endless faith in our efforts, commitment; their love, affection and appreciation drive us to write what is relevant today and needed for future to enhance skill as learning never ends.

The theme: Best patient care and safety is the single most important benchmark for progress

Contributors

Prakash H Trivedi MD DGO DNB FCPS
Diploma in Pelvic Surgery, Germany
Advanced Hysteroscopic Surgery, France
Fellowship in ART, Australia
Director of National Institute of Laser and Endoscopic Surgery and Aakar IVF Centre
Mumbai, Maharashtra, India
Professor and Head
Department of Obstetrics and Gynecology
Rajawadi Municipal Hospital
Mumbai, Maharashtra, India
Gynecological Endoscopist and Urogynecologist and Advanced Infertility Consultant
Jaslok and Bhabha Atomic Research Centre (BARC) Hospital, Mumbai, Maharashtra, India

PG Paul
Paul's Hospital
Kochi, Kerala, India

Co-authors
Indranil Chaudhuri, Shreevidya G, Anita Budania, Pravin Thakare
Paul's Hospital
Kochi, Kerala, India

Dinesh Bajani MD DA
Specialized in Anesthesia for Endoscopic Surgery
Mumbai, Maharashtra, India

Gopinath N Shenoy MD LLM
PhD (Law) DGO DFP FCPS MNAMS
KJ Somaiya Medical College
Mumbai, Maharashtra, India

Ajay Rane MBBS MSc MD FRCS FRCOG FRANZCOG CU FICOG (Hon)
Chair and Head
Department of Obstetrics and Gynaecology
James Cook University
Consultant Urogynaecologist
Mater Pelvic Health Education and Research Unit and Townsville Hospital
Townsville, Queensland, Australia

Jay Iyer MBBS MD DNB MRCOG FRANZCOG
Senior Lecturer
Department of Obstetrics and Gynaecology
James Cook University
Consultant Obstetrician and Gynaecologist
Mater Pelvic Health Education and Research Unit and Townsville Hospital, Townsville, Queensland, Australia

Deepika Desai MD DA
Specialized in Anesthesia for Endoscopic Surgery, Mumbai, Maharashtra, India

Shyam V Desai MD DGO DFP FCPS MNAMS
Endoscopist, Obstetrician and Gynecologist
Mumbai, Maharashtra, India

S Krishnakumar
Kumars' Maternity and Surgical Nursing Home, Dombivli, Nirmiti Fertility and IVF Center, Thane, Mumbai, Maharashtra, India
Fortis Hospitals
Mumbai, Maharashtra, India

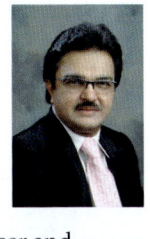
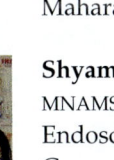
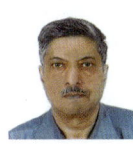
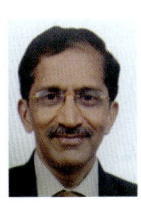

Pravin Patel
Director
Pulse Women's Hospital
Pulse Women's Hospital Pvt Ltd
Ahmedabad, Gujarat, India

Co-authors
**Manish Bankar, Sujal Munshi,
Dipesh Sorathia**

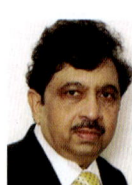

Mahendra Borse
Gynecological Endoscopist
Dinanath Mangeshkar Hospital
Pune, Maharashtra, India

Aditi Singhi
Consultant Obstetrician, Gynecologist, Endoscopic Surgeon and Infertility Specialist
Godrej Memorial Hospital Research Centre and The Apollo Clinic, Mumbai, Maharashtra, India

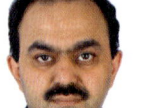

Atul Ganatra
Obstetrician Gynaecologist and Endoscopist
Ganatra Nursing Home, Fortis, HMN and Gurunanak Hospital

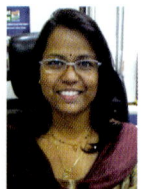

Maya Prasad
ICOG Certificate Course, NILES and Aakar IVF, ICSI Centre, Mumbai, Maharashtra, India

Sunita Tandulwadkar MD FICS
FICOG
Diploma in Endoscopy
Head of Department
Department of Obstetrics and Gynecology
Chief, IVF and Endoscopy Centre, Ruby Hall Clinic, Pune, Maharashtra, India

Co-authors
Rahul Gore, Pooja Lodha, Anuja Joshi

B Ramesh
Endoscopist and Infertility Consultant, Bengaluru, Karnataka, India

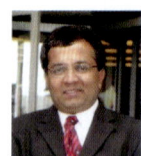

Sanjay Patel MD
Diploma in Endoscopy, Germany
Director, Mayflower Women's Hospital Ahmedabad, Gujarat, India
Endoscopic Surgeon Infertility and IVF Specialist

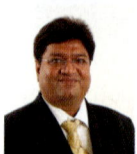

Pandit Palaskar
Deogiri Nursing Home
Aurangabad, Maharashtra, India

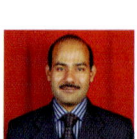

Anthony Lewis
Ex-Senior Technologist (OT)
Jaslok Hospital and Research Centre, Mumbai, Maharashtra, India

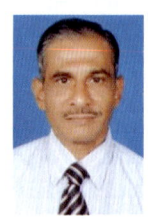

Shaily Jain
Clinical Assistant, NILES and Aakar IVF, ICSI Centre
Mumbai, Maharashtra, India

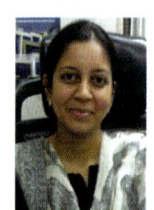

Neha Rani
ICOG Certificate Course, NILES and Aakar IVF, ICSI Centre
Mumbai, Maharashtra, India

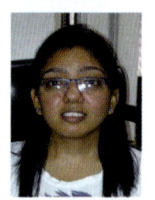

BV Bharathi
Endoscopist, B Ramesh Hospital
Bengaluru, Karnataka, India

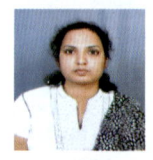

Anjali Gupta
ICOG Certificate Course, NILES and Aakar IVF, ICSI Centre
Mumbai, Maharashtra, India

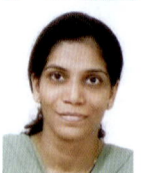

Foreword

There is no drug without side effects;
there is no surgery without complications.

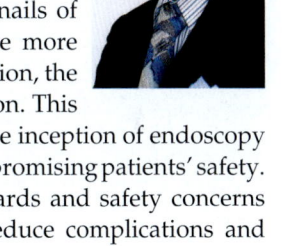

Endoscopic surgery is well entrenched in gynecological practice. In many situations, it is the best option. With proper selection and skilled execution, it is optimum care for the patient. Many books are available emphasizing the efficacy of endoscopic surgery. This outstanding book additionally focuses on the safety of endoscopic surgery.

No surgical procedure is free from complications. If you pare the nails of a thousand persons, the occasional ones will develop paronychia. The more complex a surgical procedure and higher the skill demanded in its execution, the greater the possibility of something going wrong ending in a complication. This applies to any surgery. Endoscopic surgery is no exception. Ever since the inception of endoscopy when it was a mere diagnostic tool, endoscopists faced complications compromising patients' safety. As endoscopic surgeries became more and more complicated, the hazards and safety concerns grew exponentially. Endoscopic surgeons are perpetually trying to reduce complications and make surgery safer by adequate training, acquiring experience, developing skills and employing better instruments and technology. Three pillars of safe surgery are good training, use of proper equipment and dedication to patient safety.

Professor Prakash H Trivedi is a master Endoscopist, ideal Teacher, and a prolific medical Writer with numerous publications and many books to his credit. His present book deals with all aspects of each and every endoscopic surgery. But in addition, it especially deals with prevention of every possible complication that can occur compromising patients' safety. It is remarkable that he is able to get the topmost experts in endoscopic surgery to spare their precious time to contribute valuable chapters to this book. The writing is simple but efficient and is well supported by excellent photographs. Every endoscopist, beginner or expert, will find this book very useful and indispensible. I congratulate Dr Trivedi on producing a much-needed authentic book which like his earlier books is sure to become highly successful. Lastly, we must remember that even a great surgeon is capable of doing anything wrongly and compromising patient care.

Mahendra Parikh
Professor Emeritus
Nowrosjee Wadia Maternity Hospital
Past President
Indian Association of Gynaecological Endoscopists
Editor Emeritus
The Journal of Obstetrics and Gynecology of India

Foreword

Words that enlighten are more precious than jewels

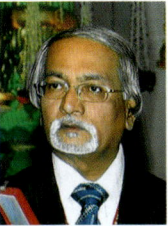

It is indeed my great pleasure to write the foreword of the book *Safe and Effective Gynecological Endoscopic and Minimal Access Surgery* edited by a person, whom I have known for more than two decades. Even as a student, he had an unusual flare, supreme confidence and different method of expressing the knowledge which convinced people and developed an improbable faith in his abilities. I have witnessed the release of some of his outstanding books with involvement of best talents from various countries. The contents express his relentless passion of sharing accurate knowledge, the flame of that candle— Dr Prakash H Trivedi has spread light of knowledge to young and old in all corners.

The contents of this book and the experts involved in contribution have been meticulous and precise to the need of the hour. In this year, when I am the president of Indian Association of Gynecological Endoscopy, I feel if there was any time when such a book was to be released, then, this is the right time.

There are pioneers who are extraordinarily skilled, some who are immensely popular but very few cross all the barriers set as benchmark as the most productive skilled intellectuals when, they convert their knowledge, skills, values and commitment as a responsibility which they owe towards their patients and peers, one of them is Dr Trivedi.

I am sure you will enjoy and enrich by reading this book as I enjoyed writing this foreword. May God bless him and his passion and relentless efforts.

PK Shah
President
Indian Association of Gynaecological Endoscopy
President Elect-FOGSI
Professor and Head
Unit Obstetrics and Gynecology, KEM Hospital
Mumbai, Maharashtra, India

Preface

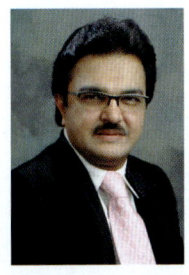

In today's time, it is not possible for a person who is busy in private practice with multiple superspecialities, is a part of major organization or society which deals with health care to come up periodically with books which are relevant, keeping future insight.

Endoscopy and minimal access surgery are done in every corner of world with skills and experience of the surgeon's varying. Access to instruments, technologies is no more difficult, to get patients for defined purpose is also possible, but to have a keen sense of patient's safety, understanding the problems in different situation needs decades of experience.

A desire to share their expertise, skill and knowledge are left with very few. We have a bunch of committed contributors who give their unselfish donations of time and pen down chapters with practical values that go a long way in today's knowledge-based society. In this book, an attempt is made by such contributors to focus on the patient's safety for gynecological endoscopist and minimal access surgery.

I am sure that this effort of ours will make all readers; whether experts or amateurs, interested or disliking endoscopic surgery, shift to a virtual set-up with a feeling of 'de-ja-vu', saying 'Yes these are the problems we face!' The experts have precisely clarified those points which make, gynecological endoscopy and minimal access surgery, safe and effective.

I am indebted to all the contributors, and the team of young, mature and enthusiastic doctors working with us—Dr Maya Prasad, Dr Shaily Jain, Dr Neha Rani, Dr Anjali Gupta, Dr Sachin Bhosale, Dr Manpreet Patel and Ms Riddhi Kapadia, who have helped me to make each chapter more specific. I owe every academic contribution of mine to every learning readers and especially my wife Priti and son Soumil who keep igniting my relentless passion to share with responsibilities which never dies.

Prakash H Trivedi

Acknowledgments

We are indebted to all the eminent contributors, and the team of young, mature and enthusiastic gynecologists working with us, Dr Maya Prasad, Dr Shaily Jain, Dr Neha Rani, Dr Anjali Gupta, Dr Sachin Bhosale, Dr Manpreet Patel and Ms Riddhi Kapadia, Mr CM Chhabra who have helped me to make each chapter more specific. I especially thank my wife Priti and son Soumil who keep igniting my relentless passion to share with responsibilities which never dies. Finally, I owe every academic contribution of mine to every learning reader and our followers.

Contents

1. **Is Safety an Option or Necessity in Endoscopic Surgery?** 1
   Prakash H Trivedi

   Philosophy 1

2. **Operation Theater Set-up for Safe Gynecological Endoscopy** 3
   PG Paul

   Operating Theater 3
   Postanesthesia Care Unit 5
   Operation Theater Set-up 6
   Operation Table 6
   Video Monitors 7
   Static Posture 7
   Laparoscopic Vision—Limited View 7
   Less Efficient Instruments 8
   Surgeon's Fatigue 8
   Record Keeping 8

3. **Selecting Optimum Instruments for Safe Gynecological Endoscopic Surgery** 10
   Aditi Singhi

   Major Equipment for Laparoscopy and Hysteroscopy 10
   Laparoscopy Instruments 13
   Newer Instruments 21
   Hysteroscopy Instruments 21

4. **Patient Selection for Gynecological Endoscopic Surgery to Make it Safe** 24
   Atul Ganatra, Maya Prasad

   Background 24
   Problem 24
   Relevant Anatomy 25
   Umbilicus 25
   Endoscopic Surgery—A Rule 26
   Ectopic Pregnancy 26
   Management of Ectopic Pregnancy 26
   Tubal Factor 27
   Proximal Tubal Occlusion 27
   Intrauterine Adhesions 28
   Uterine Anatomical Defects 28
   Hysteroscopic Myomectomy 30
   Ovarian Cysts 31
   Fibroids 31
   Endometriosis 32
   Postmenopausal Bleeding 32
   Miscellaneous 32

5. **Safe Anesthesia for Gynecological Endoscopic Surgery** 35
   Dinesh Bajani, Deepika Desai

   Anesthesia for Hysteroscopy   35
   Anesthetic Management   36
   Anesthesia for Gynecological Laparoscopic Surgery   36
   Complications   37
   Problems   39
   Anesthesia Management   40

6. **Operative Laparoscopic Surgery Step by Step for Achieving Safety** 42
   Shaily Jain

   Interaction with Patient and Proper Consent   42
   The Beginning of the Surgery   44
   Introduction of Veress Needle and Trocars   47
   New Energy Sources, Vessel Sealing Devices a Brief Clear Concept   49
   Golden Rules of Each Person in Endoscopic Surgery   50
   Documentation and Explaining Patients After Surgery   51

7. **Making Laparoscopic Myomectomy Safe** 52
   Sunita Tandulwadkar

   Practical Tips of Myomectomy   52
   Strengthening of Myoma Scar   56

8. **Ectopic Pregnancy: How to Make it Safe for Patient, Tubes and Fertility** 58
   Pandit Palaskar

   Etiology of Ectopic Pregnancy   58
   Conservative Medical Therapy of Ectopic Pregnancy   60
   Surgical Management   60
   Comparison of Surgical and Medical Therapy   64

9. **How to Make Laparoscopic Surgery Safe for Advanced Endometriosis** 70
   PG Paul

   Preoperative Assessment   70
   Technique   70
   Mild Endometriosis   71
   Moderate to Severe Endometriosis   71
   Correction of Retroflexion of Uterus   72
   Salpingo-ovariolysis   72
   Cystectomy   74

10. **How to Make Total Laparoscopic Hysterectomy Safe?** 78
    Prakash H Trivedi, Shaily Jain

    Indications of Laparoscopic Hysterectomy   78
    Philosophy of Patient's Safety in Laparoscopic Hysterectomy   79
    Contraindication for Laparoscopic Hysterectomy   79
    Debulking of Uterus   83

11. **Safe Laparoscopic Surgery for Prolapse in Young Patient and Vault Prolapse** 89
    Pravin Patel

    Preoperative Preparations   89
    Surgical Technique   90
    Anterior   90
    Uterine Prolapse   91
    Sacrocervicopexy   91
    Vaginal Vault Prolapse   91

Sacrocolpopexy 92
Enterocele 93
Complications 93

12. Laparoscopic Adenomyomectomy 96
Sanjay Patel

Transvaginal Ultrasonography 96
Adenoma on Laparoscopy 97
Adenoma on Hysteroscopy 97
Coexisting Pathologies 97
Preoperative Adenoma Mapping 99
Aim of Adenoma Resection 99
Technique of Adenomyoma Resection 99
Technique of Endosuturing: Intracorporeal Slip Knot Technique 100

13. Safe and Efficient Laparoscopic Suturing 104
Mahendra Borse

Patient's Position 104
Instruments 104
Port Placement 105
Needle Insertion 106
Ipsilateral Suturing 107
Contralateral Suturing 108
Needle Removal 108
The Art of Camera Holding 108
Needles 108
Suture Material 108
Barbed Suture 109
Microsurgery 110
Extracorporeal Knot 110

14. Hysteroscopy—An Art to Achieve Excellence with Safety 112
S Krishnakumar

Hysteroscopic Anatomy of the Uterus 112
Distending Media for Hysteroscopy 113
Distending Media Delivery 114
Technique of Panoramic Hysteroscopy 117
Procedures (Technical Nuances) 118
Metroplasty 118
Lateral Metroplasty 120
Lysis of Intrauterine Adhesions 120
Leiomyomas and Endometrial Polyps 120
Endometrial Resection (TCRE) 122
Complications and Prevention 122
Do's and Dont's in Hysteroscopic Surgery 124

15. Safe Management of Female Urinary Incontinence 126
Prakash H Trivedi, Maya Prasad, Neha Rani

Magnitude of the Problem 126
Safety Points for Laparoscopic Burch 127
Trivedi's Adjustable Tape 131

16. Performing Safe Multicompartment Mesh Replacement Surgery 134
Ajay Rane, Jay Iyer

General Considerations for Mesh Surgery 134
Mesh Extrusions/Erosions/Sexual Dysfunction 138
Specific Considerations for Mesh Surgery 138

17. **Training and Credentialing in Endoscopic Surgery** 141
    Shyam V Desai

    Objectives of a Training Program   141
    Course Contents   143

18. **Conquering Complications of Laparoscopic and Urogynecologic Minimal Access Surgery to Make it Safe for Patients** 147
    Prakash H Trivedi, Shaily Jain, Anjali Gupta

    Complications of Veress Needle   147
    Complications of Trocar-cannula   148
    Electrosurgical/Cautery Complications   150
    Bleeding and Poor Hemostasis   151
    Technical Complications with Instruments   152
    Conversion to Open Surgery   153
    Medical, Anesthesia or Non-gynecological Reasons   154

19. **Resist Temptation or to Try New Techniques for Experience Before Evidence** 155
    B Ramesh, BV Bharathi

    Is SILS Future of Minimally Invasive Surgery   155
    Vessel Sealing Devices   156
    Barbed Sutures   157
    Morcellators: Gynecare vs RotoCut G1   159
    Stress Urinary Incontinence   159
    Company Pressure/Temptation   160

20. **How to Make Ambulatory Endoscopist's Surgery Safe?** 163
    Prakash H Trivedi, Neha Rani, Anjali Gupta

    Consent, Expectation and Counseling   163
    Complications   165
    Deficiency   165
    Medicolegal Aspects—Mortality, etc.   166

21. **Maintenance and Sterilization of Endoscopic and Minimal Access Surgery Instruments and Equipment** 167
    Anthony Lewis

    Maintenance and Sterilization   167
    Carrying Steam Sterilized Instruments Outside the Hospital   169

22. **Medical Law—What is What and What is not Medical Negligence** 172
    Gopinath N Shenoy

    Negligence and Rashness   172
    Standard or Degree of Skill and Care   173
    Criminal Negligence   173
    Accidents; Misadventures; Mishaps   174
    Error of Judgment   174
    Inherent Risks of Treatment   174
    Choice of Treatment—Discretion   174
    Guarantee and Warranty   175
    Vicarious Liability   175
    Deficiencies in Statutory Requirements   175

Index 177

CHAPTER 1

Is Safety an Option or Necessity in Endoscopic Surgery?

Prakash H Trivedi

Chapter Outline
- Philosophy

*"Talents hits a target no one else can hit,
Genius hits a target, no one else can see"*

PHILOSOPHY

Endoscopic surgery came with promises beyond the expectations of the instruments and skills of surgeons especially in gynecology where pathologies are diverse. Vaginal surgeries in the hands of experts are safe and so are abdominal surgeries, but they have their own share of complications.

As endoscopic surgery is and was viewed to be competing and replacing open surgery, a resistance from gynecologist and surgeon was obvious, which was overcome by tall claims made by few endoscopic surgeon, but the truth lies 'in-between'.

In the hands of expert, endoscopic or vaginal surgery is less invasive than open surgery. However, if every endoscopist feels he/she is the expert endoscopist or every gynecologists feels he/she is a great vaginal surgeon, this gives the patient a false expectation that except miracles no complication can take place with gynecological endoscopy and minimal access surgery.

Thus, it becomes imperative that safety is a necessity and not an option in gynecological endoscopic and minimal access surgery.

The pioneers of gynecological endoscopic surgery in world and in India have spent sffi-cient unselfish donation of time to enhance their skills, increase their knowledge and also give faster recovery to the patient promising safety. Simultaneously the assistants, anesthetist, operation theater staff also had to upgrade their standards of understanding new technology, equipment, limitations and difficulties of each surgery in this group.

"Habits are safer than rules you don't have to watch them or keep them either. They keep you."

Further a gynecological endoscopist needs to be organized and also a good conventional surgeon, otherwise having great instruments in their hands, can expose only their limitations, problems or inability to convince the observing gynecologist, surgeon, urologist and patients.

The fear of safety and longer duration of advanced endoscopic surgery prevented thousands of skilled gynecologists and surgeons not to venture into a never ending exciting field of gynecologist endoscopy and minimal access surgery.

"Be not afraid of growing slowly, be afraid of standing still. Minds are like parachutes they work best when open".

These new surgeries also glamorized the younger group of average surgeons and gynecologists to take upon endoscopic or minimal access surgery beyond their capacity. Thus, to run down good endoscopic surgery became easy, but as this is the true consumer driven advance on demand of patients either the gynecologist themselves had to do the surgeries or call somebody else to do at their own place. The biggest groups are fertility enhancing endoscopic surgery, benign gynecological pathology, myomectomy, hysterectomy, urinary incontinence surgery. Thus, many gynecologists (but not all) could pick up good cases for gynecological endoscopic surgery in their own center for a visiting expert. The lacuna it created was a gap between the requirements of proper instruments and assistants in many operation theaters in addition to cutting-cost and corners. The meticulous endoscopist overcame this by carrying their own instruments, expert assistants or even operation theater staff.

A phenomenal number of live endoscopic and minimal access surgery made these surgeries reach into the heart and minds of patient and doctors. Hence, person from smaller places and smaller center with skills could match the expectations.

However, universal application of these techniques by poorly trained surgeon or one with inadequate experience always added catastrophic proportion of morbidity or mortality.

As endoscopic surgery is seen on a big screen surgeons skills were observed, whereas few were fanatic about the timings, few about the number of cases, weights, sizes, number of ports, multiple conventional ports or single port or single incision multiple ports and few accepting any new technology before even evidence proved their superiority of safety.

To add fuel to fire the companies promoted products through good role model gynecologists and surgeons, few experts withhold this temptation but many fell for 'me-first' philosophy.

Gynecological endoscopy and minimal access surgery today in India, is poised on the gateway of excellence in the hand of skilled experienced endoscopist with outstanding safety, yet the neoendoscopist trying to cross the gates in hurry to prove the supremacy of success in a short-time fell into an equal division of achieving and others complicating.

In summary, as India is blessed by skilled vaginal, abdominal, laparoscopic, hysteroscopic and urogynecological surgeons, its imperative for a surgeon ensuing this as a superspeciality to do proper course of training, not only from one center but more than one expert, not only mastering one or two common surgeries but the wide plethora which gynecology provides safely.

After more than two decades of endoscopic surgery in India, now you have to remember about a silent friend and admirer who is impressed with everything you do—he slips in your consulting room impressed with your power of convincing patient for right surgery, meticulous investigations, sonography, proper counseling you do, he also in present prior to your talk to the relatives before starting surgery. In operation theater he watches and admires your set up, team, anesthetists, and your own mastery to show excellence in even difficult cases or handling crisis. After the surgery he is your shadow when you explain patients and relatives about how the surgery went, what postoperative care they should take in the hospital and at home. Restriction, if any of food, bath, walk, resumption of work and when to aim at desired outcome like pregnancy. He is most impressed with your DVDs, photo demonstrations, books, teaching DVD's, busy schedules.

You always wonder why he is not seen, but the moment you affect the safety, morbidity or mortality of the patient he makes his appearance felt and that's the lawyer. So, if you want to take chance keep safety as an option but if you want to deliver the best keep safety as necessity in gynecological endoscopy and minimal access surgery. It's the mind that stimulates you to do new surgery, it's your hands which develops the skills, it's your heart which is concerned about safety to the patient and it's the soul which tells you that you have succeeded in the endeavor finally.

"Ability is what you are capable of doing, motivation determines what you can do, attitude determines how well you do it, and courage is grace under pressure".

CHAPTER 2

Operation Theater Set-up for Safe Gynecological Endoscopy

PG Paul

Chapter Outline

- Operating Theater
- Postanesthesia Care Unit
- Operation Theater Set-up
  - Surgical Team
  - Instrument Cart
- Operation Table
- Video Monitors
  - Suction Irrigation Equipment
  - Ergonomics in Laparoscopy
- Static Posture
- Laparoscopic Vision—Limited View
- Less Efficient Instruments
  - Fixed Ports, Longer Instrument and Fulcrum Action
  - Equipment Organization
- Surgeon's Fatigue
- Record Keeping

INTRODUCTION

Operative laparoscopy and hysteroscopy have become an integral part of gynecological surgery. Endoscopic surgery needs a number of gadgets like monitors, camera, insufflators, light generator, etc. It also needs extra space for gas cylinders, cables, tubing and suction irrigation system. Majority of gynecologists perform endoscopic surgeries in their regular gynecological operation theater which is not designed for endoscopic surgery. Naturally there is overcrowding of equipments in a chaotic manner. Inappropriate use of these equipments can result in operative inefficiencies and safety problems for both patients and staff. Proper operation theater set-up, use of appropriate equipment and techniques can greatly add to patient's safety and satisfaction. The aim of this article is to give general idea about setting up an operation theater for safe gynecological endoscopic surgery.

OPERATING THEATER

An organized and well equipped operating theater is essential for successful laparoscopic surgery. The set-up should be designed to optimize efficiency using a team concept.

The operating room should be sufficiently large to accommodate a variety of equipments, preferably 20 × 20 feet (**Fig. 2.1**). Smaller cent-

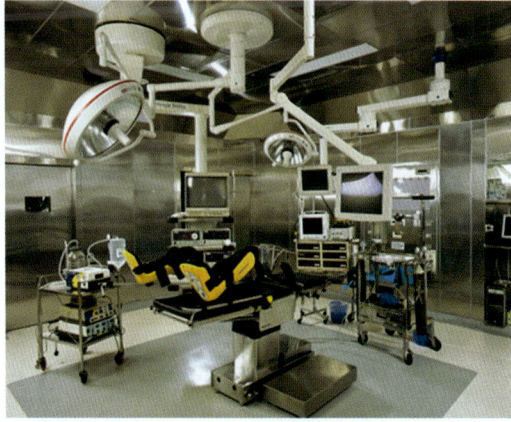

Fig. 2.1: Operation theater

ers can manage with a 15 × 15 feet room. Ceiling mounted instrument carts avoid gas tubing and electrical wires on the floor. Modern operation theater needs false ceiling for installing the operation theater lights, ceiling mounted instrument carts and plenum type air conditioning. So room height should be at least 12 feet to provide space for the false ceiling.[1]

Operation theater walls and floor should be washable, scrubable and nonpermeable. Epoxy coating is suitable for this purpose. But if the walls have a potential to get wet, epoxy coating can bleb or peel off. Steel or aluminum paneling with sealed joints are suitable in these situations. We have used epoxy on the floor, steel paneling of the walls and roof in one operation theater. Other operation theater have epoxy floor, polyurethane coating on the walls and steel false-roof. The floor and the wall should not meet at right angles, as this creates an area that is difficult to clean. Rather, the floor should continue seamlessly up the wall for 4 to 6 inches **(Fig. 2.2)**. The door size is also very important. It should be large enough to allow a patient bed to be brought in. Two-part door with large main door and smaller second door works well because the entry way can be enlarged when needed **(Fig. 2.3)**. Sliding automatic doors are ideal.

Central air conditioning is the most suitable one for operating theater. There should be at least 15 air changes per hour; at least three of these exchanges should be fresh outdoor air. The air supply should be from the ceiling near the center of working area. Fitting HEPA filters at the air supply give cleaner air. The return air outlet must be from the floor level. There should be at least 2 return outlets located as remotely from each other.

There should be enough number of electrical plugs on the walls. UPS plug sockets should be of different design, so that, it is easily identifiable. All endoscopy equipments, anesthesia monitors should be supplied by UPS, so that, surgery will not be interrupted during generator change over. The operating theatre lights should have independent switches so that some can be turned off during endoscopic surgery.

Anesthesia gases should be brought to the operation theater through pipes. There should be at least two oxygen, one nitrous oxide, two vacuum outlets, and one air outlet available at the head of the table. There are different methods by which gas connections can be brought to the room. The options include wall outlets, fixed columns or multiservice articulated arms **(Figs 2.4 and 2.5)**. Carbon dioxide and vacuum

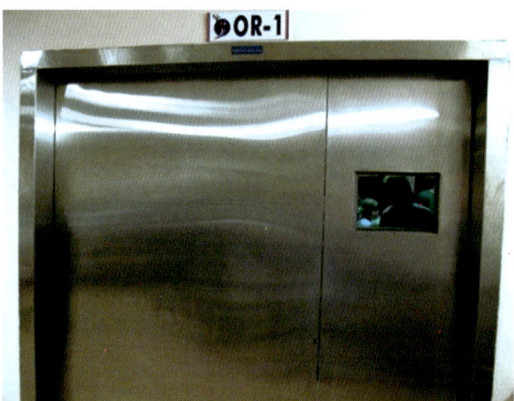

Fig. 2.3: Two-part door

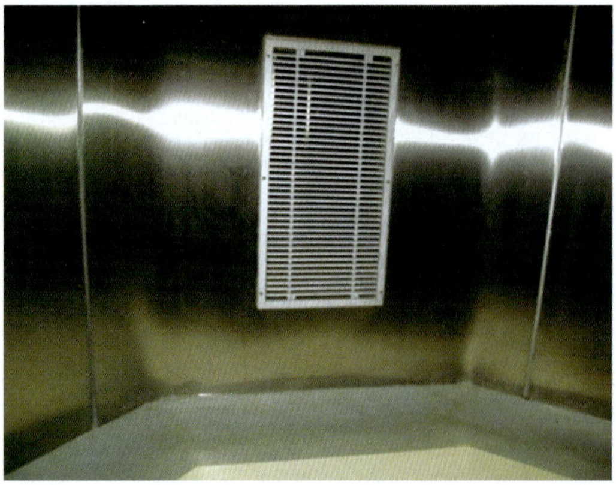

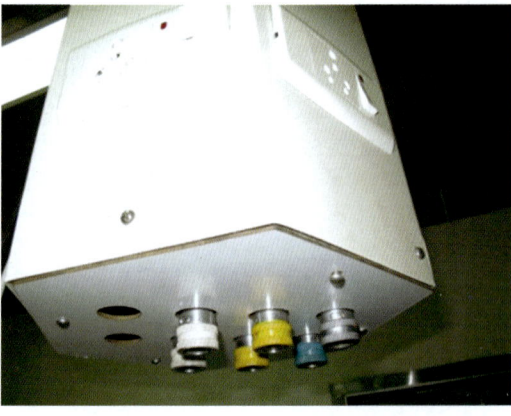

Fig. 2.2: Seamless corners

Fig. 2.4: Fixed column gas outlet

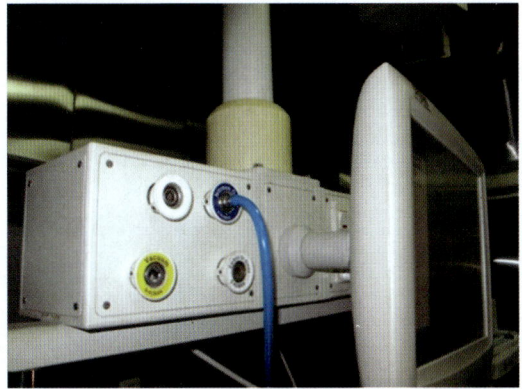

Fig. 2.5: Anesthesia pendent

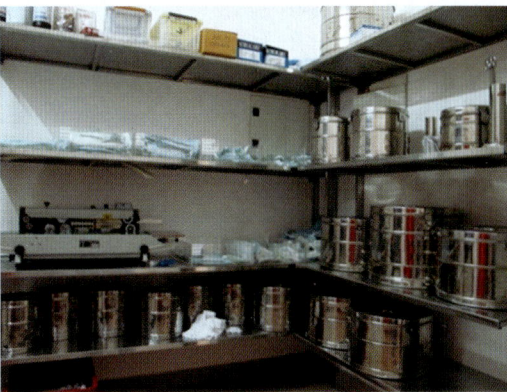

Fig. 2.8: Sterile store station

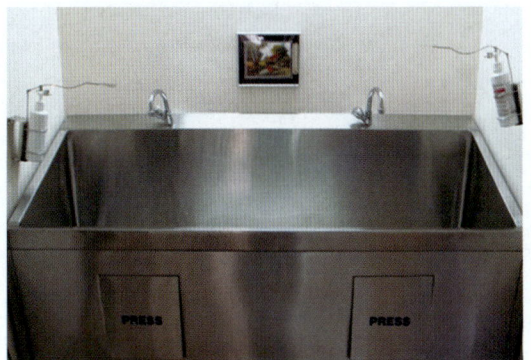

Fig. 2.6: Knee operated scrub sink

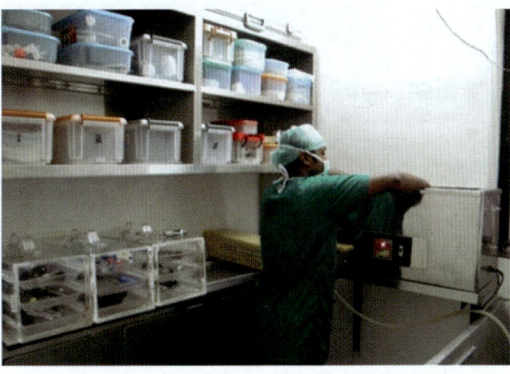

Fig. 2.9: Endoscope cleaning and storing

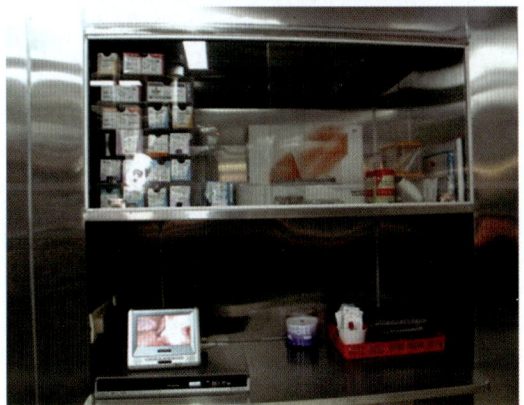

Fig. 2.7: Storage inside the operation theater

outlets should be available on the equipment pendent or trolley. This avoids bringing a carbon dioxide cylinder in the operation theater for the insufflators.

Different types of scrub sinks are available. Knee operated or sensors with timers are available **(Fig. 2.6)**. It can be located between two operation theaters.

Storage space is one of the most important requirements for modern operating room. Only few items like sutures, meshes and essential disposables are kept in the operation theater **(Fig. 2.7)**. Other sterile items are kept in the adjacent room **(Fig. 2.8)**. Cleaning and disinfection of telescopes and hand instruments are done in the intervening room between two operation theaters **(Fig. 2.9)**. These delicate instruments are not mixed with the open surgery instruments in the regular cleaning area.

POSTANESTHESIA CARE UNIT

This room is kept adjacent to the operation theater because it provides instant access to essential resources and equipments **(Fig. 2.10)**. Moreover anesthesiologist and surgeon can supervise the operated patients. The number of beds depends

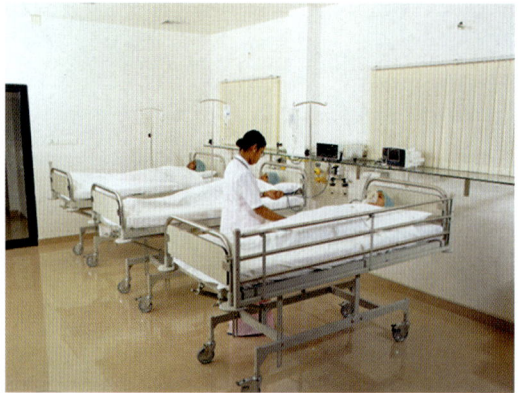

Fig. 2.10: Postanesthesia care unit

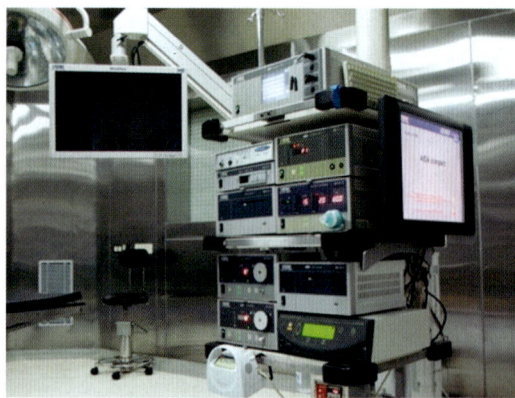

Fig. 2.12: Ceiling mounted instrument carts

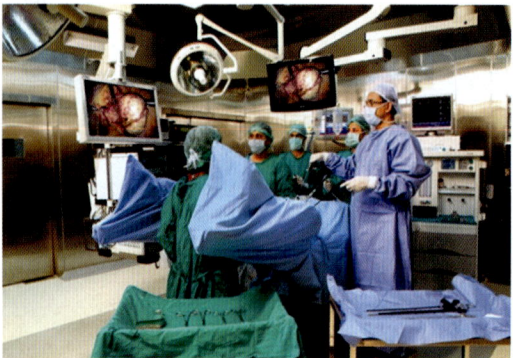

Fig. 2.11: Laparoscopy team

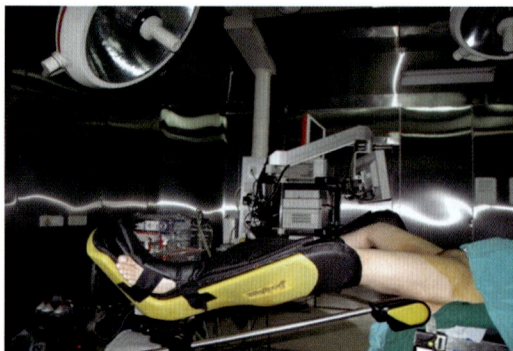

Fig. 2.13: Patient positioning

on the average number of surgeries performed on a day.

OPERATION THEATER SET-UP

Surgical Team

Surgeon and assistant view the ceiling mounted high definition digital monitor placed at the foot end of the table on the right side **(Fig. 2.11)**. The operation theater nurse standing between the legs of the patient views the ceiling mounted digital monitor at the head end of the patient. One trolley for vaginal instruments kept at the leg end of the patient and another for laparoscopy instruments.[2]

Instrument Cart

The hardware laparoscopy equipments are usually kept on a mobile cart. Electrical cables, gas and suction irrigation tubing on the floor make it very difficult to move. The instrument panels should always be visible to the surgeon for safe surgery. The ceiling mounted instrument cart is very convenient although costly. Our instrument cart has a Diathermy (Autocon II 400), Enseal, Image 1HD digital camera, AIDA video capturing system, Morcellator, carbon dioxide insufflators, Xenon light sources, Harmonic generator, SCB computer for controlling the equipments remotely and pneumatic sequential compression device for DVT prevention **(Fig. 2.12)**.

OPERATION TABLE

The patient is positioned in a semilithotomy position. The legs must be properly padded and supported. The legs are positioned in such a way that the thigh makes 160 degree with the abdomen. This will allow free movement of operating instruments. The modern stirrups like OR direct allow easy positioning of legs by the surgeon **(Fig. 2.13)**.

The table should have capabilities for at least 45 degrees Trendelenburg and reverse Trendelenburg position, preferably motorized. The height of the table should be in the lowest position so that, the patient's abdomen is below the waist of the surgeon. Short surgeons may still need stepping stools to achieve this.

VIDEO MONITORS

The quality of the surgery image depends not only on camera but monitor also. Monitor resolution should be equal to that of the camera for best picture quality. 14 and 20-inch size monitors are commonly used. High Definition digital LCD monitors are easier to handle **(Fig. 2.14)**. Digital cameras have DVI output and this can be connected to the LCD monitors with DVI/HDMI cable. LCD televisions (HD or HD ready) are cheaper alternatives to medical grade LCD monitors. They have S-Video and HDMI inputs and depending on the type of camera any of these connections can be used.

Suction Irrigation Equipment

There are different types of pumps to deliver the fluid for irrigation. Some of them pressurize the saline bottle with air to get a jet of fluid. They are usually noisy. We prefer to use a peristaltic pump which works only when the irrigation is used. This type of pumps allows the saline bottle to remain warm in the fluid warmer **(Fig. 2.14)**. Peristaltic pump can be used for both hysteroscopy and laparoscopy.

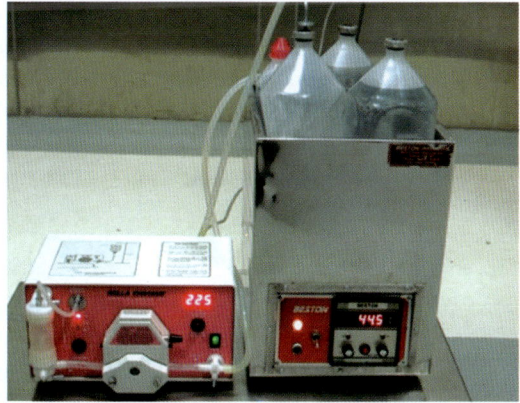

Fig. 14: Irrigation with fluid warmer

Ergonomics in Laparoscopy

There are many ergonomic difficulties experienced during laparoscopic surgeries.

STATIC POSTURE

One of the main and basic ergonomic problems during laparoscopy is the surgeon's non-neutral posture during laparoscopy. Surgeons hold postures that are more static during laparoscopic surgery than during open surgery because they move about less and hold still longer-during laparoscopic surgery. The static postures have been demonstrated to be more disabling and harmful than dynamic postures. The surgeon should be relaxed and take the assistants help when prolonged holding of instruments are required.

LAPAROSCOPIC VISION—LIMITED VIEW

The laparoscopic surgeon typically views a 2-dimensional video image of the operating field on a video monitor placed at a distance of 5 to 8 feet. Surgeon has to compensate for the loss of 3rd dimension by experience since binocular depth cues are lost. Laparoscopic image depends on many factors like distance of telescope from the tissue, its color and amount of bleeding. Closer the telescope to the tissue, higher the magnification **(Fig. 2.15)**. This magnification can be used for fine dissection when required. Too close-up view should be avoided when diathermy is used as it can give a false safety to the surgeon even though the vital structures are very close. A balance of panoramic and close-up view should be used for safe surgery.[3]

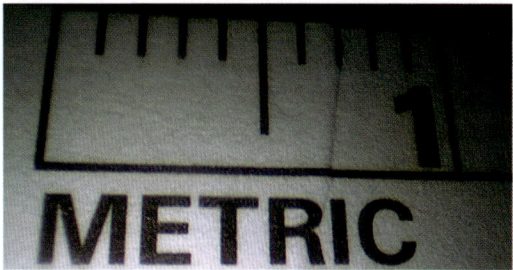

Fig. 2.15: Close-up view of a 1 cm on a scale almost fills 3/4th of the 50 cm screen

LESS EFFICIENT INSTRUMENTS

Laparoscopic instruments are designed to work through small ports 3 to 10 mm in size. This results in more complex internal mechanical movements that decrease the efficient transmission of force from the surgeon's hand to the instrument tip. The surgeon must therefore work about 6 times as hard to accomplish the same grasping task with the laparoscopic instrument. This problem becomes magnified when handle of the instrument is too big for the small hand of the surgeon.

Fixed Ports, Longer Instrument and Fulcrum Action

Laparoscopic surgery involves fixed operating ports and so port placement is very critical for accessibility to the operating site. The handling of instrument is also different from open surgery as the instruments are longer and movement is fulcrum type. Only 4 degree-of-freedom of movement (rotation, up/down angulations, left/right angulations, in/out movement) are possible. So planning the port site is very critical when organs are enlarged or there is history of previous surgery. Instrument exchanges during laparoscopic surgery are laborious and distracting to the surgeon. Using multifunction instruments can circumvent this problem.[4]

Equipment Organization

Unexpected bleeding is difficult to control in laparoscopic surgery. So instruments for hemostasis like bipolar forceps, atraumatic grasper should be kept close at hand. A suction irrigation instrument with properly connected tubings should also be kept ready.

SURGEON'S FATIGUE

Surgeon's fatigue can compromise the safety of the patient. Operation theater setup should aim at improving the comfort of the surgeon. The screen should be kept below the eye level of the surgeon. The OT table should be kept low so that, the surgeon's elbow touches his body. Short surgeons can stand on a foot step to achieve the same effect **(Fig. 2.16)**. This position

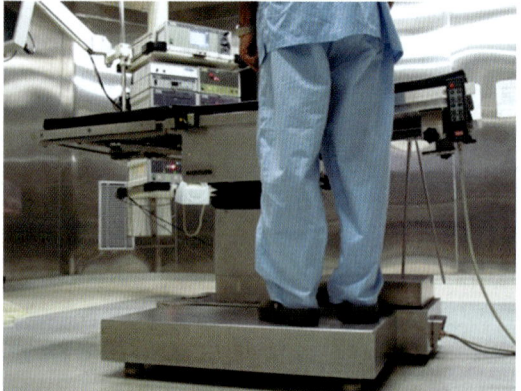

Fig. 2.16: Large foot step

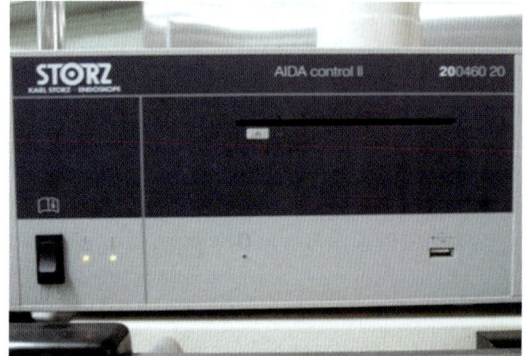

Fig. 2.17: AIDA video capturing system

will allow the surgeon to make movements at the level of elbow or wrist.

RECORD KEEPING

Record keeping is an essential part of surgical practice. Video recording of the laparoscopic procedure is a standard practice in most endoscopic units. We record all our procedures with AIDA control II **(Fig. 2.17)**. This recording system allows recording of videos in 1,024 × 768 resolution and still pictures in 1,920 × 1,080 (HD) resolutions. Recording can be done directly by an assistant or using the camera head buttons by the surgeon himself. The still pictures can also be captured from the videos already recorded. The unedited videos are then written on DVDs, named and stored. It should be done on the same day. Delay can result in losing the recorded data. Edited video is given to patient on request. Still pictures are printed and given to patient along with discharge summary.[5]

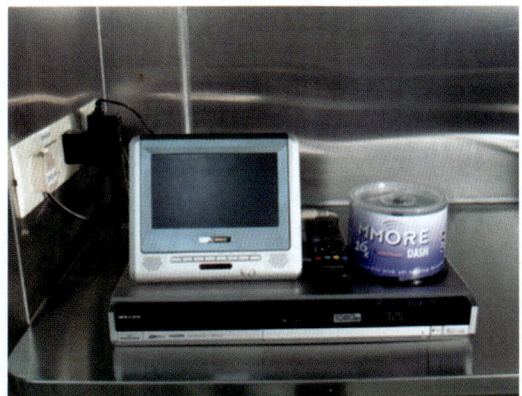

Fig. 2.18: DVD writer

We simultaneously record the surgery on a DVD recorder with a hard disk as a standby. On many occasions when the recorder malfunctions this can be used. It can store up to 40-50 surgeries depending on the size of hard disk **(Fig. 2.18)**. The detailed surgical notes are prepared by the assistant immediately after the surgery. Surgeon should verify it for accuracy.

REFERENCES

1. Operating room Design Manual: Jan Ehrenwerth (Ed). American Society of Anesthesiologists, 1999.
2. Manual of operative Laparoscopy: Paul PG, 1998.
3. A practical manual of laparoscopy: Resad P Pasic, Ronald L. Levine (Eds). Publisher: The Parthenon Publishing Group, 2002.
4. Operative Laparoscopy: The masters' techniques in gynecological surgery: Soderstrom (Ed). Lippincott-Raven, 1998.
5. ESHRE guidelines for training, accreditation and monitoring in gynaecological endoscopy. Human Reproduction 1997;12(4):867-8.

CHAPTER 3

Selecting Optimum Instruments for Safe Gynecological Endoscopic Surgery

Aditi Singhi

Chapter Outline

- Major Equipment for Laparoscopy and Hysteroscopy
- Laparoscopy Instruments
- Newer Instruments
- Hysteroscopy Instruments

INTRODUCTION

The precise and functioning instruments are the key for any successful surgery. Selecting optimum instruments rather than the fancy ones with the knowledge of their use and limitations are of primary importance. For any surgeon who is going to start endoscopic surgery, selection of proper instruments is the first step. All instruments should be functioning properly with no insulation break, proper sharpness, adequate lubrication and appropriate handle attached. This chapter is an attempt to give you the knowledge of basic and specialized instruments, which are needed for safe gynecological endoscopic surgery.

MAJOR EQUIPMENT FOR LAPAROSCOPY AND HYSTEROSCOPY

Endovision Camera

The function of camera is to pick up a video image of whatever is seen through laparoscope. This image is transmitted through a cable to video processing unit, which converts it into picture, which can be seen on TV monitor. Three types of laparoscopic cameras are available:
 i. Single chip camera
 ii. Three chip camera
 iii. High definition camera

The primary advantage of three chip camera **(Fig. 3.1)** as compared to single chip camera is that, in the former color reproduction is more natural. A prism is located in the camera head which splits incoming lighted image into three primary colors which fall on three different chips in three chip camera. Each of the three CCD chips has sensor cells, which convert this light into electrical charge. Then, it forms an integrated image. Some three chip cameras have higher resolution than single chip camera. The optical zoom in the camera is advantageous as it has no negative effect on image resolution.

Both single chip and three chip cameras have standard definition resolution, which are 640*480 pixels with 4:3 aspect ratio (sometimes

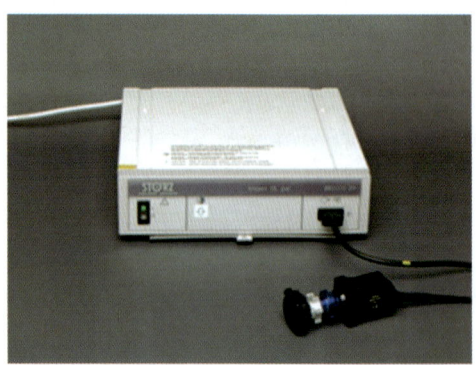

Fig. 3.1: Three chip camera

720*576 with either 4:3 or 16:9). On the contrary, high definition cameras have resolution of 1920*1080 pixels with 16:9 aspect ratio or 1280*720 pixels also with 16:9 aspect ratio. This corresponds to approximate 2 megapixel video. This high resolution is native from the chip and not interpolated by camera. 16:9 HD monitoring gives the benefit of more natural image and a panoramic view. As normally in human beings, horizontal view is wider than our vertical view, 16:9 monitors provide more vision laterally, which gives much wider vision of surgical field.

While selecting the camera, few important points should be kept in mind:
- Affordability
- Camera head should be light in weight
- Picture should be good at low light intensity without any granularity
- There should not be any reflection or glare while viewing white structure
- Auto iris should be able to reduce the glare if light intensity is high.

3D cameras were introduced in early 1990's but ultimately had only little application. They were developed to provide the depth perception, which is lacking in routine 2D laparoscopic surgery. It requires the special glasses to be worn by the surgeon during surgery.

Video Monitor

Ordinary TV sets can be used for routine operative work. The TV set should have video jack to allow video input. The high-resolution medical monitors are better as color display is more accurate but they are expensive.

Light Source

Cold light source are xenon, halogen or mercury bulbs. Xenon bulbs give high intensity of pure white light and last longer but they are expensive. They are available commonly with 150,175 and 300 watts power. The life of a xenon bulb is approx 500 hours. When the lifetime rating of a bulb is exceeded, the subsequent performance of light source becomes unpredictable, i.e. the surgeon is not able to produce a well lit view despite the fact that light is seen coming out of laparoscope.

The completion of life of bulb is shown by the red bulb sign on the light source. The xenon light source (Fig. 3.2) is very powerful and if the tip of light cable with light on comes in contact with skin or drapes, it leads to burn in 20-30 sec. So light should always be kept in standby mode when not in use during surgery.

The halogen bulb is cheap and produces yellow light. Proper white balancing is a must while using it. The life of halogen bulb is around 250 hours.

Light Cable

The fiberoptic light cables are needed to transmit cold light from light source to endoscope. The light carrying capacity depends upon the number of functioning fiberoptic bundles within the cable .The fiberoptic bundles get damaged due to bending of the cable. If more than 45 percent are damaged, it is advisable to change the cable to avoid overheating. The cables can be thick or thin. The thick cables (Fig. 3.2) are used for laparoscopy and thin can be used for hysteroscopy.

Fluid light cables are also available but they are heavy and stiffer and less flexible but they can transmit light with much more intensity as compared to fiberoptic light cables.

CO_2 Insufflators (Fig. 3.3)

CO_2 insufflators of a standard company with parameters like preset abdominal pressure, real

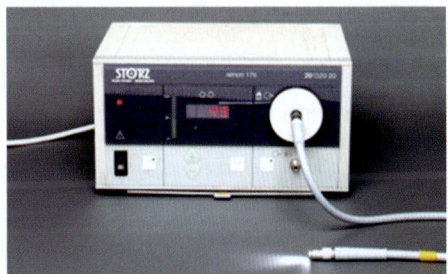

Fig. 3.2: Xenon light source with thick cable

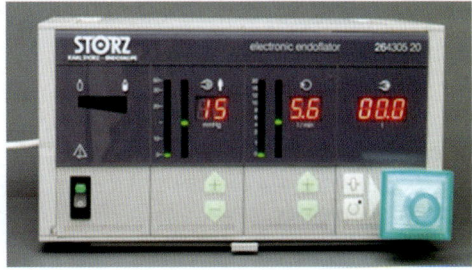

Fig. 3.3: CO_2 insufflator

abdominal pressure, real flow and total gas consumption is a must.

CO_2 insufflators with thermostat for temperature regulation of CO_2 are also available. It reduces the chill effect of high flow rate and reduces telescope fogging.

CO_2 insufflator is connected to CO_2 cylinders with long metal tube with PSI adjusted valve (pressure reducing valve) as gas in cylinders is under very high pressure. CO_2 from insufflators goes to Veress needle via a tube through filter. The pressure should be kept at 15 mm Hg. It can be increased to 20-25 mm Hg at the time of insertion of trocar if required and especially during insertion of morcellator. After insertion, pressure should be reduced back to 15 mm Hg. The initial flow rate at the insertion of Veress needle should be low at less than 1 lit/min. Once the intraperitoneal insertion of Veress is confirmed, flow rate is increased to 4-6 lit/min. When about 3 liters of CO_2 has gone in peritoneal cavity, trocar insertion is done. Then flow rate can be increased further if needed. In some cases flow rate can be increased to maximum in operative laparoscopy keeping pressure constant at 15 mm Hg. This helps in avoiding the interference in visualization due to gas loss during operative laparoscopy requiring repeated use of suction cannula.

Endomat (Fig. 3.4)

This is controlled irrigation and suction apparatus used for mainly operative hysteroscopy and also laparoscopy. The two domes, each for hysteroscopy and laparoscopy are available which when connected to the machine, the endomat, acts accordingly. It has settings to control inflow rate, inflow pressure and suction pressure.

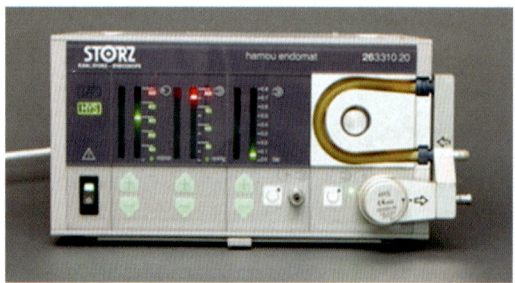

Fig. 3.4: Endomat with hysterodome attached

It has important implication for operative hysteroscopy like submucous fibroid resection and TCRE where absorption of 1.5 percent glycine beyond the critical level may cause serious health hazard. In operative hysteroscopy, flow rate is kept at 200-300 ml/min and pressure 100-150 mm Hg and suction pressure is kept less than 50 mm Hg. In few cases like hysteroscopic adhesiolysis, further increase in pressure up to 200 mm Hg might be needed.

The strict charting of fluid inflow and outflow should be kept during operative hysteroscopy to find out the amount of fluid absorbed. If fluid absorbed is between 500-1000 ml (less if patient is medically compromised), surgeon should be informed and surgery should be finished as soon as possible. Injection furosemide should be given as prophylactic to avoid fluid overload and Foley's catheter should be placed if not already put. If fluid absorption exceeds 1000 ml, blood should be sent for serum electrolytes and the surgery should be temporarily stopped and fluid status should be ascertained. If fluid absorbed is around 1500 ml or serum sodium is <125 mmol/lit, procedure should be immediately terminated and patient treated for hyponatremia and fluid overload.

In laparoscopic surgeries, the suction pressure is usually kept at or below 300 mm Hg as higher suction pressure can cause loss of pneumoperitoneum and subsequent loss of vision. Higher suction pressure can also be traumatic for intra-abdominal structures like bowel, etc.

Electrosurgical Units

The cautery machine with separate bipolar and monopolar connections and their respective footswitches is essential equipment needed for endoscopic surgery.

It works on the principle that heat is generated due to electrical resistance of tissues when high frequency waves of current pass through it. The bipolar coagulating units **(Fig. 3.5)** are attached to Kleppinger or spatulated forceps and it helps in coagulating the tissue or blood vessels in between the prongs. Usually, the cautery is kept at setting of 25-30 watts.

The monopolar cautery is connected to the hand instruments like spatula, puncture needle, scissors, etc. to cut the tissue along with coagulation. It should be used with caution as lateral spread is more than bipolar cautery. While using monopolar current, patient's plate should be properly connected.

The cutting current is usually kept at 80-100 watts and coagulating current at around 60 watts. The footswitches should be kept at preassigned fixed position, at a comfortable distance from the foot to avoid confusion and pressing of wrong foot switch during surgery.

LAPAROSCOPY INSTRUMENTS

Endoscope

Laparoscope may vary from 2-12 mm in diameter and angle of view may range from 0-70 degree. Laparoscope has attachment for light cable and endoscopic camera. The most commonly used laparoscopes are 0° for straight view and 30° for oblique view with 10 mm diameter for all operative as well as in most diagnostic procedures **(Fig 3.6)**.

5 mm 0° laparoscope is extremely useful during operative laparoscopy when specimen retrieval has to be done through 10 mm port. In such situation 5 mm laparoscope is inserted from left lower trocar and specimen is removed under vision through 10 mm trocar **(Fig. 3.7)**.

3 mm laparoscope is used in microlaparoscopy. This is 3 mm rod lens scope which is used with other 3 mm hand instruments for minor operative procedures like PCO drilling. The disadvantage with this scope is lesser illumination and smaller field of vision.

For hysteroscopy 30° Hopkin's II scope is used for all diagnostic as well as operative surgeries. The Bettocchi design of microhysteroscope is 30° with 2.6 mm diameter. The advantage with it is very less dilatation of cervix is required and can be tried in cervical stenosis cases.

Veress Needle

It can be reusable **(Fig. 3.8)** or disposable. It comes in large, medium or small size. Large sized needle is used in obese patients with thick abdominal wall and small needle in thin patients. Veress needle works on spring mechanism, as soon as it is pushed against skin perpendicularly, due to the resistance offered by skin, subcutaneous tissue and rectus sheath, blunt end of needle retracts and sharp end helps in piercing the tissues. As it enters peritoneal cavity, blunt end comes out as there is no resistance and protects the bowel. The confirmation of intraperitoneal entrance of needle should be done by checking

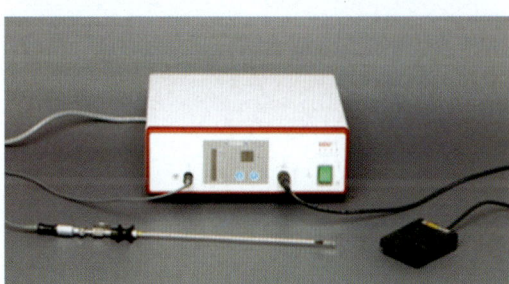

Fig. 3.5: Dedicated bipolar unit

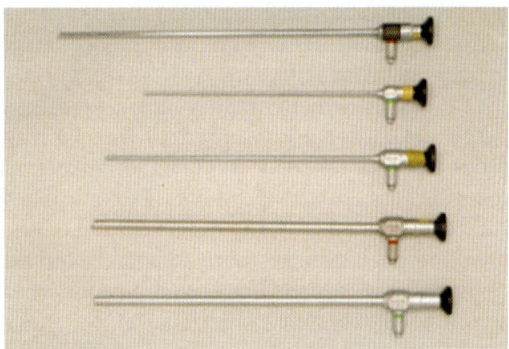

Fig. 3.7: Types of laparoscopes

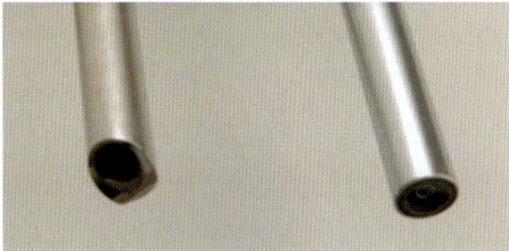

Fig. 3.6: 30° and 0° laparoscope

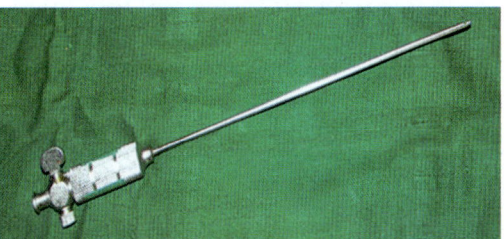

Fig. 3.8: Metallic reusable Veress needle

the pressure and flow rate with negative pressure display and either of various methods like aspiration test, syringe test, drop method, etc. The initial flow rate should be kept low at less than 1 litres/min. so as to avoid inadvertent flow of gas into blood vessel accidentally.

The new Veress needle has other additional safety features like a hanging ball and red and green mark which further help in confirming the proper placement of Veress needle.

The 'open entry' in laparoscopic surgery avoids use of Veress needle.

Trocars and Cannula

Primary Trocars and Cannula (Fig. 3.9)

They are usually metallic reusable trocars with multifunction flap valve. This valve prevents the leakage of gas when scope or other instruments are removed. It also helps in removing the specimen by pressing the valve. Usually blind nonvisual trocars are used but optical trocars are also available. Despite their ability to optically display tissue layers on the monitor during entry, these instruments retain the conventional push through trocars and cannula insertion dynamics. Serious entry injury still can occur with their use, especially when the operator is not familiar with safe use of these systems and fails to interpret or recognize the displayed images. Nonvisual trocars with sharp cutting pyramidal tip are better than conical ones as less perpendicular force is required for its trajectory propulsion, so less chances of inadvertent bowel or vessel injury due to overshoot. The conical trocars have pointed sharp tip but no cutting edges, therefore, significantly more force is required as tissue layers are not transected but parted to accommodate cannula's outer diameter.

In closed laparoscopy, pneumoperitoneum is created first followed by entry of primary trocar. However, open laparoscopy first secures peritoneal entry through minicut down, followed by insertion of Hassan trocar and finally peritoneal insufflation.

Secondary Trocars (Fig. 3.9)

Like primary trocars, they can also be disposable or reusable. They can be metallic or plastic with variable sizes. We prefer to use threaded plastic 5 mm reusable apple trocars. These trocars allow easy laparoscopic suturing without thread entrapment and because of serrations they are less likely to come out again and again during surgery while removing the hand instruments. They are reusable after sterilization, so reduce the cost or surgery.

7 mm metallic trocar and cannula are useful in double puncture laparoscopic tubal ligation surgery. 10 to 5 to 3 mm reducers **(Figs 3.10A and B)** are available which when connected to 10 mm

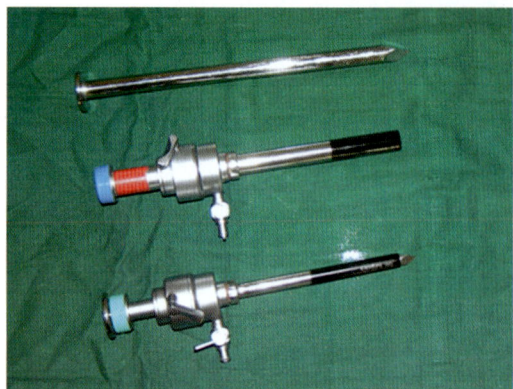

Fig. 3.9: Metallic 10 mm primary trocar and 7 mm secondary trocar

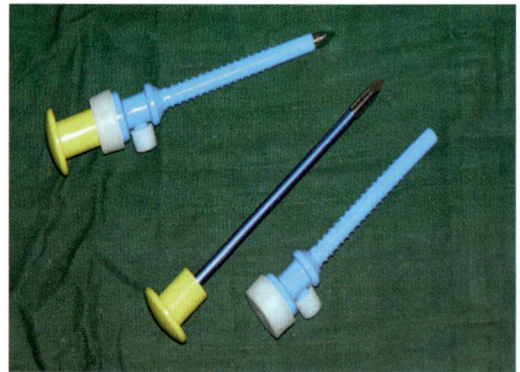

Fig. 3.10A: Plastic 5 mm apple trocar

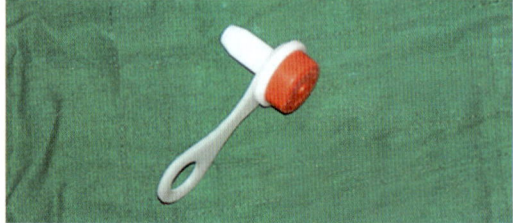

Fig. 3.10B: 10 mm to 5 mm reducer

trocar, help in inserting 5 mm or 3 mm instrument without leak of pneumoperitoneum.

Fenestrated Hrasper (Fig. 3.11)

It is an atraumatic grasper available in two sizes viz. long and short. As it is without tooth and minimal serrations, it holds the tissues softly without damaging. The handle attached to it should not have lock for soft catch. It is used in holding and retracting bowel, fallopian tubes, excision of cyst wall, grasping the thread during endosuturing, etc.

Claw Forceps (Figs 3.12 and 3.13)

It is also available in long and short sizes. It has tooth to have a firmer hold of the tissues. So it is called as traumatic grasper also. It is used to hold the specimen side of the tissue as in ovarian cyst wall excision, myoma enucleation or to retrieve the specimen from the abdomen. It is available in both 5 mm and 10 mm sizes.

Tenaculum Forceps

It looks like tenaculum of open surgery, used in holding the tissue at specific point. It is used in holding and pulling the cervix during circumferential colpotomy in laparoscopic hysterectomy.

Spoon Forceps (Fig. 3.14)

10 mm spoon forceps are useful in holding and retrieving soft tissues like chorionic tissues, tubes in ectopic pregnancy and also the clots.

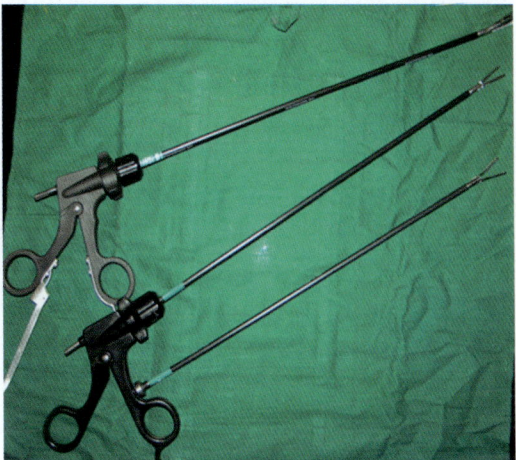

Fig. 3.11: 5 mm atraumatic grasper

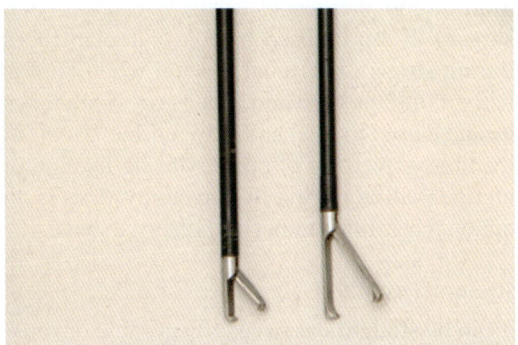

Fig. 3.13: Claw forceps

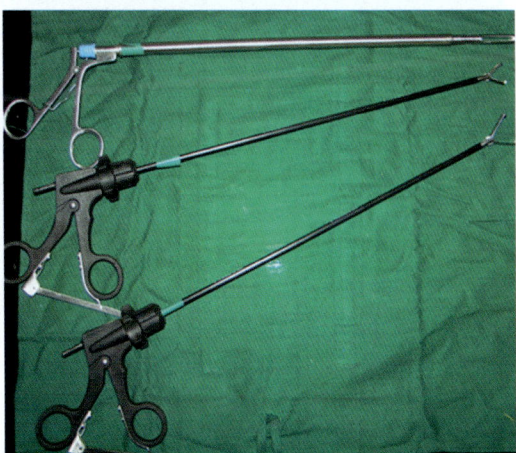

Fig. 3.12: 10 mm and 5 mm claw forceps

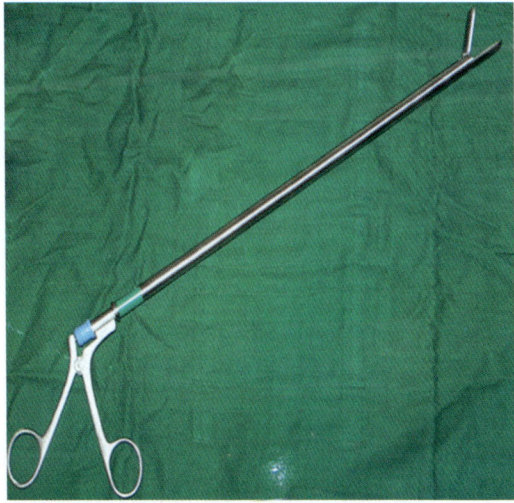

Fig. 3.14: 10 mm spoon forceps

Maryland Grasper (Fig. 3.15)

It functions like curved artery forceps of open surgery. 5 mm Maryland grasper is useful in holding UV fold while cutting it during hysterectomy. It functions like a good dissector also.

Dissecting Forceps

Various dissecting forceps with angulated tip, angle may vary from 60° to 90° like Mixter forceps are available. It is useful in ureteric and uterine dissection.

Alligator Forceps

The jaws have deep serrations which help in providing good grip. It is mainly used in holding the appendix during appendicectomy.

Babcock/Oval Grasper (Fig. 3.16)

5 mm atraumatic grasper just like Babcock of open surgery. It can be used to hold fallopian tubes during surgery like tubal ligation when knot is tied around the loop and tube is cut. Sometimes it can be used to hold and grip uterine vessels at the time of piercing of needle during ligation of uterine pedicle during hysterectomy. This is an optional instrument not compulsory to have.

Scissors (Fig. 3.17)

It can be straight or curved, disposable or reusable. It is used during adhesiolysis, cutting of thread, separating firmly attached ovarian cyst wall from its bed. Few scissors have adapter to attach monopolar cautery to achieve coagulation while cutting the tissues. But use of cautery reduces the sharpness of scissors. The most commonly used scissors are curved Metzenbaum type.

Monopolar Puncture Needle (Fig. 3.18)

This needle is used for polycystic ovarian drilling, cyst puncture, for incising the fallopian tube during salpingostomy in unruptured ectopic pregnancy. It is also used for spray coagulation of oozing surface. It is attached to monopolar current through an adapter. It has a spring control at the finger grip which prevents the surrounding structures from accidental piercing during its use.

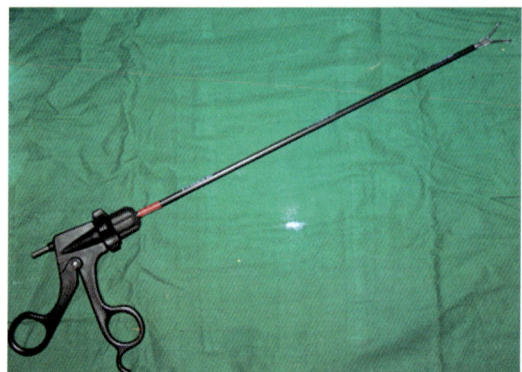

Fig. 3.16: 5 mm oval grasper

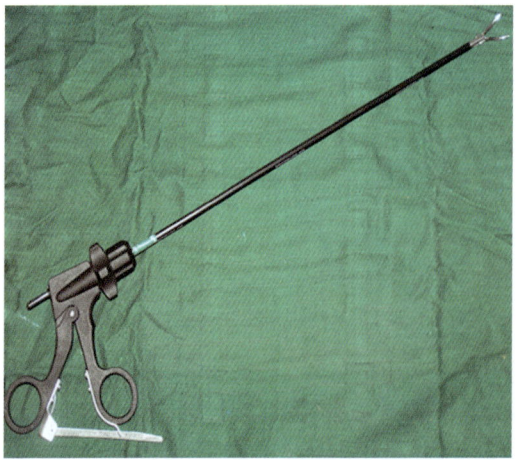

Fig. 3.15: 5 mm Maryland grasper

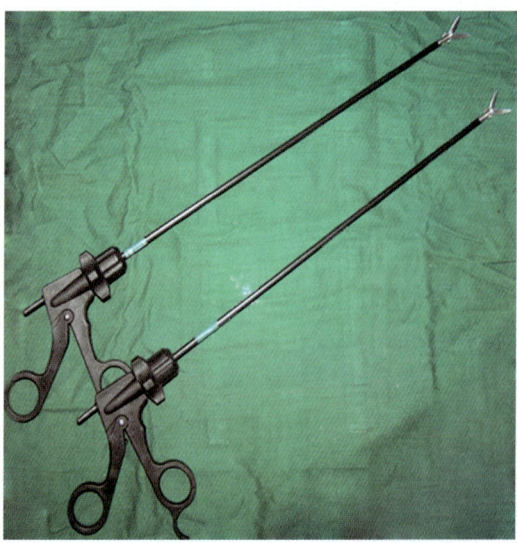

Fig. 3.17: 5 mm scissors (thick and fine)

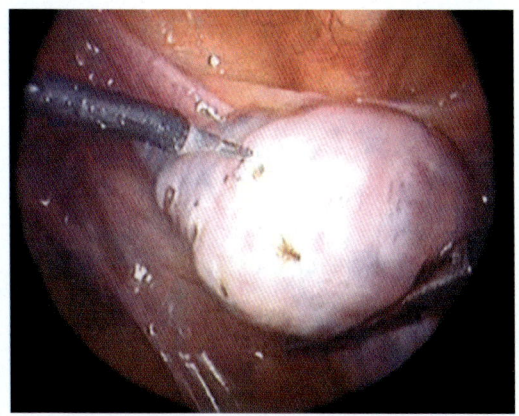

Fig. 3.18: Monopolar puncture needle

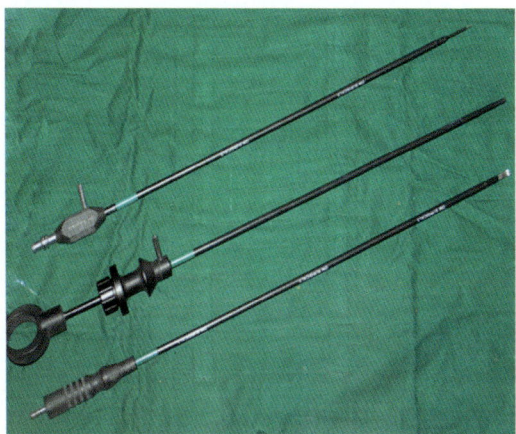

Fig. 3.19: Injection needle (upper), puncture needle (middle), spatula (lower)

Aspiration Needle

It is 16-gauge needle to aspirate the fluid from peritoneal cavity or from cyst when attached to needle or suction. The fluid can be collected for cytological evaluation. It should always be in the field of vision while introducing it into abdominal cavity as it is pointed wide bored and without any spring control.

Injection Needle

It is 22-gauge needle. It is used to inject dilute vasopressin into myometrium at the site of myoma and its base during myomectomy. It is also used for injecting dilute vasopressin in mesosalpinx and antimesenteric border of fallopian tube during salpingostomy in ectopic pregnancy. This should also be under constant vision as like aspiration needle during its use.

Spatula (Fig. 3.19)

The distal end is spoon shaped. It has adapter for connection with monopolar cautery. It can be used with or without current depending upon the need during surgery. It is very helpful in incising the uterine wall during myomectomy when used with cutting current. It also helps in dissecting and enucleating the myoma from its bed. Its curvature helps in dissecting and pushing the bladder down during hysterectomy.

It is also used for colpotomy and also cutting the large specimen into pieces before removing them out from abdomen.

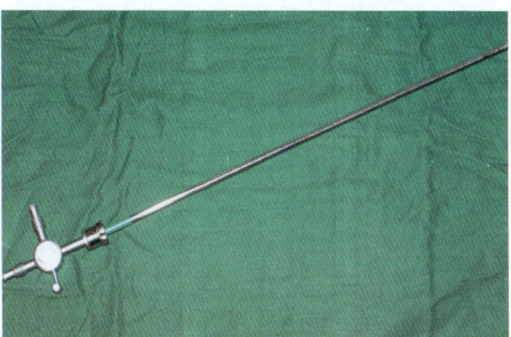

Fig. 3.20: 5 mm suction and irrigation cannula

Irrigation/Suction Cannula (Fig. 3.20)

It is available in 3 mm, 5 mm and 10 mm size. Various designs of distal end as well as finger grip are available. By moving the knob at hand control grip, it can function as suction cannula or irrigation cannula. It is used to clear the operative field from blood and clots, helps in localizing the spurter, also washing the lens of laparoscope intra-abdominally to clear vision without removing the scope out from abdomen. This also helps in dislodging and detaching the chorionic tissue from tubal mesothelium in ectopic pregnancy during salpingostomy. In accidental rupture of dermoid cyst during surgery, continuous irrigation and suction helps in cleaning the peritoneal cavity and reduces the chances of peritonitis. After puncturing the chocolate cyst, it is used to aspirate the contents and irrigate the cyst.

It is also used as a dissector in aquadissection. The suction force should be adjusted at the main unit according to the need as too much of suction force can be traumatic.

Palpation Probe/Rod (Fig. 3.21)

This is a 5 mm rod with various demarcating marks on it, corresponding to 1 cm each. This helps in estimating the size of any structure inside the abdomen like fibroid, etc. It has rounded blunt tip, so by palpation helps in knowing the consistency of the tissue to some extent.

Myoma Screw (Fig. 3.22)

This is available in 5 mm and 10 mm sizes. The distal end may have closer or distant spirals. The screw with closer spirals is better as it gives good grip on the tissue. It is extremely useful instrument to apply traction during fibroid enucleation. This is also used in stabilizing the uterus during laparoscopic hysterectomy or subtotal hysterectomy.

Knot Pusher

This is 5 mm instrument used to push extracorporeally tied knot into laparoscopic surgical field. Various designs of knot pushers are available like Clarke-Reich knot pusher, SWEC and Trivedi's knot pusher **(Fig. 3.23)**, etc. A Scissor-knot pusher has also been developed which helps in cutting the thread after pushing and tying the knot without the need for separate scissors. The knot pushers are reusable and can be sterilized by ETO, formalin, glutaraldehyde or autoclave.

Needle Holders (Fig. 3.24)

Two needle holders, one curved and other straight are essential for laparoscopic suturing. The curved is usually parrot beaked with or without tooth. The tooth gives additional advantage of gripping the edge of the tissue while needle is passed with the help of another needle holder. Sometimes flamingo tip needle holder is useful especially when the thread is small. The needle holders are available with various types of handles attached. The needle holder with simple lock and release mechanism should be chosen. In ipsilateral intracorporeal

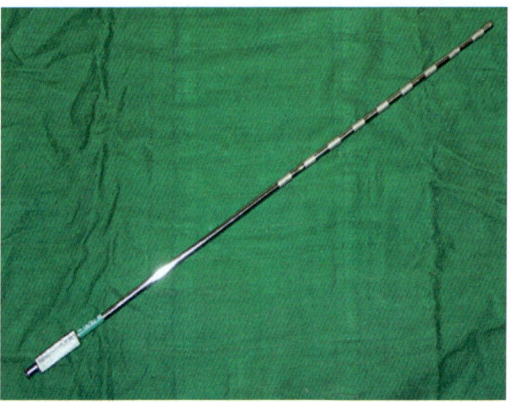

Fig. 3.21: 5 mm palpation rod

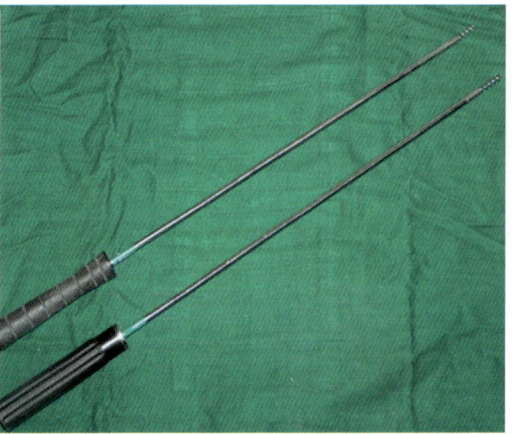

Fig. 3.22: 5 mm myoma screw (with and without central needle)

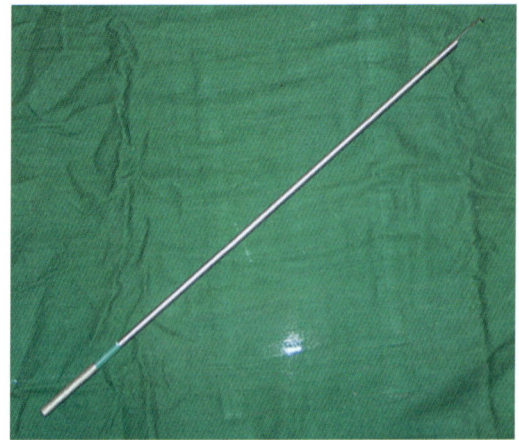

Fig. 3.23: 5 mm Trivedi's knot pusher

suturing, it is preferable to insert curved needle holder through left lower port and straight one through left upper port.

Bipolar Forceps (Fig. 3.25)

It could be Kleppinger or spatulated forceps. The spatulated forceps are broad so useful in holding and coagulating pedicles in hysterectomy. Bipolar forceps with different handle and gripping mechanism are available. The robust bipolar forceps (ROBI of KARL STORZ) has insulation covering at outer surface of prongs which minimizes accidental thermal injury if touched to any important tissue. A good functioning bipolar is essential in operative laparoscopy.

Vaginal Tube (Fig. 3.26)

This is cylindrical tube available in various diameters ranging from 3 to 5 mm. They are made up of materials like silicone or polyvinylchloride. The other end has a lid or is closed with 10 mm channel having flower valve which allows insertion of 10 mm instrument through it to hold the cervix if required during hysterectomy while doing circumferential colpotomy over the tube. This prevents leakage of pneumoperitoneum while incising the vagina. The most commonly used tube is McCartney's tube.

CCL trocar (Colpo-Chirurgie Lausuane, Karl Storz) (Fig. 3.27)

It has rounded ball like attachment at its end which is 35- 40 mm in diameter. It is passed into the vagina and makes posterior vagina prominent and bulging to help in incising it during hysterectomy (colpotomy). This also has a channel through which a 10 mm instrument like claw forceps can be passed to retrieve the tissue without leakage of gas.

Sometimes anterior colpotomy is needed and can be done using wet gauze on sponge holder making anterior vagina prominent.

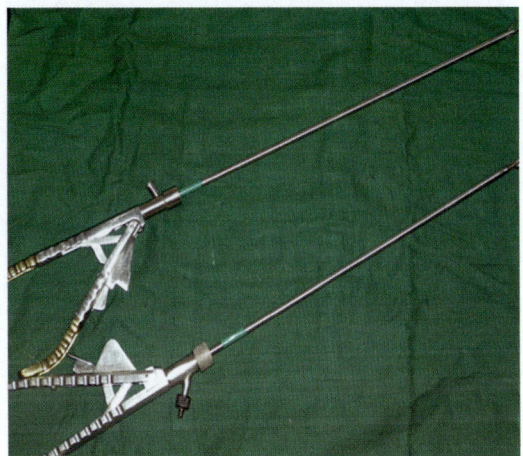

Fig. 3.24: 5 mm straight and curved needle holders

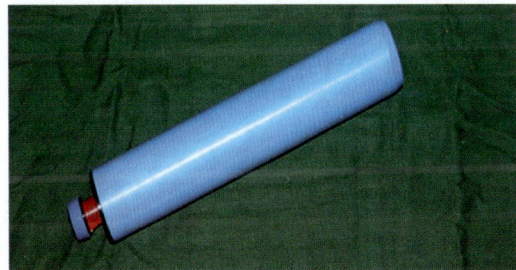

Fig. 3.26: Vaginal tube with 10 mm channel

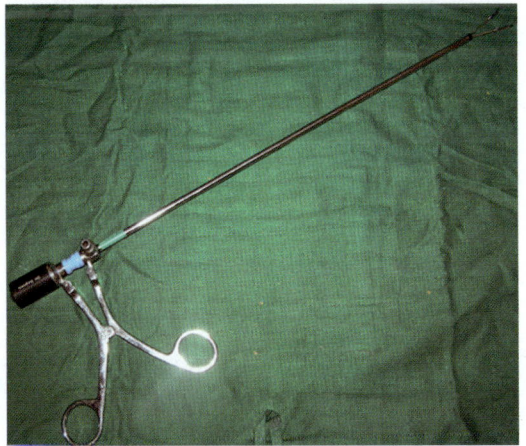

Fig. 3.25: 5 mm spatulated bipolar forceps

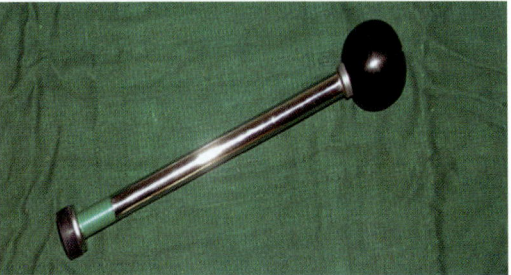

Fig. 3.27: CCL trocar

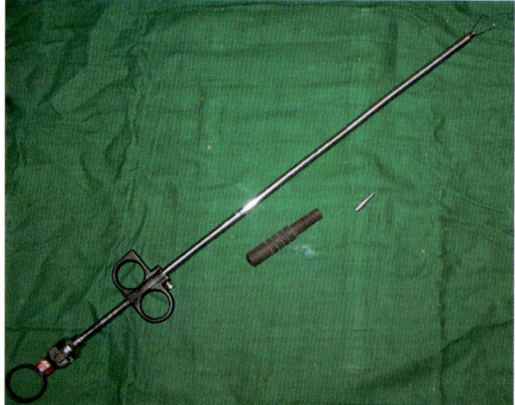

Fig. 3.28: Silastic ring applicator with loader

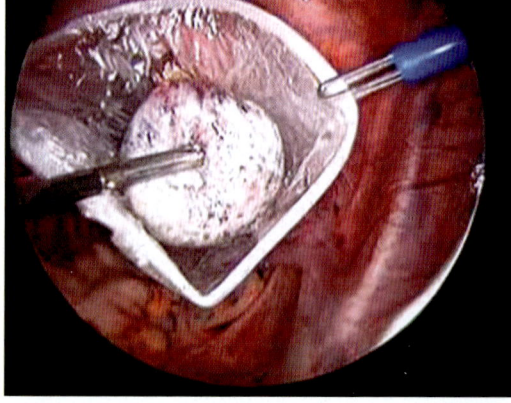

Fig. 3.29: Lapsac

Silastic Ring Applicator (Fig. 3.28)

This instrument has tongs to hold the fallopian tube, which is pulled inside the instrument and silastic ring (Falope ring) is slipped over the loop of tube for tubal sterilization. It has a rotating knob with adjustment slot at other end. This helps in loading 2 rings initially and pushing one ring at a time. The handle has spring mechanism to pull and push the prongs in and out.

Clip Applicator

This is available in 5 mm and 10 mm size. This can be used to clamp medium sized vessel. The reusable single clip applicator and disposable loaded clip applicators are available.

Laparoscopic Retrieval Bags

Different types with different mechanisms of retrieval bags are available. This is used to take out the soft and cystic tissue from abdomen laparoscopically without spillage of the contents. It is especially useful to retrieve dermoid cyst after separating from the ovary and in suspected or proven malignancy to prevent spillage of its contents. The bag is transparent which allows visualization of its contents during puncturing and breaking it into pieces. The bag is made up of nontoxic material with good tensile strength. Some of the retrieval bags are Endobag, Endopouch, Lapsac **(Fig. 3.29)**, Endocatch, etc.

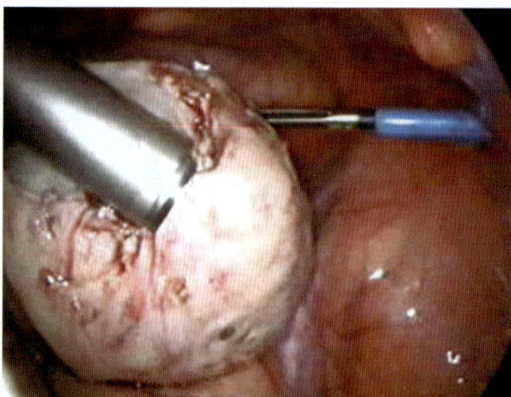

Fig. 3.30A: Morcellator

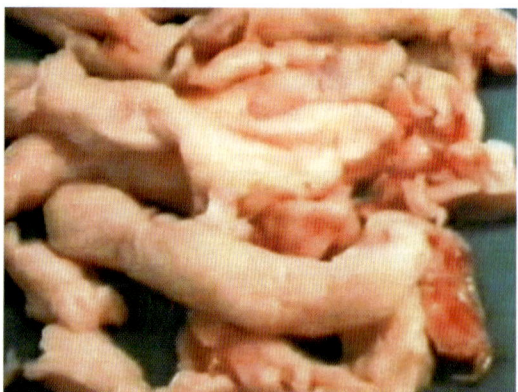

Fig. 3.30B: Morcellated fibroid

Morcellators (Figs 3.30A and B)

It is used for cutting, coring and extracting firm tissues out of abdomen in operative laparoscopy. The tissues come out in the form of thin strips. It has rotationally fixed and axially movable inner tube with foot control switch. It is used in removal of fibroid after enucleation, removal of uterus in supracervical hysterectomy and sometimes in total laparoscopic hysterectomy when size of uterus is big and can not be removed vaginally. It has the advantage of greatly reducing the surgical time and keeping laparoscopic surgery as minimal invasive without the need of increasing the size of incision for removal of tissue. The instrument should be used under continuous laparoscopic vision to prevent accidental injury to other tissues. The various types of morcellators are Rotocut, Gynaecare, Sawalhe's, etc.

NEWER INSTRUMENTS

Single Port Access Surgery Instruments (SPA)

Also known as single incision laparoscopic surgery (SILS), one port umbilical surgery (OPUS) and laparoendoscopic single site surgery (LESS). This is a newer technique and has been developed with the aim of still less post operative pain, faster recovery, less blood loss, better cosmetic outcome as compared to multi-port entry. A 2 cm incision is taken at umbilicus and whole surgery is done through that port. There is no separate postoperative scar (as umbilicus is naturally scarred structure). SPA equipments are broadly divided into access ports and hand instruments. The access port has openings for CO_2 connection, laparoscope and 2 hand instruments. The hand instruments can be rigid or articulating. The rigid are the standard hand instruments used for laparoscopic surgery. The articulating instruments overcome the main problem of SILS which is decreased triangulation of instruments but they are expensive.

HYSTEROSCOPY INSTRUMENTS

Diagnostic Sheath

This can be single channel with only inflow or double channel **(Fig. 3.31)** with inflow as well as outflow. The outflow can be connected to suction apparatus. The vision in double channel is better than single channel as outflow is in surgeon's control. It is 6 mm in diameter.

Operative Channel Sheath (Fig. 3.32)

This is 7.5 mm in diameter with a special channel for passing instruments like hysteroscopic scissors, graspers **(Fig. 3.33)**, tubal catheter, etc. The grasper is used for foreign body removal or removal of CuT with broken thread. The scissors are used for adhesiolysis. The tubal catheter is used for tubal cannulation. This procedure is done in proximal tubal block mainly due to plugs or debris.

The operative sheath has bilaminar flow of fluid. It has two connections each for inflow and for outflow but has single channel for fluid medium.

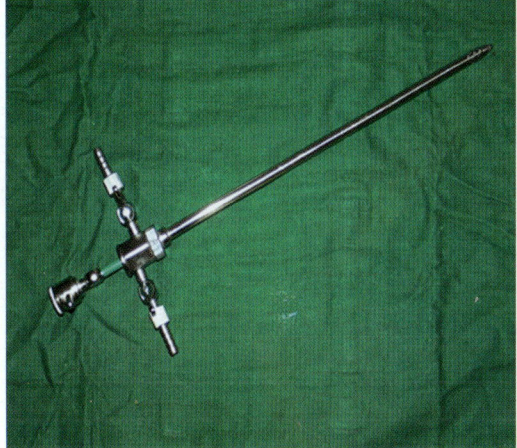

Fig. 3.31: Double channel diagnostic hysteroscopic sheath

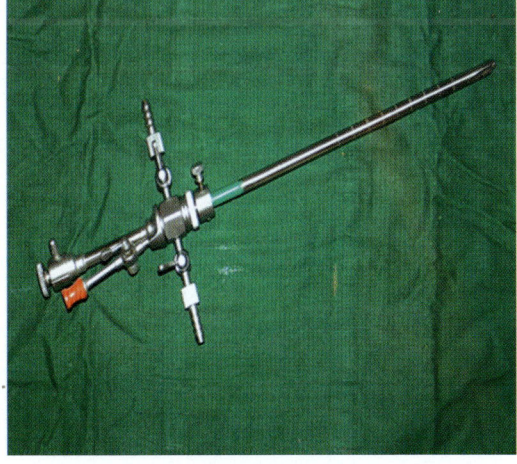

Fig. 3.32: Operative hysteroscopy sheath

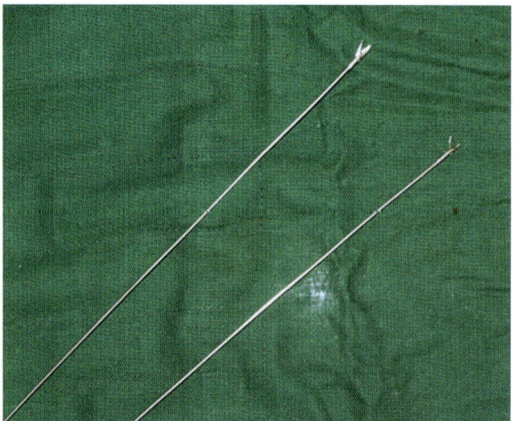

Fig. 3.33: Scissors and grasper for operative channel

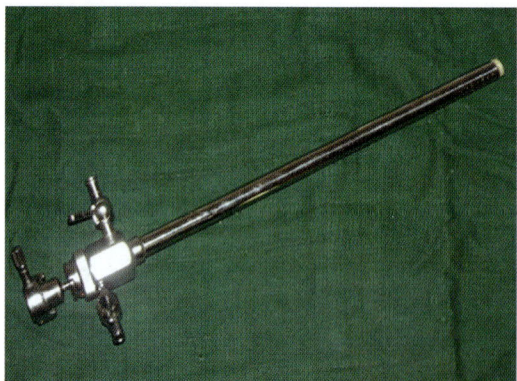

Fig. 3.34: Resectoscope sheath with obturator

The versapoint can also be passed through this sheath and be used for septal incision and adhesiolysis with normal saline as distension medium as it uses bipolar energy. This avoids the need for extradilatation of cervix and use of resectoscope which utilizes monopolar energy and 1.5 percent glycine as distention medium.

Resectoscope Sheath (Figs 3.34 and 3.35)

This is 9 mm in diameter. This includes inner sheath, outer sheath, obturator and working element. The inner channel is connected to inflow and outer channel connected to outflow. This double channel flow helps in keeping field clear during operative hysteroscopy.

First the sheath with the obturator is passed through cervix after dilatation. The obturator has blunt rounded tip which helps in smooth entry and minimizes risk of perforation. Then obturator is removed and working element with electrode and hysteroscope is inserted.

The resectoscope is used for procedures like submucous fibroid resection, polyp resection, TCRE, etc. The working element is connected to the respective electrode which in turn is connected to monopolar cautery. This utilizes non ionic 1.5 percent glycine as distention medium.

The resectoscope handle mechanism can be active when the electrode is outside the resectoscope sheath at rest or passive when it remains inside the sheath at rest. The passive handle mechanism is preferable as it reduces the risk of accidental uterine perforation.

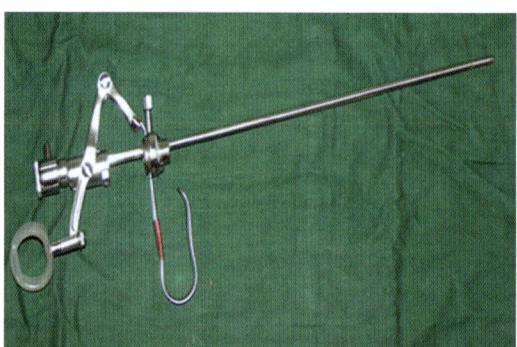

Fig. 3.35: Working element

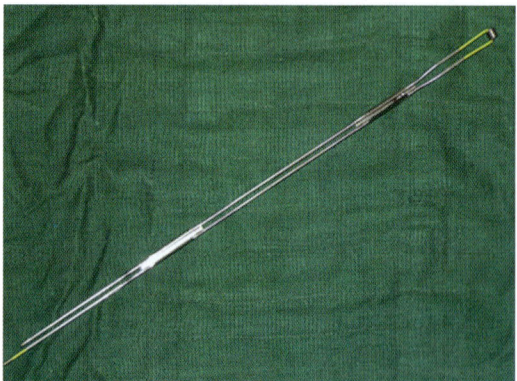

Fig. 3.36: Monopolar cylindrical electrode for resectoscope

Electrodes/Loop

These are connected to the working element for operative hysteroscopy.

Ball or cylindrical electrode is used for coagulation. Smaller ball is especially useful for cornual coagulation and cylinder **(Fig. 3.36)** has wider area of contact so useful for coagulation of uterine walls.

Collin's knife is used for septal incision, lateral metroplasty and adhesiolysis.

The loops can be forward angle with 135° and backward angle with 45° angle. The forward angle loop is used for mainly cornual and fundal resection of endometrium and backward angle for remaining endometrium in TCRE. The backward angle is mainly used in submucous fibroid and polyp resection.

Bettochi Operative Hysteroscopic Sheath

It is very thin and has a very thin 2.6 mm diameter rigid hysteroscope. It has the advantage that less cervical dilatation is required and the same hand instruments like grasper and versapoint can be passed through it also.

CONCLUSION

The endoscopic instruments should be simple, functioning properly and to their best utilization by the surgeon. The instruments should be regularly checked by biomedical engineer for wear and tear and regular maintenance.[1] There should be constant upgradation and acceptance of newer equipments and technology with its through knowledge and awareness of their limitations to keep pace with newer development and utilize them in their best way.

REFERENCE

1. Anusch yazdani, Hannah Krause. The Journal of Minimally Invasive Gynecology Volume 14, Issue 2 , Pages 2007; 228-32.

CHAPTER 4

Patient Selection for Gynecological Endoscopic Surgery to Make it Safe

Atul Ganatra, Maya Prasad

Chapter Outline

- Background
- Problem
  - Indications
- Relevant Anatomy
  - Abdominal Scars
  - Abdominal Wall Thickness
- Umbilicus
  - Abdominal Wall Vessels
- Endoscopic Surgery—A Rule
- Ectopic Pregnancy
- Management of Ectopic Pregnancy
  - Medical Management
- Tubal Factor
- Proximal Tubal Occlusion
- Intrauterine Adhesions
- Uterine Anatomical Defects
- Hysteroscopic Myomectomy
- Ovarian Cysts
- Fibroids
- Endometriosis
- Postmenopausal Bleeding
- Miscellaneous
  - Posthysterectomy Adhesiolysis
  - Clinical Dilemma

Strange how much you got to know before you know how little you know—Anonymous

BACKGROUND

During the last 35 years, gynecologic laparoscopy has evolved from a limited surgical procedure used only for diagnosis and tubal ligations to a major surgical tool used to treat a multitude of gynecologic indications. Today, laparoscopy is one of the most common surgical procedures performed by gynecologists.

For many procedures such as, removal of an ectopic pregnancy, treatment of endometriosis or, ovarian cystectomy, laparoscopy has become the treatment of choice. Compared with laparotomy, multiple studies have shown laparoscopy to be safer, cost-effective and to have a shorter recovery time.

PROBLEM

Laparoscopy is a hybrid surgical approach that shares characteristics of both minor and major surgery. To patients, laparoscopic procedures often seem to be minor surgery because of the small incisions, relatively small amount of postoperative pain, and short convalescent period. In minor laparoscopic surgeries (e.g. diagnostic laparoscopy, tubal fulguration), both postoperative discomfort and the risk of complications may more closely resemble a minor procedure than a major procedure.

At its essence, laparoscopy remains an intra-abdominal procedure. Therefore, it shares all intraoperative and postoperative risks of laparotomy, including infection and injury to adjacent intra-abdominal structures. When major intra-abdominal procedures are performed laparoscopically the resultant postoperative pain and morbidity are still significant. However, because a large abdominal incision is unnecessary, the postoperative pain and morbidity are always less significant than similar major surgery performed by laparotomy.

Laparoscopic procedures have unique risks, which are related to methods used for the placement of abdominal wall ports and to the pneumoperitoneum required for laparoscopy. The use of energy within the abdominal cavity likewise introduces risk. These risks include injury to bowel, bladder, or major blood vessels and intravascular insufflation. In addition, increased intra-abdominal pressures associated with laparoscopy increase anesthesia-related risks such as aspiration and increased difficulty ventilating the patient. Although, the risk of blood loss is relatively low for most procedures, potentially massive blood loss may occur and is complicated by the fact that control of blood loss may be delayed by the time taken to perform an emergency laparotomy.

Indications

Minor procedures	Major procedures
Diagnostic laparoscopy	Myomectomy
Tubal sterilization	Treatment of endometriosis
Adhesiolysis	Laparoscopic hysterectomy
Treatment of ectopic pregnancy	Oncologic procedures
Ovarian cystectomy	
Oophorectomy	

RELEVANT ANATOMY

Anterior abdominal wall anatomy should receive special attention prior to laparoscopy because many laparoscopic complications result from trocar placement.

Abdominal Scars

Previous surgery is associated with a greater than 20 percent risk of adhesions of bowel or omentum to the anterior abdominal wall, for this reason, many laparoscopists adjust their techniques in these patients to minimize the risk of bowel injury. Of special concern are incisional scars immediately adjacent to the umbilicus because bowel adherent underneath the umbilicus may be at risk for injury regardless of the technique used. Although, Pfannenstiel and abdominal incisions distant to the umbilicus may also be associated with adhesions, in many laparoscopists' experiences, these incisions appear to represent less of a risk than incisions near the umbilicus.

In addition to location, the width and depth of the scar should be evaluated because a wide or retracted scar may suggest that a postoperative wound infection had occurred. Common wisdom dictates that postoperative infections may be associated with an increased risk of intra-abdominal adhesion formation. If the dome of the bladder is involved in the infectious process, it may cause progression of the bladder dome higher behind the anterior abdominal wall, thus increasing the risk of bladder injury at the time of suprapubic trocar placement.

Abdominal Wall Thickness

Although abdominal thickness correlates with patient weight, short stature or truncal obesity may increase abdominal wall thickness out of proportion to patient weight. Routine evaluation of the abdominal wall prior to laparoscopy is important because the success of trocar insertion may depend on altering the technique based on abdominal wall thickness.

UMBILICUS

The umbilicus should be examined for signs of umbilical hernia. Techniques for trocar insertion should be adjusted, and closure of the defect should be considered. In the absence of incarcerated bowel, the skin over the hernia can be carefully incised and the peritoneal cavity entered using an open technique. Closure of a small defect can be performed with interrupted sutures at the completion of the laparoscopic procedure. For ideal cosmetic results, larger defects may require the assistance of a surgeon experienced in umbilical hernia repair.

Abdominal Wall Vessels

The anterior abdominal wall contains two sets of bilateral vessels, the superficial and the inferior (deep) epigastric vessels. These arteries originate from the femoral and external iliac arteries, respectively, and are accompanied by a large vein in most cases. Immediately above the symphysis pubis, they are both located an average of 5.5 cm from the midline and course slightly more laterally at points more cephalad. In order to avoid injuring these vessels during lateral trocar placement, the superficial vessels should be visualized by transillumination and the inferior vessels should be laparoscopically visualized whenever possible. The use of conical trocars and not pyramidal tipped trocars can also decrease the risk of injury to these vessels.

ENDOSCOPIC SURGERY—A RULE

- Ectopic pregnancy
- Treatment of endometriosis in infertility
- Adhesiolysis
- Tubal cannulation
- Intrauterine septum
- Submucous myomas and polyps
- Asherman's syndrome

ECTOPIC PREGNANCY

Incidence of ectopic pregnancy is rising, this rise has been attributed to an overall increase in sexually transmitted disease (STD), late child bearing, increased infertility and ART, surgical interference and improvement in diagnosis modalities. Modern management of ectopic pregnancy is one of medicine's greatest success stories.

Advanced technology has enabled us to diagnose ectopic pregnancy before significant hemorrhage occurs. Transvaginal sonography can pick up early, unruptured ectopic pregnancy **(Fig. 4.1)**.

Laparoscopy remains the gold standard in the detection and management of ectopic pregnancy **(Fig. 4.2)**.

MANAGEMENT OF ECTOPIC PREGNANCY

Medical Management

Medical treatment should be preferred if the patient has undergone surgery many times previously, has extensive pelvic adhesions, a contraindication to general anesthesia, a cornual pregnancy, and after failure of a conservative laparoscopic treatment. Medical treatment is

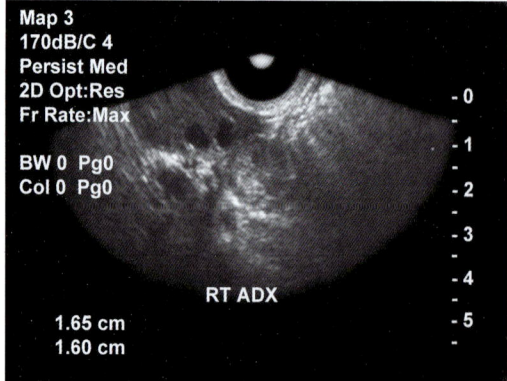

Fig. 4.1: TVS—ectopic mass

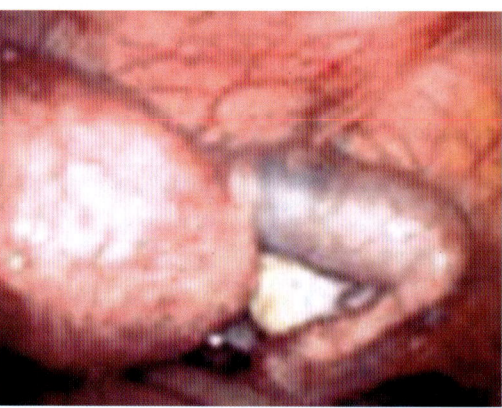

Fig. 4.2: Laparoscopic—unruptured tubal pregnancy

possible if serum β-hCG is below 10,000 mIU/mL, if the ectopic pregnancy is less than 4 cm in diameter. Medical treatment should be preferred if the patient has no pain and ectopic pregnancy cannot be visualized at ultrasound.[1]

Laparoscopic treatment[2,3] is indicated when the patient has provided informed consent, she is hemodynamically stable, the surgeon has the required equipments and operative laparoscopy experience, and intraoperative bleeding can be controlled. Early diagnosis with serum β-hCG levels and pelvic ultrasonography increases the feasibility of a laparoscopic approach.

Treatment may involve linear salpingostomy, segmental tubal resection, or salpingectomy. Linear salpingostomy should be done if the ectopic mass is less than 5 cm in the ampulla or 2 cm in the isthmus, the woman desires future fertility, and if the tube is healthy.

Patients who have had a salpingectomy have a 50 percent chance of eventually achieving a viable pregnancy, and those having linear salpingostomy have a 60 to 65 percent chance. Both have a 10 to 15 percent probability of a recurrent ectopic pregnancy.[4,5] A laparoscopic procedure for ectopic pregnancy, therefore, offers comparable or improved results, with a much lesser operative procedure, less morbidity, a shorter recovery time, and reduced cost.

TUBAL FACTOR

Tubal factor is responsible for up to 40 percent of female infertility. The most common etiology being pelvic adhesions, mostly due to previous surgery or as a sequel of PID. Other conditions include endometriosis, hydrosalpinx and proximal tube obstruction due to complications of salpingitis.[6]

Diagnosis can be done by HSG, but laparoscopy facilitates easy visualization of the fallopian tubes and ovaries and also picks up any pelvic adhesions, and gives an idea regarding the tubal patency by chromopertubation and has an added advantage of absence of radiation and eliminates false negative test due to tubal spasm.

Combining hysteroscopy along with laparoscopy aid in further assessment of the uterine cavity as well. Mild operative procedure can be carried out in the same sitting.

Management of tubal infertility can be safely and effectively carried out with endoscopic procedures. Tubal block or adhesions treated with conventional surgery have shown poor results than laparoscopic management.

Status of the tubal mucosa is shown to be the most powerful prognostic factor in predicting pregnancy outcome.[7] Poor results are seen in badly damaged tubes.

Prognosis of laparoscopic adhesiolysis in mild pelvic adhesions is good with 68 percent pregnancy rate in 24 months. Adhesiolysis which cannot be managed by laparoscopy are better treated by IVF. Adhesiolysis by laparotomy not indicated as far as infertility management is concerned.

PROXIMAL TUBAL OCCLUSION

It accounts for 10 to 25 percent of tubal factor infertility. Tubal block is mostly because of inflammatory process or endometriosis which leads to local fibrosis. Functional obstructions are due to mucosal plugs.

Diagnosis is by HSG **(Fig. 4.3A)**, fluoroscopy or hysteroscopy. Diagnostic tubal catheterization **(Fig. 4.3B)** by selective salpingography to eliminate artifacts of conventional chromopertubation.

Traditional treatment of uterotubal implantation or tubocornual anastomosis has 10 to 15 percent results proximal tubal occlusion can be treated by transcervical catheter recanalization or falloposcopy.

Functional obstructions due to mucosal plugs can be treated by cannulation **(Fig. 4.3C)**,

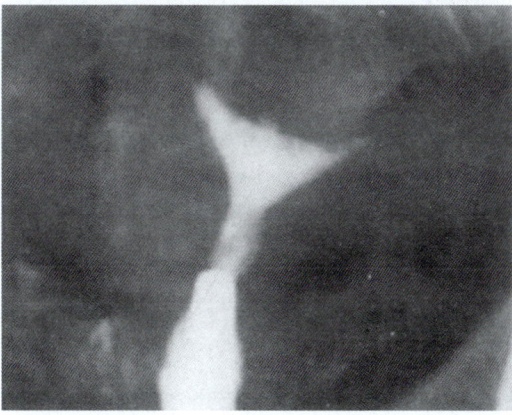

Fig. 4.3A: HSG—bilateral proximal tubal occlusion

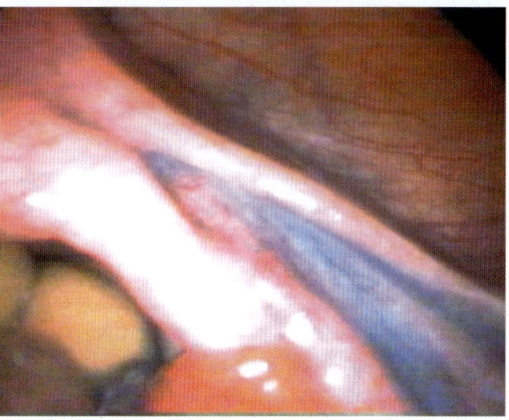

Fig. 4.3B: Hysteroscopic tubal cannulation

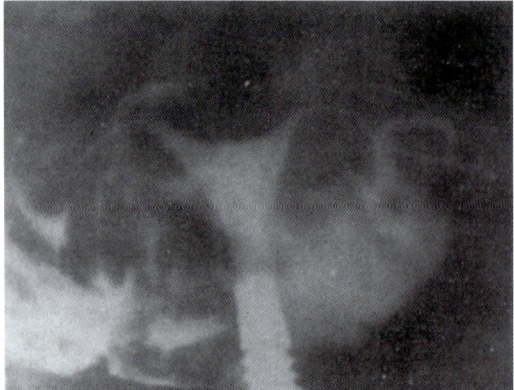

Fig. 4.3C: Postcannulation HSG

with success rate of 83 percent. Results of tubal surgery are inversely related to damage that exists prior to surgery. Development of adhesions remains a problem. Patients with operated tubes are at increased risk for ectopic pregnancy.[8,9]

INTRAUTERINE ADHESIONS

Most useful screening test for intrauterine adhesions is HSG **(Figs 4.4A and B)**. However, final diagnosis is determined by direct visualization with hysteroscopy because about 30 percent of abnormal HSG findings may be excluded and corrected by hysteroscopy **(Fig. 4.5)**.[10]

Endoscopy is the rule for treatment of intrauterine adhesions. In cases of primary amenorrhea menstruation restored is almost in 90 percent patients. Second-look scopy shows a newly formed endometrium. Fertility depends upon the extent of disease and associated tubal pathology.

UTERINE ANATOMICAL DEFECTS

The overall incidence of müllerian defects has been estimated to be between 0.1 percent and 3.5 percent.

The worst prognosis may be in women with a single uterine horn or a bicornuate uterus. Postabortion office hysteroscopy[11] is a simple and efficient tool in the early diagnosis of congenital and acquired uterine pathologies. Diagnostic hysteroscopy can be performed after the first miscarriage in order to determine congenital and acquired uterine pathologies. Hysteros-

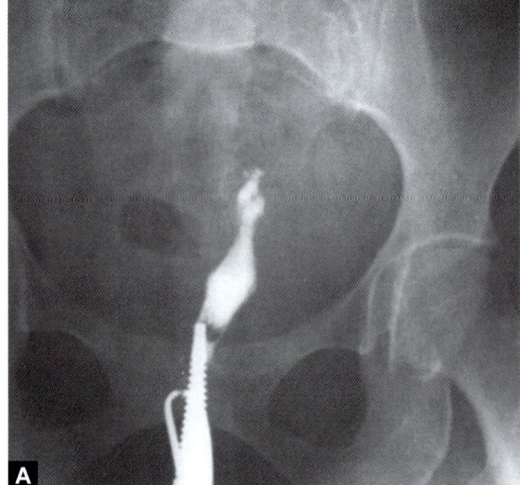
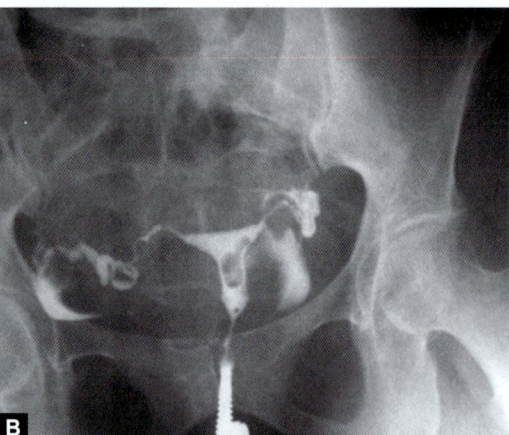

Figs 4.4A and B: HSG—intrauterine adhesions

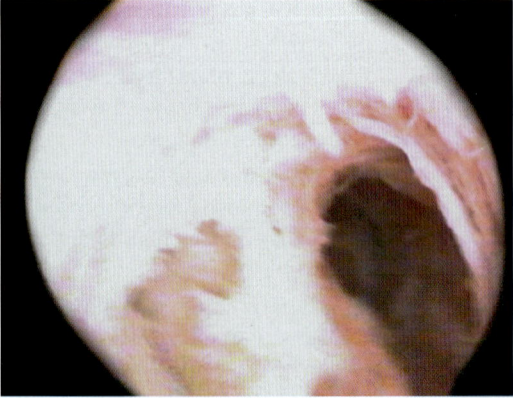

Fig. 4.5: Hysteroscopy—intrauterine adhesions

copy may be justified following two spontaneous pregnancy losses.

Uterine septum: One-third of patients with habitual abortion have a septate or subseptate uterus. The incidence of repeated spontaneous abortion in cases with low-grade anomalies is as high as the incidence among cases with more severe anomalies. Uterine septum can be picked-up on HSG **(Fig. 4.6A)**, USG **(Fig. 4.6B)** and confirmed on Hysteroscopy **(Fig. 4.6C)**.

There is uniform agreement in the literature on the benefits of hysteroscopic septal resection **(Fig. 4.6D)** in patients with reproductive wastage.

The presence of a residual uterine septum of 0.5 to 1 cm as shown by ultrasonography does not appear to worsen the reproductive prognosis as compared with that in women in whom the septum has been completely or almost completely corrected.

Intrauterine septum can be cut hysteroscopically with scissors, resected using a resectoscope or monopolar/bipolar current. Septum incision is done under laparoscopic control. Postoperatively pregnancy should be avoided for three months.

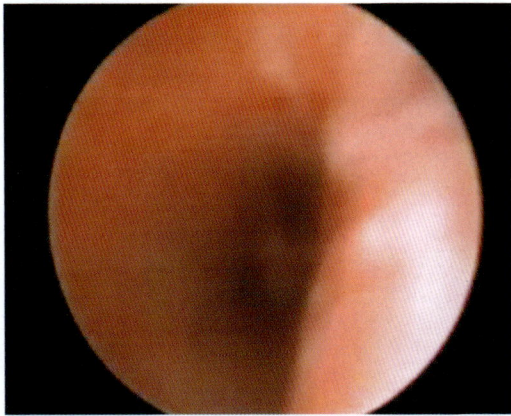
Fig. 4.6C: Hysteroscopy—uterine septum

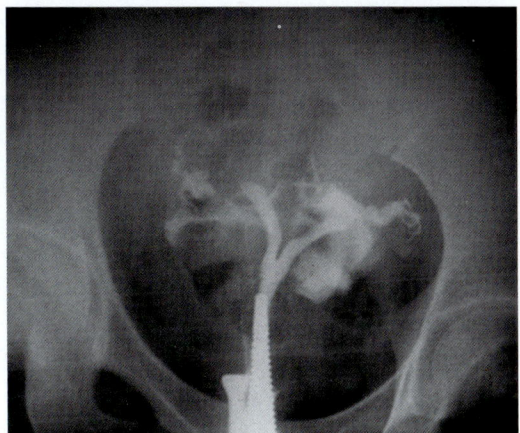
Fig. 4.6A: HSG—septate uterus

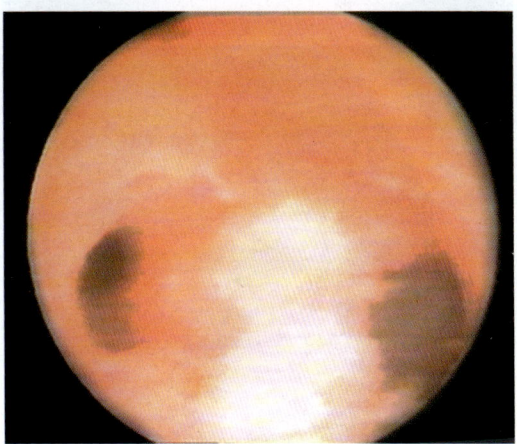
Fig. 4.6D: Hysteroscopy—septal resection

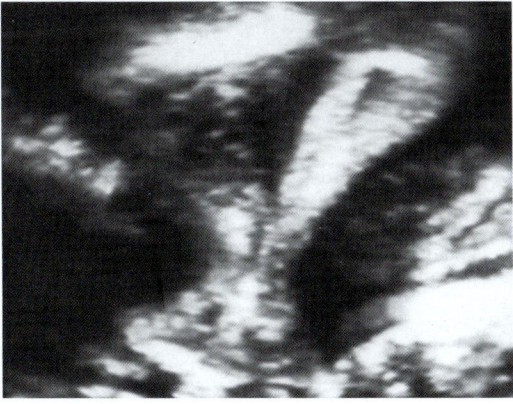
Fig. 4.6B: USG—septate uterus

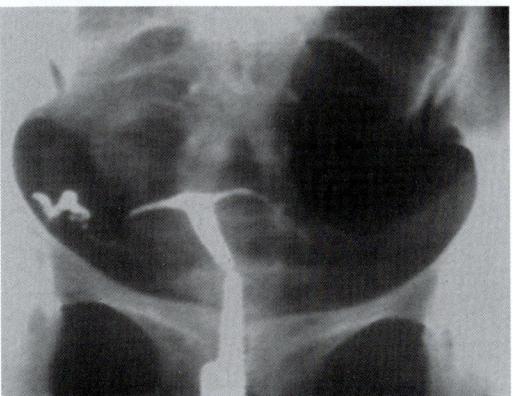
Fig. 4.7: HSG—T-shaped uterus

T-shaped uterus: T-shaped uterus diagnosed on HSG **(Fig. 4.7)** usually on the work up of primary infertility.

Treatment can be done endoscopically-lateral metroplasty **(Figs 4.8A to C)**, which is less invasive then the traditional surgical metroplasty. Risk to the uterine vessels is negligible. And the outcomes reported in literature have been fairly good.

HYSTEROSCOPIC MYOMECTOMY

Single fibroid less than 5 cm and protruding more than 75 percent of its volume into uterine cavity can be resected in one-step procedure and if more than 5 cm and protruding 50 to 75 percent within the cavity can be managed with GnRH agonists suppression before procedure followed by single-step procedure. Underwater bipolar technology has an advantage of using saline as medium Hysteromyomectomy.

Removal of fibroids that distort the uterine cavity may be indicated in infertile women, where no other factors have been identified, and in women about to undergo *in vitro* fertilization treatment.[12]

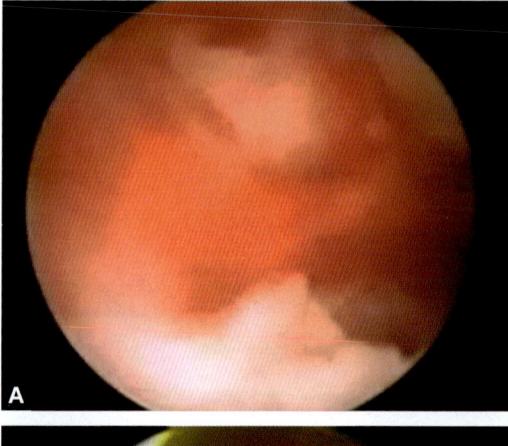

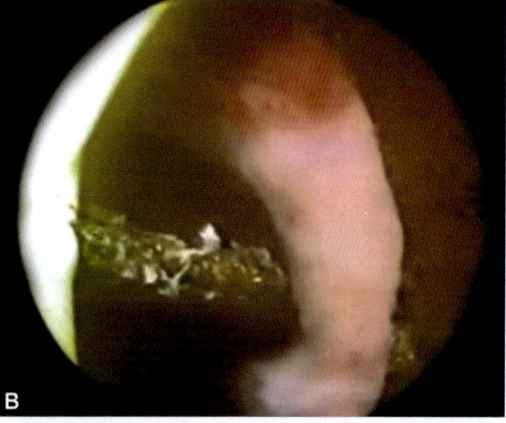

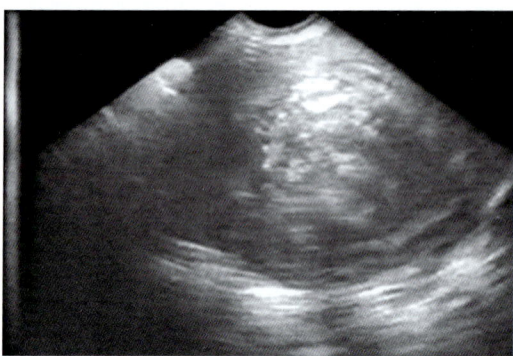

Fig. 4.9A: TVS—submucous fibroid

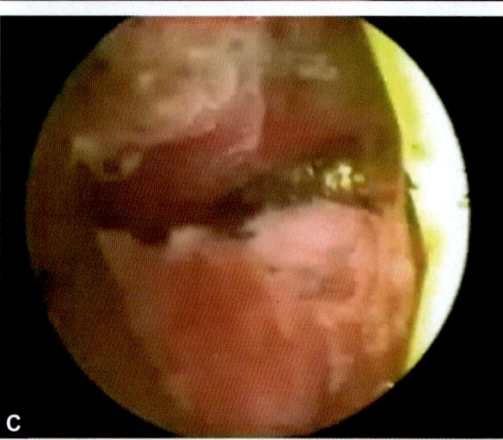

Figs 4.8A to C: Hysteroscopic-lateral metroplasty

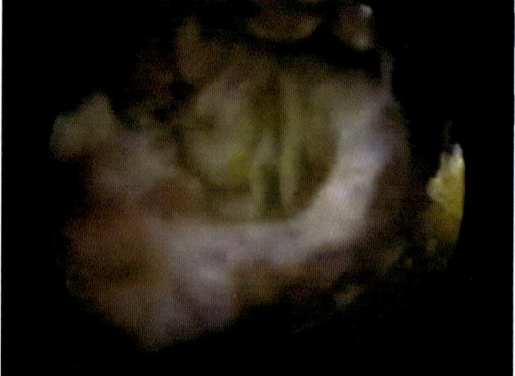

Fig. 4.9B: Hysteroscopy—submucous fibroid

OVARIAN CYSTS

Eighty to eighty-five percent of ovarian cyst can be managed laparoscopically **(Fig. 4.10)**.

An ideal ovarian cystectomy consists of removal the intact cyst with limited trauma to the residual ovarian tissue. Alternatively, cyst fluid may be drained to minimize spillage and to facilitate removal.

Advantages and disadvantages of techniques of cystectomy:

	Advantages	Disadvantages
Punctured cyst	Small ovarian incision	Spill of fluid contents
	No size limit	
	Faster to perform	
Intact Cyst	No fluid spill	Larger ovarian incision
		Size limit
		Longer to perform
		Accidental rupture
		Extraction difficult

Main difficulty is in the identification of early malignancy in young women. Risk of spreading the cancer in event of rupture of ovarian malignancy may compromise patient's survival unless chemotherapy is given or immediate laparotomy is performed.

Benign cystic teratomas **(Fig. 4.11)** comprising of 13 percent of all ovarian tumors with a malignant potential one to three percent, can also be managed laparoscopically. It can often be excised intact, but if it ruptures, the result will be poor than it would if the cyst were opened and aspirated. The contents should be removed with an endobag followed by copious lavage.

FIBROIDS

Myoma of 5 to 8 cm subserosal or intramural can be managed laparoscopically **(Figs 4.12A and B)**. Size of > 8 cm and multiple myomas

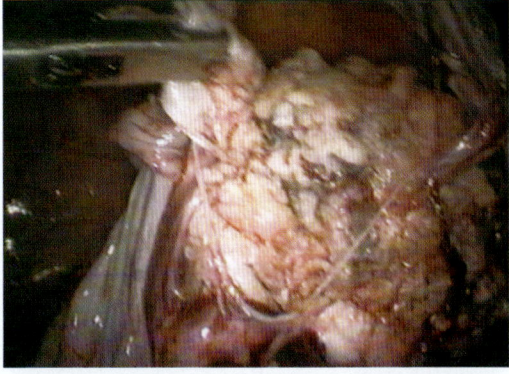

Fig. 4.11: Laparoscopy benign cystic teratomas

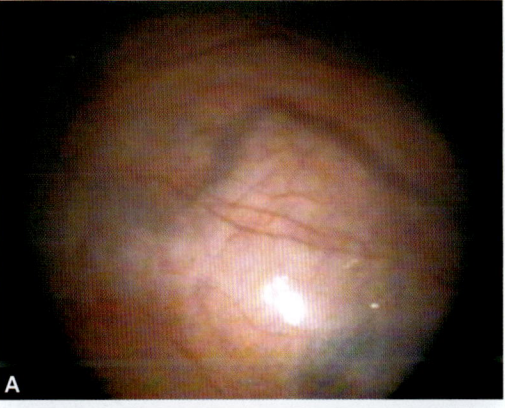

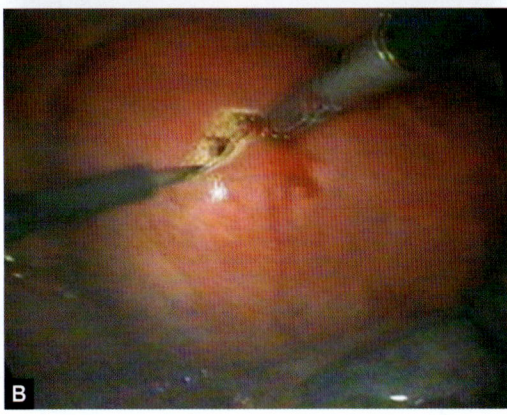

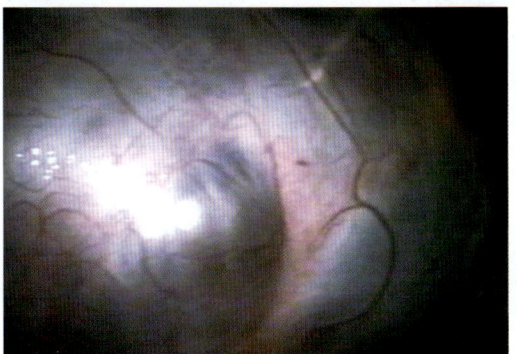

Fig. 4.10: Laparoscopy—ovarian cyst

Figs 4.12A and B: Laparoscopy—uterine fibroid

(>3) should be done by laparotomy. Laparoscopic experts may have higher cut offs.

A hysteroscopy is always done before starting laparoscopy to exclude a sub mucous myoma.

Myoma of >5 cm should be removed by colpotomy if an electronic morcellator is not available.

Laparoscopic myolysis may present an alternative to myomectomy or hysterectomy for selected women with symptomatic intramural or subserous fibroids who wish to preserve their uterus but do not desire future fertility.[13]

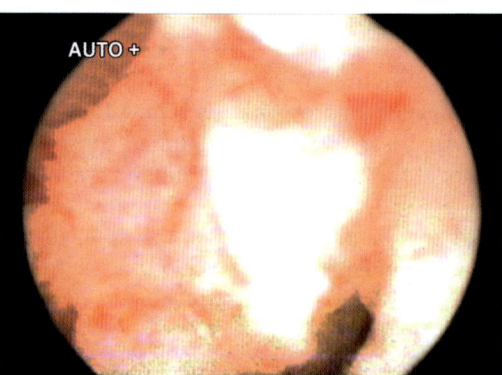

Fig. 4.14: Endometrial carcinoma (Frozen section)

ENDOMETRIOSIS

Laparoscopic assessment in combination with histologic examination of the excised lesion remains the gold standard for diagnosis of endometriosis **(Fig. 4.13)**. An increase awareness of the variations in the appearance of the endometriotic lesions has resulted in an almost two fold increase in the diagnosis. Even an expert laparoscopic surgeon can miss 7 percent or underdiagnose 50 percent of cases of endometriosis.

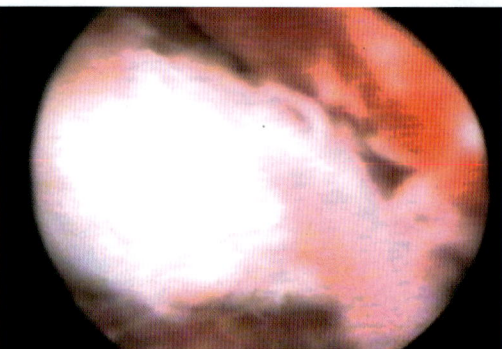

Fig. 4.15: Endometrial polypectomy

POSTMENOPAUSAL BLEEDING

Endometrial cancer presents as abnormal bleeding in approximately 93 percent of cases. Transvaginal sonography may rule out most intrauterine pathologies, but diagnostic hysteroscopy with targeted biopsy is the gold standard **(Figs 4.14 and 4.15)**.

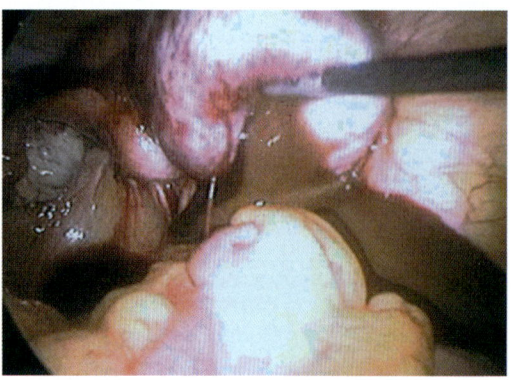

Fig. 4.13: Laparoscopy endometrioma

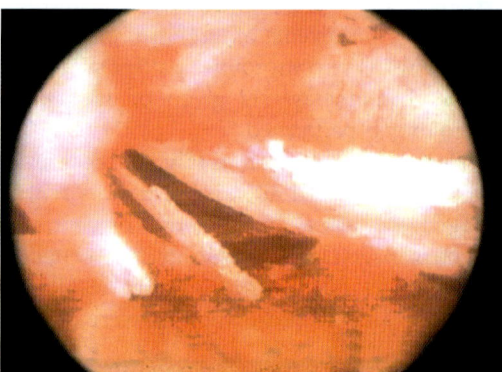

Fig. 4.16: Hysteroscopy—postabortion fetal bone

MISCELLANEOUS

Removal of foreign body, misplaced IUCD, post abortion fetal bones **(Fig. 4.16)** can be identified and removed hysteroscopically.

Posthysterectomy Adhesiolysis

Proper history and clinical evaluation necessary. Diagnosis by process of exclusion **(Figs 4.17A and B)**.

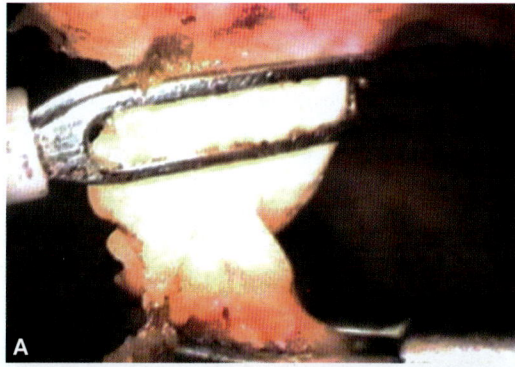
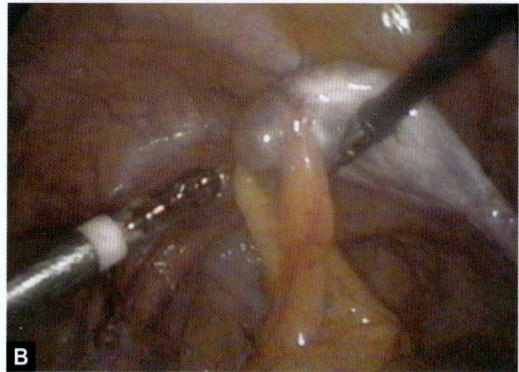

Figs 4.17A and B: Laparoscopy—posthysterectomy adhesions

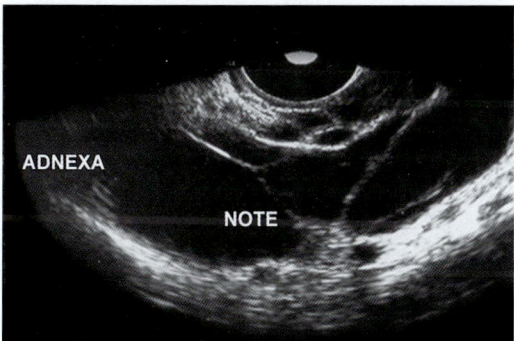

Fig. 4.18: USG-multiseptate ovarian tumor

Clinical Dilemma

Multiseptate Ovarian Tumor—On Table Loculated Ascites (Fig. 4.18)

Patient referred with USG diagnosis of ovarian tumor.

On laparoscopy, it was found to be loculated ascites, hence emphasis should be on detailed history taking and proper clinical examination.

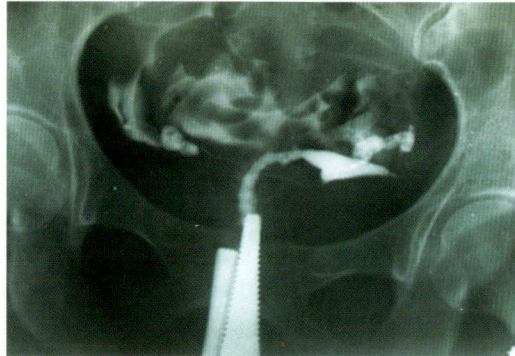

Fig. 4.19: HSG—postlaparoscopy round ligament plication

Laparoscopic Round Ligament Plication

Patient with history of 15 years infertility and unexplained infertility conceived following laparoscopic round ligament plication **(Fig. 4.19)**.

Know thyself
— *Socrates*

REFERENCES

1. Canis M, Savary D, Pouly JL, Wattiez A, Mage G. Ectopic pregnancy: criteria to decide between medical and conservative surgical treatment? J Gynecol Obstet Biol Reprod (Paris). 2003 Nov; 32(7 Suppl):S54-63.
2. Brumsted J, Kessler C, Gibson C, et al. A comparison of laparoscopy and laparotomy for the treatment of ectopic pregnancy. Obstet Gynecol 1988;71:889-92.
3. Leach RE, Ory SJ. Modern management of ectopic pregnancy. J Reprod Med 1989;34:324-38.
4. Mecke H, Semm K, Lehmann-Willenbrock E. Results of operative pelviscopy in 202 cases of ectopic pregnancy. IntJ Fertil 1989;34:93-4,97-100.
5. Vermesh M. Conservative management of ectopic gestation. Fertil Steril 1989;51:559-67.
6. Otolorin EO, Ojengbede O, Falase AO. Laparoscopic evaluation of the tuboperitoneal factor in infertile Nigerian women. Int J Gynaecol Obstet. 1987; 25(1):47-52.
7. Yu SL, Yap C. Investigating the Infertile Couple Ann Acad Med Singapore 2003;32:611-4.
8. Sulak PJ, Letterie GS, Hayslip CC, Coddington CC, Klein TA. Hysteroscopic cannulation and lavage in the treatment of proximal tubal occlusion. Steril Fertil 1987;48:493-4.

9. Mohapatra P, Swain S, Pati T. Hysteroscopic Tubal Cannulation: Our Experience. J Obstet Gynaecol Ind 2004;54(5):498-9.
10. Valle RF, Sciarra JJ. Current status of hysteroscopy in gynecologic practice. Fertil Steril. 1979;32:619-32.
11. Cogendez E, Dolgun ZN, Sanverdi I, Turgut A, Eren S Eur J Obstet Gynecol Reprod Biol. 2011;156 (1):101-4. Epub 2011 Mar 2.
12. Lefebvre G, Vilos G, Allaire C, Jeffrey J, Arneja J, Birch C, Fortier M, Wagner MS. Clinical Practice Gynaecology Committee, Society for Obstetricians and Gynaecologists of Canada.
13. The management of uterine leiomyomas. J Obstet Gynaecol Can. 2003 May; 25(5):396-418; quiz 419-22.

CHAPTER 5

Safe Anesthesia for Gynecological Endoscopic Surgery

Dinesh Bajani, Deepika Desai

Chapter Outline

- Anesthesia for Hysteroscopy
  - Positioning
  - Monitoring
  - Complications
  - Glycine Toxicity
- Anesthetic Management
- Anesthesia for Gynecological Laparoscopic Surgery
  - Preoperative Considerations
  - Premedication
  - Monitoring
- Complications
  - Cardiovascular
  - Respiratory
  - Gastrointestinal
  - Renal
  - Surgical Trauma
  - Others
- Problems
  - Pneumoperitoneum
  - Insufflating Gas and its Effect
  - Position of Patient
- Anesthesia Management
  - Regional Anesthesia
  - General
  - Combination of Regional Anesthesia (Using Epidural Catheter) and General Anesthesia
  - Extraperitoneal Laparoscopic Surgery

INTRODUCTION

Anesthesia for gynecological endoscopy includes both hysteroscopic and laparoscopic procedures. Range of surgical procedures vary from short, simple diagnostic endoscopy to advanced, lengthy surgical operations.

This technique requires distension of uterus in hysteroscopy and of peritoneum in laparoscopy resulting in significant pathophysiological repercussions related to the reabsorption of liquid or gas used. There could be additional effects on hemodynamics due to trendelenberg position and diaphragmatic compressions.[1]

These repercussions depend on the condition of the patient, operative skills of the surgeon and competence of the anesthetist.

ANESTHESIA FOR HYSTEROSCOPY

After careful selection and optimum preparation of the patient, anesthesia can be planned as per the surgical requirement.

Positioning

Due care must be taken when positioning the patient to avoid popliteal and/or sciatic nerve compression in the leg restraints.

Monitoring

Routine monitoring includes parameters like pulse, NIBP, SpO_2, ECG and E_TCO_2. Specific monitoring includes monitoring of temperature as there can be considerable heat loss due to the use of copious, cold irrigating fluid. Strict monitoring of the input and output of distending fluid is indispensable. Any deficit of 1 liter or more should be dealt with by giving injection frusemide 10 to 20 mg. Procedure must be interrupted, if the discrepancy reaches 2 liters.

Anesthetist must also monitor the rate and pressure at which the distending fluid is administered. Sudden, rapid distension of uterus may cause bradycardia or arrhythmias. Auscultation of chest to detect earliest signs of pulmonary overload is also called for. Clinically, patient's sensorium can be checked, if patient is under local or regional anesthesia, which may help detect early glycine toxicity. Catheterization of bladder is required when frusemide is given. Intrauterine pressure should be monitored and it should not be more than 150 mm Hg.

Complications

There is no substitute for vigilance by the competent anesthetist. Strict, vigilant monitoring can help prevent as well as detect the earliest signs of complications requiring intervention and safe outcome.

Glycine Toxicity

Acute intoxication with glycine occurs when large quantities of glycine have been reabsorbed.[2,3] The toxicity leads to:
- Intracellular hyperhydration and hyponatremia leading to circulatory overload and pulmonary edema
- The neurological symptoms because of metabolism of glycine leading to increase serum ammonia levels. They may present with simple confusion progressing to agitation to coma. Sometimes visual disturbances or focal conversions may be the presenting signs
- Cardiovascular symptoms range from bradyarrhythmias to collapse with ECG changes.

ANESTHETIC MANAGEMENT

Minor diagnostic and operative procedures can be managed using total intravenous anesthesia (TIVA) or mask anesthesia (including use of LMA). For lengthy operative procedures endotracheal intubation with controlled ventilation is indicated.

Regional anesthesia can be given in case of medically compromised patients. Early signs of vascular overloading and glycine toxicity can be detected by observing the sensorium of the patient. Though, because of the increased vascular capacitance, signs of fluid overload can be masked during the surgery. When the effect of regional anesthesia wears off, these signs may come up in postoperative period.

Hence, anesthetic management continues into the postoperative period.

ANESTHESIA FOR GYNECOLOGICAL LAPAROSCOPIC SURGERY

Preoperative Considerations

For the safe outcome of the surgery, thorough preoperative assessment of the patient is required. Complete evaluation includes relevant laboratory investigations and speciality consultation as indicated. Preoperative visit by the anesthetist is of help to counsel the patient and reduce the anxiety and fear about anesthesia.

Proper informed consent for laparoscopic surgery and anesthesia including possibility of conversion to conventional open surgery and longer duration of hospitalization should be taken. Blood may be kept ready for major surgery with anticipated bloodloss.

Premedication

As a routine, anxiolytic drugs along with antisialogogue can be ordered before surgery. Applying prilox/emla cream before venepuncture for its local anesthetic effect actually gives some confidence to the patient regarding pain free anesthesia and surgery. Patient must continue all other medications, if any, for the systemic medical problems.

Tablet clonidine in the dose range of 0.1 to 0.2 mg/kg can be added.

Monitoring

With more and more advanced, complicated surgical procedures being undertaken, need for superior anesthesia machines and monitors cannot be stressed less.

Along with the upgradation of laparoscopic surgical instruments and gadgets, there is a need for upgrading of anesthesia delivery systems and multiparameter monitoring device for superior care of the patient.

- Precordial stethoscope is an integral part of monitoring for diagnosis of gas embolism as well as equality of ventilation, trendelenberg position may lead to selective intubation
- SpO_2: Longer surgery along with steep head low and increased intra-abdominal pressure will compromise the respiratory function leading to some decompensation and reduction in SPO_2
- ECG monitoring enables detection of arrhythmias due to hypercapnia, use of halothane may also lead to tachyarrhythmia
  Change in ECG voltage can be early sign of subcutaneous emphysema or pneumomediastinum
- NIBP monitoring is preferred on the hand other than the one used for intravenous fluid and SpO_2 monitoring to avoid false alarms.
- Temperature monitoring: Intraperitoneal insufflation of dry unheated gas, irrigation with cold liquids, cold intravenous fluids, and dry unhumidified gases (if so) and cold operation theater environment can all lead to hypothermia requiring mandatory monitoring of core temperature
- Monitoring of intraperitoneal pressure is an integral part of anesthesia monitoring. The insufflators must have preset pressure limit control and automatic cut-off facility
- During insufflation by Verres needle, any extraperitoneal collection leading to subcutaneous emphysema should be vigilantly observed
- End tidal CO_2 monitoring is a MUST during any laparoscopic procedure. Any sudden increase or decrease in $ETCO_2$ is a sign of complication. Physiological consequences of surgery leading to gradual increase in $ETCO_2$ can be dealt with by adjusting the ventilation.
  Sudden drop in $ETCO_2$ is suggestive of gas embolism requiring urgent intervention with appropriate measures.

COMPLICATIONS[4]

Cardiovascular

Cardiac Arrhythmias

Pneumoperitoneum causes rise in systemic and pulmonary vascular resistance and there by decreases cardiac index by 20 to 40 percent.[5] There is an increase in preload, which is akin to chronic heart failure. This is essentially due to release of catecholamine, renin and aldosterone during laparoscopy.

Stretching of peritoneum during pneumoperitoneum and pulling of viscera during dissection can cause strong vagal stimulation leading to severe bradycardia or a systole.

Blood Pressure

- Hypertension: There is almost always increase in blood pressure during pneumoperitoneum. Besides release of catecholamine, raised blood level of carbon dioxide and painful stimuli would cause rise in blood pressure. Therefore preoperative oral clonidine (100-200 mcg 1 hr prior) or preinduction IV clonidine 20 to 50 mcg would help. Addition of propofol—fentanyl-sevoflurane or isoflurane would keep the BP undercontrol. Only undercertain situation you may have to start NTG drip to control hypertension.
- Hypotension during induction phase usually indicates pre-existing dehydration. Intraoperative hypotension can be because of bleeding. In laparoscopy, dissection is usually by cautery and irrigation of fluid, therefore it may be little difficult to judge the actual loss of blood. While considering bloodloss fluid used for irrigation should be considered.
  On creating pneumo, if there is hypotension, it is possibly because of very high IADP. (>30 mm Hg) On releasing the IADP usually hypotension is corrected.

Venous Gas Embolism

This is usually not seen where open puncture method is selected to create pneumoperitoneum. Though it is rare, it is life-threatening complication and prognosis depends essentially on prompt detection and treatment.

Vigilant monitoring of sudden drop in ETCO$_2$, pulse rate, SPO$_2$ and BP during pneumo is the signal for venous gas embolism.[6] If the insufflating gas is CO$_2$ it is safer. It requires 5 times higher volume of CO$_2$ to create the symptoms of embolism and being a blood gas which is highly soluble in blood, the prognosis of patient is better.

Treatment: Immediate aspiration of gas by putting central line, left lateral and head low position, 100 percent oxygenation and IPPV and other supportive treatment is necessary.

Respiratory

There is alteration in respiratory mechanics when trendelenberg position (head low) is given for pelvic surgery. Head low, lithotomy and pneumoperitoneum cause reduction in lung compliance, FRC and vital capacity. Ninety percent of compression atelectasis occurring intraoperatively persists up to 1 hr, so this explains the importance of spirometry intraoperatively. In patients with COPD, preoperative nebulization should be considered.

In order to compensate for reduced lung compliance you need to increase overall minute ventilation. It can be best taken care off by using newer low flow anesthesia machines with ventilator.

Gastrointestinal

The incidence of nausea and vomiting during conventional surgery is higher after endoscopic surgery. It can be prevented and treated by giving antiemetic drugs like ondancetron and metoclopramide.

Renal

With intra-abdominal distension pressure (IADP) of 15 mm Hg there is 60 percent reduction in renal cortical perfusion by direct compression. This leads to 50 percent reduction in GFR and reduction in urine output.

On release of pneumoperitoneum, renal cortical perfusion returns to normal almost instantaneously, but reduction in urine output persist for another 1 to 2 hours. This suggests the role of hormonal factor in prolongation of oliguria (caused by release of aldosterone and ADH. This oliguria is transient and in healthy patients it is reversible within a period of 2 hours.

Patients with borderline cardiorespiratory problem or with diabetic nephropathy are more vulnerable to such problems.

Surgical Trauma

During laparoscopic surgery, surgical trauma can be vascular or visceral. It can be during trocar insertion or dissecting bad adhesion or due to cautery. During hemostasis you need lot of irrigation and hence anesthesiologist should keep account of actual blood loss and fluid irrigation. Timely identification of injuries and appropriate intervention in tackling problems with adequate and strict postoperative care would avoid catastrophe.

Others

Head low position during gynecological laparoscopy for 2 to 3 hours, can result in conjunctival and cerebral edema because of raised intraocular and intracranial tension. Respectively edema can cause transient visual disturbances which can be avoided and treated by eye lubrication and eye pads intraoperatively and postoperatively if required.

Mild cerebral edema occasionally delays recovery. IPPV with 100 percent O$_2$, steroids and postoperative oxygen therapy for 2 to 4 hours usually helps in recovery.

There are reported cases of brachial plexus damage because of improper shoulder blade and head low. In gynec laparoscopic surgery you need modified lithotomy position, which can strain pelvic and pubic ligaments.

Continuous insufflation of peritoneum with cold carbon dioxide, infusion of cold IV. fluids and airconditioned theaters can cause significant hypothermia. Hypothermia causes metabolic acidosis and delayed recovery. It also leads to postoperative shivering which increases oxygen demand three times. This is more significant in pediatric laparoscopic surgery. Insufflation of warm carbon dioxide, use of infusion warmer and warm air-blower would reduce hypothermia.

Peglec is used for preoperative bowel preparation and this is known to cause loss of fluid and electrolytes in addition to preoperative starvation. Insufflation of peritoneum with dry carbon dioxide and ventilation of lungs with dry anesthetic gases involves considerable insensible fluid loss causing dehydration.

PROBLEMS

Pneumoperitoneum

Creation of Pneumoperitoneum

At many centers even today, first puncture is done with Verres needle. This is a blind puncture to create pneumoperitoneum. It has several times caused visceral or vascular damage including gas embolism, which is rare, but a life-threatening complication. Severe hemorrhage is another common and serious complication. Many surgeons perform first puncture directly with trocar instead of Verres needle and hence when damage occurs it is serious and life-threatening.

Manipulation of Verres needle can cause profound vagal stimulation causing severe bradycardia and asystole, which should be kept in mind and hence diluted atropine should always be there on anesthesia trolley.

Safety precautions to minimize above problems:

- Premedicate and repeat vagolytic drugs when required
- Provide adequate abdominal wall relaxation during first puncture
- Hypos ventilate or transient apnea during actual puncture would avoid underlying structure to come near puncture site
- Proper and scientific insufflators have pressure cut-out, set initial low IADP and low flow rate (1 lit/min)
- Vigilant monitoring of patient (SPO_2- NIBP, $ETCO_2$-ECG)
- Various tests to confirm free needle tip in peritoneal cavity.

NB: Now it is a routine to do 'open puncture; which eliminates practically all problems of first puncture.

Maintenance of Pneumoperitoneum

Good gas insufflators having pressure cut-out and wide range of flow rate adjustability is excellent to keep the desired IADP (12-15 mm Hg) you have freedom to keep very high flow of about 15 to 20 liters because at set pressure the flow gets cut-off and you can easily compensate leak.

Good consistent abdominal wall relaxation is useful to keep less flow and low IADP.

Higher IADP is known to cause suppression of renal cortical perfusion and oliguria.

At higher IADP >30 mm Hg there is direct compression on capacitance vessels reducing venous return and cardiac output and creating severe hypotension and bradycardia—an untoward effect.

Insufflating Gas and its Effect

Carbon dioxide is the most preferred insufflating gas because it is highly soluble in blood, non inflammable and readily diffusible across membranes. Because of its solubility and easy excretion through lungs, prognosis of cardiorespiratory integrity is much better if carbon dioxide embolization occurs.

Raised blood levels of CO_2 can cause cardiac arrhythmias. Drugs like halothane exaggerate such possibilities.

Position of Patient

Trendelenberg (Head Low) Position

This position is useful in lower abdominal and pelvic surgery (like appendix and other gynecological operation).

In these position viscera is pushed up towards diaphragm. This along with lithotomy and pneumoperitoneum causes marked reduction in vital capacity. This impairs the respiratory mechanics and alters the gaseous exchange. This reduces tidal volume, FRC, and increases $ETCO_2$. Therefore care should be taken to rectify the changes in respiratory mechanics.

On the other hand head low will increase the venous return and hence cardiac output.

It is observed that prolonged head low position (2-3 hrs) has caused rise in intraocular and intracranial tension leading to conjunctional edema and mild cerebral edema.

Conjunctival edema and visual disturbance should be taken care off by eye lubrication and eyepad covering.

Cerebral edema is usually mild and transient and in certain patient can cause delayed recovery particularly, if it is associated with raised postoperative CO_2 level. Intravenous steroid and oxygen therapy in postoperative period is required.

ANESTHESIA MANAGEMENT

Essentially, any of the following suitable anesthesia, techniques can be selected.
  I. Regional: Spinal, epidural or both.
 II. General anesthesia with or without intubations.
III. Combined general and regional anesthesia.

Regional Anesthesia

If you are giving only regional anesthesia, following points should be kept in mind.
- The level of analgesic should be sufficiently high (i.e. up to T4-6 dermatomes) to tolerate pneumoperitoneum
- Patient should be very cooperative with excellent pulmonary function and should be able to lie in that position for 1 to 3 hours (because discomfort beyond 1 hour is quite likely)
- Intra-abdominal distension pressure for pneumoperitoneum should be as low as possible
- Insufflating gas flow rate should be low
- Head low should be minimum
- Surgeon should be aware and adjust, since the patient is spontaneously breathing
- Heavy sedation should be avoided
- Oxygen supplementation throughout laparoscopy is must
- If you are giving only spinal analgesia, then surgeon and anesthesiologist should keep time binding in mind (1-2 hr)
- Only epidural may not give required degree of abdominal wall relaxation

- Combined spinal epidural can help the anesthetist, if operation time is extended; top-up epidural is also useful in postoperative analgesia.

General

This is possibly most widely accepted choice of anesthetic technique for most of the endoscopic procedures.

Conventional anesthesia is employed keeping probable problems and complications in mind. Short duration surgeries or moderately longer procedures can be managed using LMA (laryngeal mask airway) **(Figs 5.1 and 5.2)**. Earlier, its use was regarded as risky. One has to keep in mind, the increased chances of regurgitation and aspiration.[7,8] Enhanced experience has allowed safe use of LMA quite frequently.

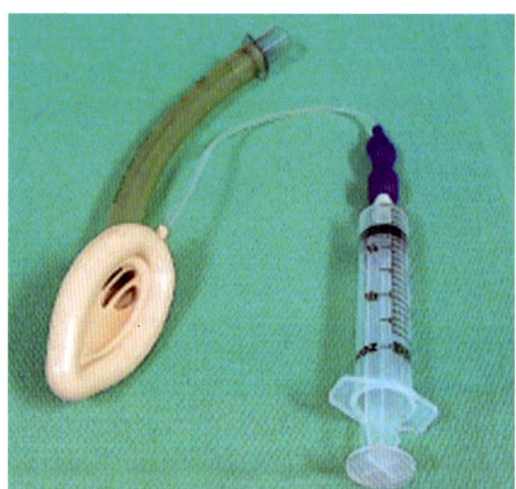

Fig. 5.1: Laryngeal mask airways (LMA)

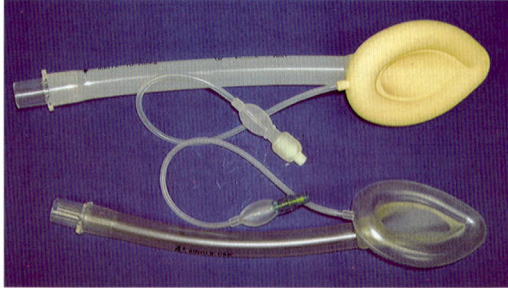

Fig. 5.2: Silicon and PVC LMA

Combination of Regional Anesthesia (Using Epidural Catheter) and General Anesthesia

It is sometimes suitable for extensive surgeries like pelvic adhesiolysis, oncosurgery, etc. where indwelling epidural catheter can be used to attenuate postoperative pain and make the patient comfortable and stress free.

Extraperitoneal Laparoscopic Surgery

Certain procedures such as Burch vaginal suspension or pelvic lymphadenectomy mean that the operating field is extended and will then include Pre or retroperitoneal space.

Extraperitoneal insufflation of CO_2 is usually accompanied by hypercapnia in proportion to the rate of rise in pressure and volume of CO_2 Insufflation. Simultaneous reabsorption may not be proportionate leading to severe acidosis. Subcutaneous or mediastinal emphysema should be diagnosed at the earliest. Anesthetist must be vigilant and must optimize the ventilation as much as possible.

CONCLUSION

Endoscopic gynecological surgery is still evolving, giving birth to newer techniques and indications. Anesthetist, as part of the team, has to evolve with these advances to preserve the safety and well-being of the patient.

REFERENCES

1. Beyond the boundaries by Dr Prakash Trivedi 2000;123-36.
2. McLucas B. Hyskon complications in hysteroscopic surgery. Obstet Gynaecol Survey 1991; 46,196-200.
3. Afzul L, et al. Transient blindness. A case report following glycine as irrigating fluid in TURP. IJA, 2002 46(3);221-3.
4. Randle S. Corfman, Micheal P Diamond, Alan H. DeCherney. Complications of Laparoscopy and Hysteroscopy 1993.
5. Cullen DJ. Eger E II. Cardiovascular effects of carbon dioxide in man. Anaesthesiology, 1974;44:1183-7.
6. Ronald DM, Anaesthesia, vol. 1 and 2, 1990.
7. DeGrood PMRM, Harbers BM, Van Egmond J. et al. Anaesthesia for laparoscopy. Anaesthsia 1987;42:815.
8. Chiu HH, Ng KH. Complication of laparoscopy under general anaesthesia. Anaesth Intensive Care, 1977;5 169-71.

CHAPTER 6

Operative Laparoscopic Surgery Step by Step for Achieving Safety

Shaily Jain

Chapter Outline

- Interaction with Patient and Proper Consent
  - Prior to Operation Theatre
  - Operation Theater set up
- The Beginning of the Surgery
- Introduction of Veress Needle and Trocars
  - Location of Standard Port Placement
- New Energy Sources, Vessel Sealing Devices a Brief Clear Concept
- Golden Rules of each Person in Endoscopic Surgery
- Documentation and Explaining Patients after Surgery
  - After the Surgery

"Wise persons learn from others mistake the otherwise learn by committing themselves"

INTRODUCTION

Operative laparoscopy is a standard procedure in almost any place in India and abroad, however every expert does with different primary steps. We will be highlighting in this chapter an accurate stepwise procedure to perform safe operative laparoscopy which is for moderate to advanced surgery like laparoscopic hysterectomy, myomectomy, ectopic pregnancy, large ovarian cyst, young patient with prolapse, vault prolapse, creating neovagina, etc.

INTERACTION WITH PATIENT AND PROPER CONSENT

As the patient expects only success or miracles from a laparoscopic surgeon, it is important to explain the operative laparoscopic procedure to the patient, close relatives, preferably by properly made photographs or small clips of video, making very clear with them regarding limitations, complications, possibility of open surgery in a subtle but clear fashion. Finally, giving a brief idea that such incidences although rare, if encountered, can be handled safely by laparoscopy or alternative methods. Further, a proper consent for anesthesia, relative risks and also elucidating history of any drug allergy or previous problems she had with any type of surgery should be taken. The consent forms though exhaustive, patient and relative should read and then sign. In certain high risk patients, a special informed consent additionally is mandatory.

Prior to Operation Theatre

The operating surgeon should have a full idea of the clinical, sonographic findings with an additional investigative details, keeping the end point desired by patient rather than what the surgeon wants.

We usually prefer to give peglec, one sachet in 2 liters of water on the day prior to surgery, one cup every half hourly till stools are watery. Post lunch, patient can have soft dinner on the day prior and is fasting on the day of surgery if scheduled in the morning, but if surgery is in the afternoon, she can have a cup of tea or coffee, six hours prior to operative procedure.

The other alternative excelyte is known to cause electrolyte disturbance, especially potassium level and occasionally excess dehydration. We have not advised liquid diet for two days to any patient, except for laparoscopic radical surgery or extensive endometriomas with bowel adhesions.

Nitrous oxide, which causes bowel distention on prolonged surgery, is best to be avoided and if possible, using an unusual combination of epidural and general anesthesia with endotracheal intubation gives a non-distended bowel and an excellent pelvic field. In selected centers, laryngeal mask apparatus (LMA) anesthesia have replaced the earlier techniques to avoid throat irritation, etc. due to endotracheal intubation.

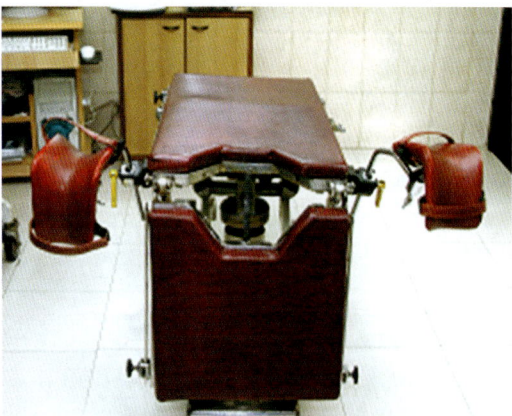

Fig. 6.2: Operation theatre table with double pelvic cut and angled padded leg rest

Operation Theater Set Up[1,2]

Before shifting the patients in the operation theater the following are mandatory:
1. A proper laparoscopic instrument trolley having all instruments needed for surgery **(Fig. 6.1)**.
2. The operating table should have a double pelvic cut to allow good manipulation of uterus **(Fig. 6.2)**.

Lithotomy padded rods which can be angled at 45° or an or direct/Allen's leg rest position of which can be changed during the surgery with sterile clothes covered **(Fig. 6.3)**.

The OT table should have padded shoulder rest and side arms to avoid patients from slipping down on head low positions **(Fig. 6.4)**. The left arm of the patient should be kept at the side of the patient, covered with green sheet, so

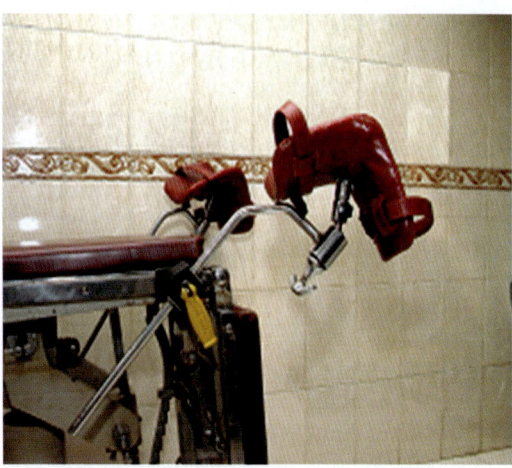

Fig. 6.3: Simple gynec operation table

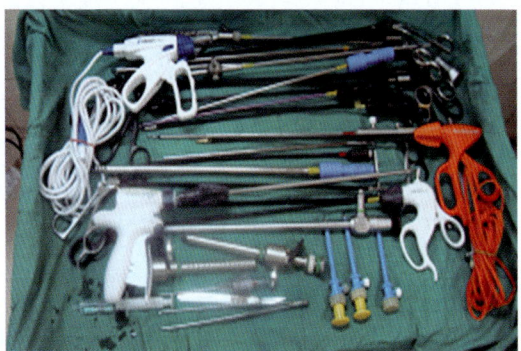

Fig. 6.1: Laparoscopic instrument trolley

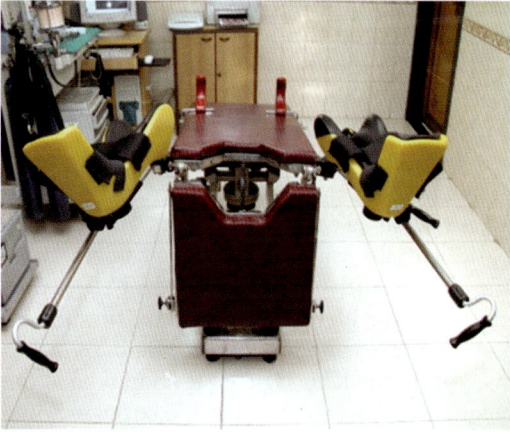

Fig. 6.4: Operation table with or direct stirrups padded shoulder rest, prominent

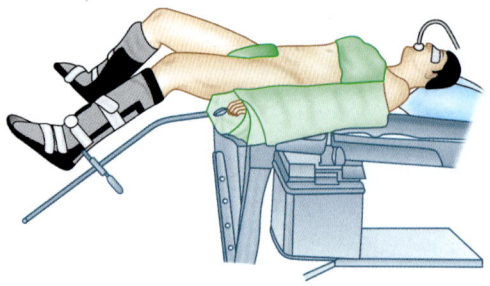

Fig. 6.5: Patient'arms positioned by the side

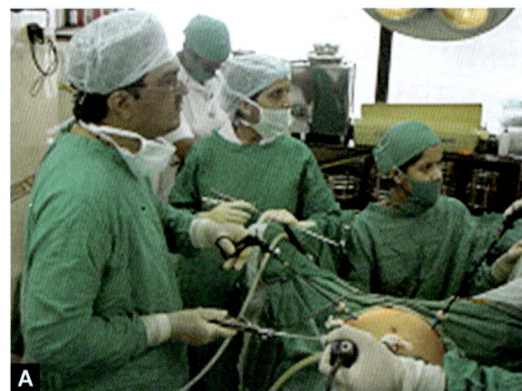

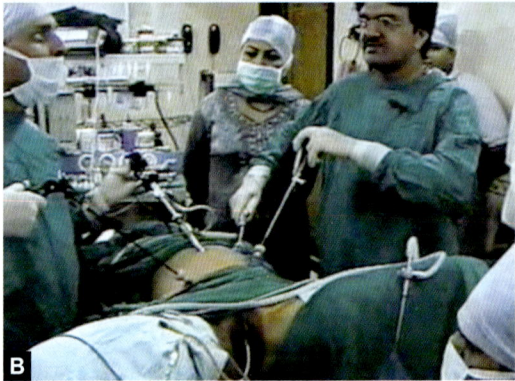

Figs 6.6A and B: Surgeon with ipsilateral ports 6" away from table and drapes with pockets

the surgeon has ample space and patient does not have any brachial plexus compression. The padded leg rests also avoids peroneal nerve pressure in popliteal fossa **(Fig. 6.5)**. Every time when the patient position is manipulated, the anesthetist is informed to take care of the endotracheal tube, side arms, multiparameter and ECG attachments remaining intact.

In some surgery like obturator sling for stress urinary incontinence patient passes urine before entering the operation theatre, catheterization is avoided. In others, a Foleys catheter 10-12 French is inserted in sterile fashion.

Equipment should be available in functioning condition, for example, in myomectomy-electronic morcellator should be functioning. Few standby instruments should be kept due to wear and tear at a busy surgical center.

A team of good assistant, OT staff and anesthetist is the key to a good laparoscopic surgery.

THE BEGINNING OF THE SURGERY

Patient is placed in a modified lithotomy position with the upper thigh at 135° from the abdomen for free movement of instruments in lower ports.

In addition, we should have long pocketed drapes to park the common instruments, from where it will be easy to pick up by the surgeon. Position of the monitors, keeping camera, cable and CO_2 insufflators tubes fixed at the working distance with free movements. The surgeon and assistant should always stand 6 inches away from the table. The table should be at the height of the flexed elbow of the surgeon while using an ipsilateral port, **(Figs 6.6A and B)** and it should be lower for using contralateral port.

The intravenous and irrigation bottles are all suspended from ceiling on a strong chain to avoid any bottlehanging stands occupying the floor space.

The instrument trolley should have optimum and not excessive instruments. The main assistant and OT staff are versatile to hold camera and give instruments sequentially before asking **(Fig. 6.7)**.

All important monitors, equipment with display should face the surgeon who subconsciously is aware without distractions **(Fig. 6.8)**.

Position of footswitches energy sources setting and irrigation suction devices.

Though there are few hand-operating instruments like harmonic scalpel, enseal vessel sealing device, and some morcellator, largely, it is controlled by foot switches which avoid you to look down every time, yet be sure of not stepping on a wrong paddle. Our foot switches are laid as follows:

Operative Laparoscopic Surgery Step by Step for Achieving Safety

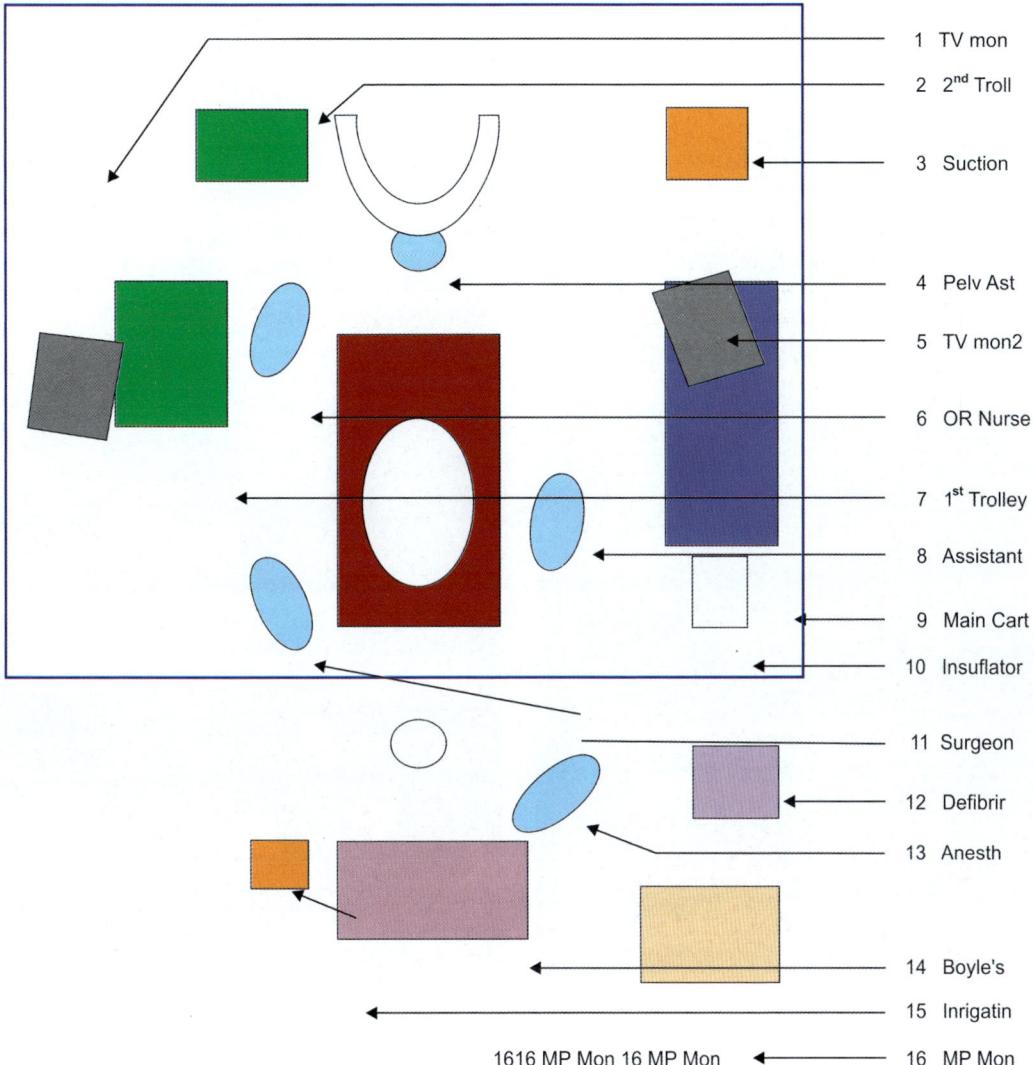

Fig. 6.7: Schematic position of all equipments, sterile instrument trolley, endoscopist, assistants, anesthetist, nurses

Closest to the operation theater table is the harmonic scalpel foot switch, followed by dedicated bipolar, vessel sealing device enseal radiofrequency/Gyrus-plasma kinetic energy.[3] The monopolar footswitch is sparingly needed today **(Fig. 6.9)**.

If morcellator is needed, it replaces one of the footswitch so that while focusing at the TV monitor the leg movement is easy. A green sheet is kept below all these footswitches to avoid them to be pushed while using. If CO_2 laser is used the footswitch is used on the right side.

The group of wires of energy sources, cable, camera wire, CO_2 insufflation tubing, inflow outflow tubing is kept in fixed position as suitable for the surgeon toward the assistants side fixed properly **(Figs 6.10A and B)**.

The setting of equipment—Monopolar current for major surgery is 80-100 watts pure cutting and 50-60 watts coagulation, bipolar dedicated cantery on 25-30 watts with matching company hand piece, if other company 35-40 watts. The setting of harmonic is no. 2 and 5 first for hemostasis and second for dissection~cutting. (Remem-

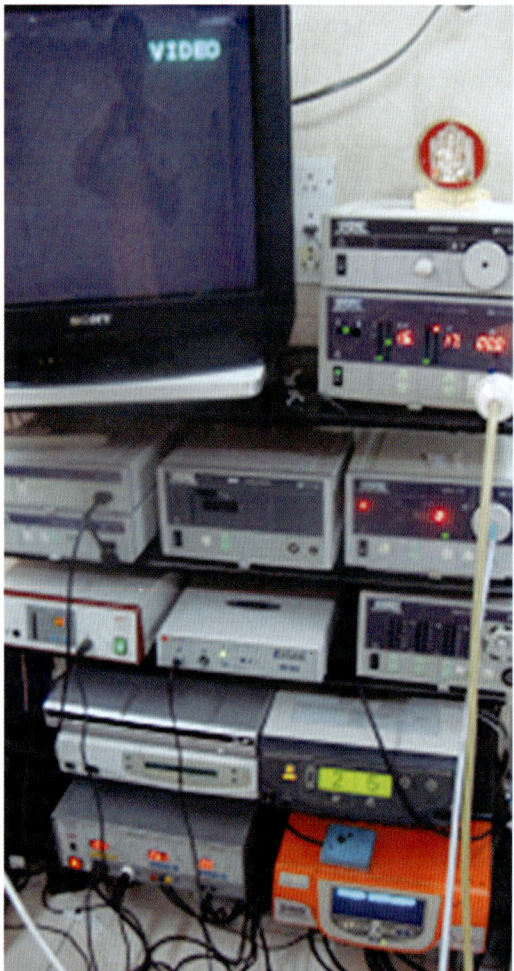

Fig. 6.8: All main equipments under vision of the surgeon

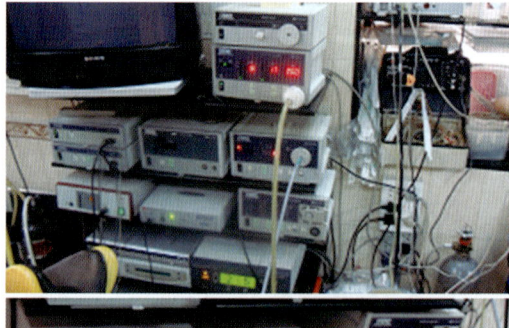

Fig. 6.10A: Set bipolar, harmonic, electrocautery, enseal and gyrus autosetting on plugging instrument

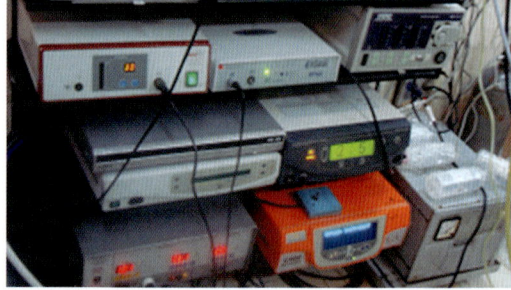

Fig. 6.10B: Electronic CO_2 insufflator

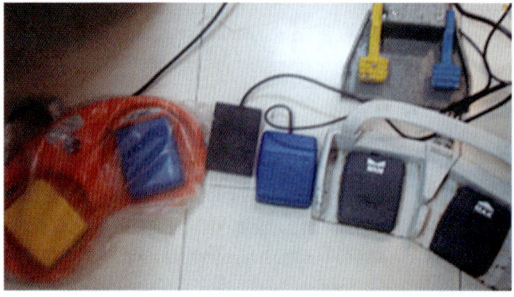

Fig. 6.9: Footswitches in standard place always

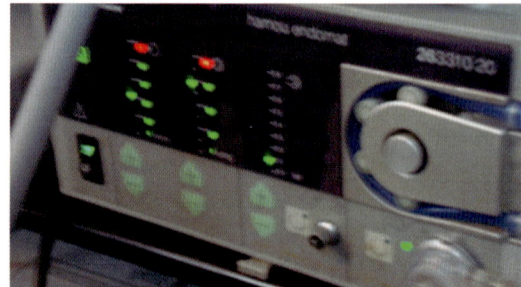

Fig. 6.10C: Endomat inflow pressure, flow and suction

ber harmonic scalpel is an excellent dissector but not a vessel sealing device). The vessel sealing devices, whether it is radiofrequency, plasma kinetic energy is set automatically on insertion of the hand piece, i.e. for sealing, cutting or morcellation. The irrigation suction can be endomat (Karl storz) at 300 ml/min flow rate and 200-300 mm of Hg by suction pressure, unless your have

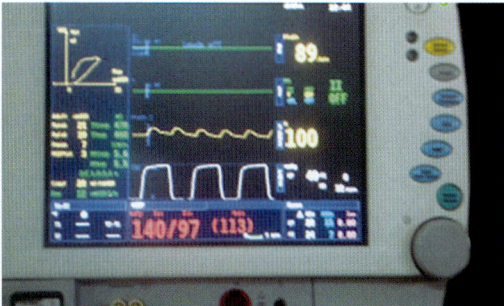

Fig. 6.11: Multiparameter monitor with display

ectopic ruptured with lots of blood or clots, the inflow is at 1litre/min flow and suction pressure of 500 mm Hg **(Fig. 6.10C)**.

The gas flow rate of CO_2 is 1-3 litre/min on starting with veress needle at 15 mm Hg pressure and then after trocar insertion the flow rate is increased from 7-8 to 20 litres/min but pressure is 15 mm Hg only. The CO_2 pressure is raised to 20-25 mm Hg for insertion of morcellator hand piece and then brought back to 15 mm Hg on insertion. In the absence of endomat, the same pressure can be set by C-infusor pressure bags with wide bore tubing and normal electronic suction at 0.05/50 mm Hg to 0.3 ~ 300 mm Hg to 0.5 ~ 500 mm Hg pressure. Adequate quantity of CO_2 cylinders, warm irrigation fluid, etc. is kept. Using heparin with saline/ringer lactate makes little difference.

The body temperature is maintained by a thermal jacket or warmer; patients have the monitoring probe and electrodes fixed at proper place for pO_2, ET CO_2, plethesmograph with ECG and body temperature **(Fig. 6.11)**.

A defibrillator is a must but respirator or spirometry is optional. A circuit busters with complete voltage transformer are mandatory and UPS/inverter backup required **(Fig. 6.12)**.

INTRODUCTION OF VERESS NEEDLE AND TROCARS

Many endoscopic surgeons have a direct trocar insertion, which we avoid by creating good pneumoperitoneum through veress needle. We use veress needle properly, vertical not oblique either disposable or reusable. A drop of fluid, which gets aspirated if in the negative pressure

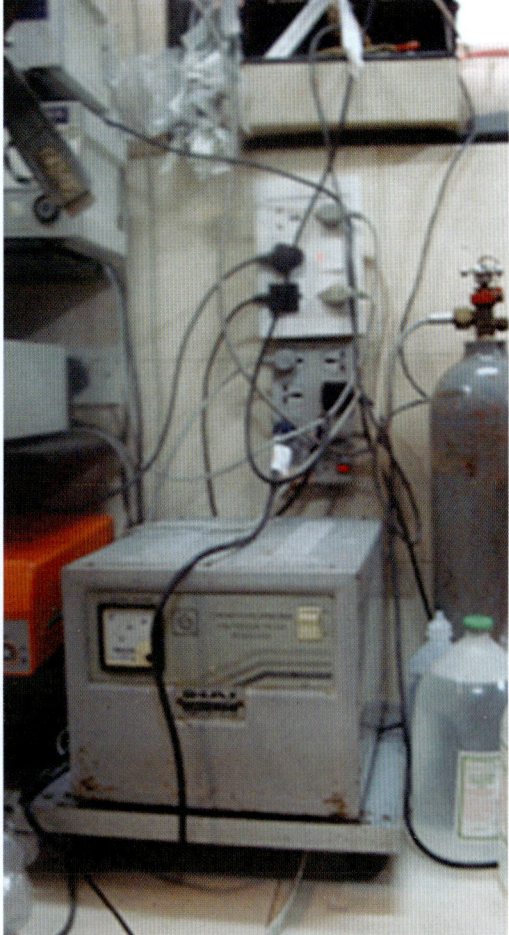

Fig. 6.12: Circuit busters and CVT complete voltage transformer

peritoneal space, identifies the confirmation of intraperitoneal space. Next a syringe with 2-3 ml is attached to the veress needle to push for clear and no resistance. Around 3-3.5 liters of CO_2 are adequate in any Asian women before first trocar insertion.

Insertion of veress needle reusable/disposable, also of primary and other trocar cannula is vertical with the index finger as a guard, preventing the instrument from sliding on the sheath obliquely **(Figs 6.13A and B)**.

Patient still in lithotomy and not with head low, increasing possible injury to iliac vessel. There are no safety trocar optiview which FDA doctors approves to be safe. However, the blunt tip termanium cannula **(Fig. 6.14)** is good

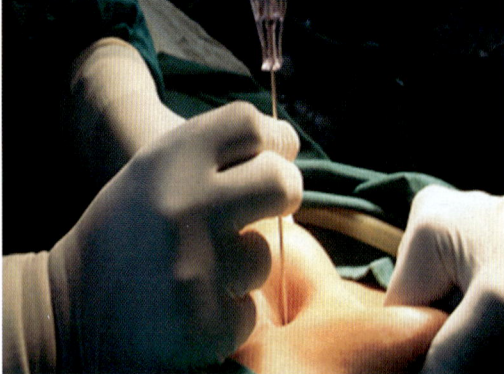

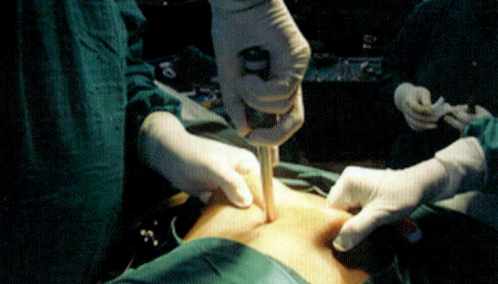

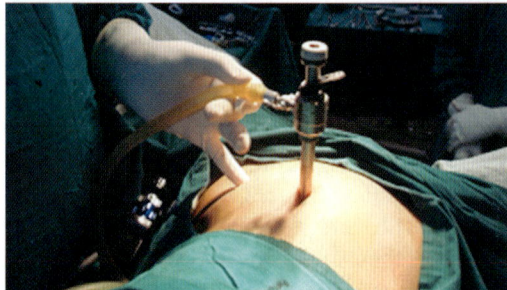

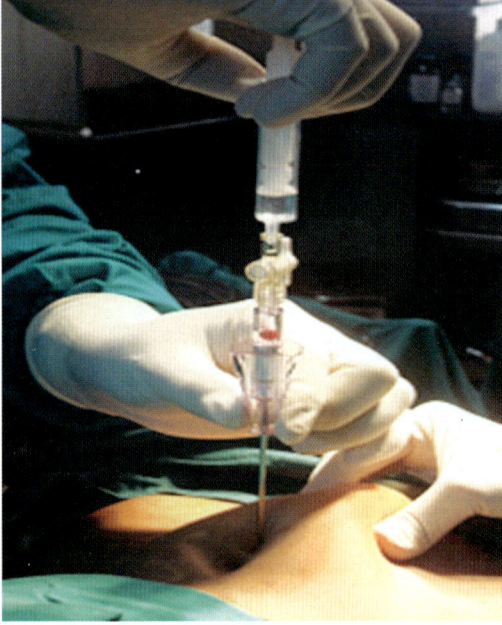

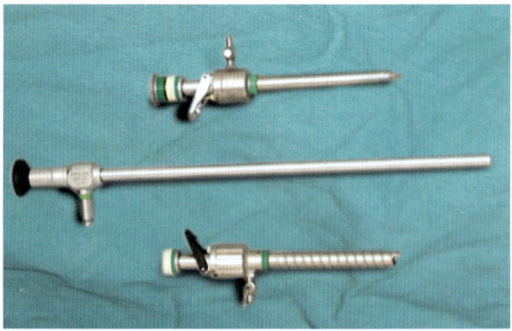

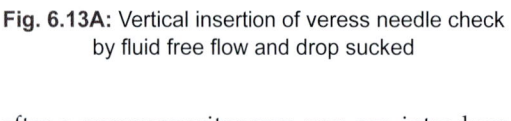

Fig. 6.13A: Vertical insertion of veress needle check by fluid free flow and drop sucked

Fig. 6.13B: Vertical insertion of reusable multifunction 10 mm trocar with pyramidal tip

Fig. 6.14: Termanium 10 mm sleeve and standard multifunction trocar cannula

after a pneumoperitoneum you can introduce the primary trocar with optics visualizing the path.

If there is a previous laparotomy scar, horizontal or vertical, the veress needle and trocar is introduced 4-5 cm above the uppermost mark of vertical incision or above the umbilicus with a nasogastric tube emptying the stomach.

The Palmer's point on the left upper abdomen below the rib cage can be used to detect adhesions. Open trocar insertion is performed by most of the surgeons but as a gynecologist that's not the routine and also you have to take a stitch to avoid gas leak or use special trocars. The primary trocar is frequently the multifunction valve trocar with pyramidal tip.

The ancillary trocars are usually 5 mm flower-valve trocar on the left and right imaginary Mc Burney's point. The left upper port is in line with the umbilicus little medial to the left lower port again introduced in vertical fashion under vision **(Fig. 6.15)**. We prefer injecting 2-3 ml of 0.25/0.5 percent sensorcaine before incising the skin to block the pain pathway, reducing

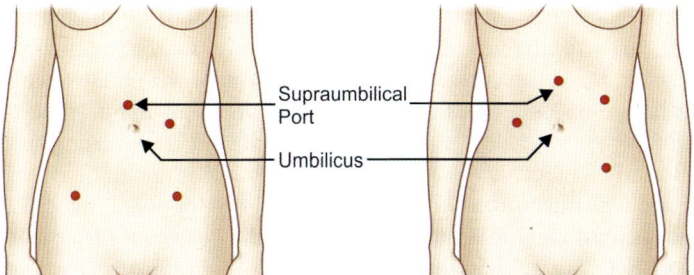

Fig. 6.15: Schematic representation of the port placement

the need for postoperative analgesia. The lower trocars are introduced lateral to the inferior epigastric umbilical vessels, avoiding injury to it.

Location of Standard Port Placement

The optic can be 10 mm 0° or 30° depending on surgeon's preference or assistant's ease of handling the camera. We have stopped using the supra pubic 5 mm trocar as it comes in the way of optics and has no advantage over the ipsilateral port placement wherein, the surgeon is comfortably not crossing hands over the patient and working like open surgery and the assistant holding the camera and instrument on assistant's side like open surgery.

The placements of trocars shift by 1-3 inches above, if the size of the uterus or fibroid is big. In cases of previous vertical scars also it is the same. The uterine manipulator is used vaginally and additionally, in cases of hysterectomy and fibroids more than 8-10 cm, we prefer a 10 mm myoma screw from the right upper port.

NEW ENERGY SOURCES, VESSEL SEALING DEVICES A BRIEF CLEAR CONCEPT

Though there are good electrocautery machines including a dedicated bipolar for a laparoscopic surgery, yet multiple change in instruments, i.e. bipolar and then to cut with scissors or suturing for hemostasis and cut with scissors. Always there was a need of instrument which can seal the vessels, cut and may be dissect tissues.

The birth of harmonic scalpel, an instrument predominantly 10 mm to start with added by 5 mm Ace; better for gynecologists, came as an excellent dissector due to one blade oscillating 55000/sec. It is a costly, disposable instrument useful for dissection, cutting, tissue separation and less for sealing vessels. It is especially useful for tissue dissection in cases of previous cesarean section, adhesions and big uterus. Setting is kept at 2/5 for moderate hemostasis and cutting. Though disposable, if used carefully it can used for 3-4 cases. When telescopes, trocars, or other instruments are not disposed after abdominal or vaginal surgery, why only these new energy sources device? It is nothing but industry driven economics of recurrent revenue to the company.

The vessel sealing device 3-what is the difference from a good bipolar? We have to remember that the amount of current delivered is the total of voltage multiplied by amperes which is the wattage. In a standard bipolar the voltage is high and amperes are low, but in vessel sealing device the voltage is low and amperes are high but wattage remains the same. This gives good dessication and vessel sealing. However, the lateral spread may depend on the size of the tip and delivery of the wattage from one electrode configuration to the other. Though each company claims to have the least lateral spread, it should be assessed and not blindly go by this claim. Finally have a combination of a good vessel sealing device with harmonic scalpel for excellent dissection and minimum instrument changes or one can do the same with scissors, bipolar and suturing main vessels like uterine arteries.

The following are the vessel sealing devices:
1. Ligasure and atlas from valley lab.
2. Martin maxim with Robi grasper.
3. Biclamp from Erbe.
4. Gyrus-plasma kinetic energy trissector and 5 mm curved sealer with dissector.
5. Harmonic scalpel 5 mm ace.
6. Enseal from Johnson and Johnson.

It was obvious that the electrocautery making companies would start with the vessel sealing devices which seals and cuts the vessel thus we had 3 vessel sealing devices from first 3 companies and others.

1. The Ligasure: Initally, when a 10 mm instrument, ligasure was introduced, for its use for cornu, infundibulopelvic ligament, up to the uterine vessels, but beyond this its use was limited as on the uterosacrals, etc. till the Atlas 5 mm came to go further.
2. Martin Maxim: The Martin electrocautery with instruments changed to vessel sealing, bipolar, cutting, etc. the combination of Martin Maxim with the Robi grasper from storz a combination works well but needs titration as Martin do not have the end hand instrument except for open surgery. Hence we have to titrate wattage for each new instrument, for cutting you have to use a Robi scissors with vessel seal.
3. The biclamp from erbe.
   Again a electrocautery making company has made 5 mm Biclamp effective through 5 mm, a lot of permutation and combination is available in terms of simple electrocautery with bipolar or cut- coagulation. A separation upgrade to vessel sealing device. Again it's more like a superior bipolar cautery till the cutting element is added.
4. The Gyrus plasma kinetic energy.
   This is a dedicated vessel sealing device initially also useful for urology and hysteroscopic surgery. The later dedicated to laparoscopic surgery only with addition of a harmonic like cutting instrument. This is available in 10 mm trissector and 5 mm curved vessel seal with a golden tip dissector. Further the brain unit can also take hand piece of a bipolar morcellator first of its type excellent instrument, but all can have lateral spread and injury to bladder or ureter. Advantages can be used for more care, than the earlier devices.
5. The Harmonic scalpel or ace.
   Basically an excellent dissector often misused at no. 1 or 2 marks for sealing vessel but it's not effective for sealing. The other functions are already highlighted.
6. The Enseal from Johnson and Johnson's. The radio frequency dedicated seal and cut instrument with relative cost-effective brain unit and had hand piece of 5 mm uterus the current flows from outer to inner cutting blade and can be used for many cases though suppose to be disposable. Perhaps has the least lateral spread may be safer than other to be proven over times to come. However still a simple dedicated bipolar is useful and safe. Monopolar should be used as per setting.

   Versapoint, plasma kinetic Gyrus and bipolar electrodes has their own use but are not necessarily less injurious to tissue. Further they have to be used through the operating channel and not continue flow resectoscopic sheath with better vision. But bipolar resectoscopes are now good and here to stay.

GOLDEN RULES OF EACH PERSON IN ENDOSCOPIC SURGERY

Endoscopic surgery is a team work hence; each person should know their role.

a. Main Surgeon: The captain should handle the main tissue dissection, suturing and every important plan is captain's job. He/she has to be organized, knows limits of assistants, sisters, instrumentation and should not be temperamental in crisis, should be cool, confident yet swift. They make the atmosphere of the operation theater responsible yet enjoyable at ease, disciplined and understanding the final mission of surgery.
b. First main assistant: To control camera movement, centralization, back up goes close as needed for the surgery. The second hand does supportive movement anticipating primary movement of surgeon.
c. Nursing staff should have organized instrument trolley, equipments, and should be well acquainted with the surgical steps. They quiet often boost the confidence of a new main assistant.
d. Anesthetist: Composed, not in hurry but will give good suggestion in crisis or decision making, should not distract the surgeon by nonspecific talks.

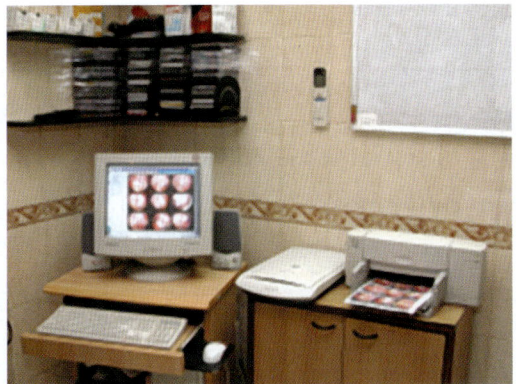

Fig. 6.16: Documentation and scanner

Hands free mobile for surgeon, too many mobile of the others should be restricted. A good music and some jokes makes a high turnover work pleasure and not stressful.

DOCUMENTATION AND EXPLAINING PATIENTS AFTER SURGERY

The future of medicine is skilled documentation of all surgery showing relevant part to the relative and the patient. Hard disc storage is very useful for the future presentation, books, DVD and medicolegal purpose. A serial photograph is an important document of each surgery given to the patient **(Fig. 6.16)**.

After the surgery all aspects are explained to the relatives, future plan of action or treatment is also explained.

In moments of crisis like bleeding or rare injury to bladder, bowel, ureter is identified treated properly, an additional support of the surgeon or urologist is useful medicolegally even if you are the best.

Periodic up gradation of operation theatre set up and each person involved in surgery is productive.

On finishing surgery port closer, analgesic suppository, color of urine, condition of patient well being is confirmed with the anesthetist. All fluid discrepancies, blood loss, etc. is well calculated.

Conversion to open is not a defeat; the set for open surgery should be always kept ready. However, this decision is taken within 2-3 minutes of introducing the laparoscope and not 1-2 hours after struggle.

A true surgical genius is not borne in crisis but they exhibit in crisis.

After the Surgery

Transfer of patient from operation theatre to the recovery room should not be taken casually. It is compulsory for a nursing staff or a qualified doctor to inform the vital parameters of the patient to main surgeon, anesthetist, checking intravenous fluid line, catheter, drainage tube if any and condition of the button hole dressing done.

Proper entry of surgical procedure and immediate postoperative notes is done by assisting surgeon and checked by the main surgeon.

REFERENCES

1. Berguer R, Rab GT, Abu–Ghaida H, et al. A comparison of surgeon's posture during laparoscopic and open surgical procedure. Surg Endosc. 1997;11:139.
2. Nezhat C, et al. Reduced fatigue and discomfort: tips to improve operating room setup. Laparosc Surg Update. 1997;5:97.
3. Landman J, Kerbl K, Rehman J, et al. Evaluation of a vessel sealing system, bipolar electro surgery, harmonic scalpel, titanium plates, endoscopic gastrointestinal anastomosis, vascular staples and sutures for arterial and venous liagation in a porcine model. J Uro 2003;169:697-700.

CHAPTER 7

Making Laparoscopic Myomectomy Safe

Sunita Tandulwadkar

Chapter Outline

- Practical tips of Myomectomy
  - Port Placement
  - Pre-operative Requisites
  - Procedure
  - Closure of Uterine Flap
  - Extraction of Myoma
  - Tips
- Strengthening of Myoma Scar

INTRODUCTION

Laparoscopic myomectomy has provided minimal invasive alternative to laparotomy for subserous and intramural myomas.[1,2] It is no longer a subject of debate[2,3] though opinion may differ in cases of large and multiple myomas among the endoscopist.[2] Number of instruments and various angles of insertion to approach surgical site are limited and therefore myomas may be technically difficult to remove laparoscopically but with experience, sound knowledge of suturing and acquiring greater skill over a period of time one can overcome these technical difficulties.[4]

It is always wise to start with smaller myomas and subserous than intramural. As experience increases the exclusion criteria relax considerably and one proceeds for more complicated cases, the comfort level expands. More one does, more number of patients he/she will be able to count as good candidates as one becomes adapt at managing large and/or multiple myomas. It is important for surgeon to know that safety of patient is more important than type of surgery (laparoscopic or open).[5] Hence, before proceeding for laparoscopic surgery it is mandatory for the surgeon to ask himself/herself –

'Is it possible for me to give the best of the result by laparoscopy in this patient with my set-up and experience'? and then proceed accordingly.

PRACTICAL TIPS OF MYOMECTOMY

Port Placement

Port placement depends upon size of myoma, its location and total number of myomas.[4] It is always wise to shift upwards towards upper abdomen as the size of myoma increases. Ancillary ports have to be taken in such a way that they can reach to the myoma without making acute angles with each other. If necessary, apart from 3 ancillary ports, one can add on more ports especially in cases of large and multiple myomas as these myomas with different location can be approached through different ancillary ports. The port of a telescope should always be at least 5-6 cm above the upper margin of myoma to have good field of vision. A 30° telescopes helps tremendously to reach difficult site myomas **(Figs 7.1A to C)**.

Pre-operative Requisites

A thorough ultrasonographic evaluation of pelvis for location, size and number of myomas is a must.[6,7] In laparoscopic surgery tactile sensation

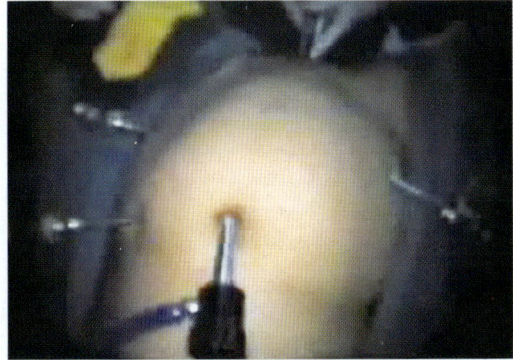

Fig. 7.1A: Routine placement up to 14 wk

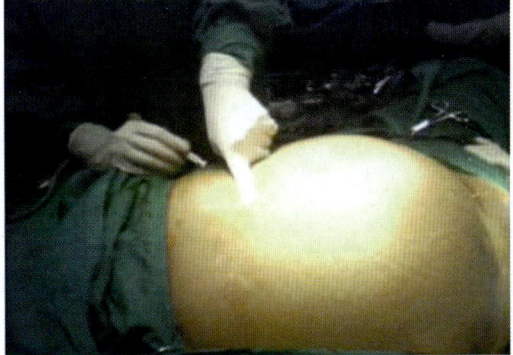

Fig. 7.1B: Veress needle at Palmer's point

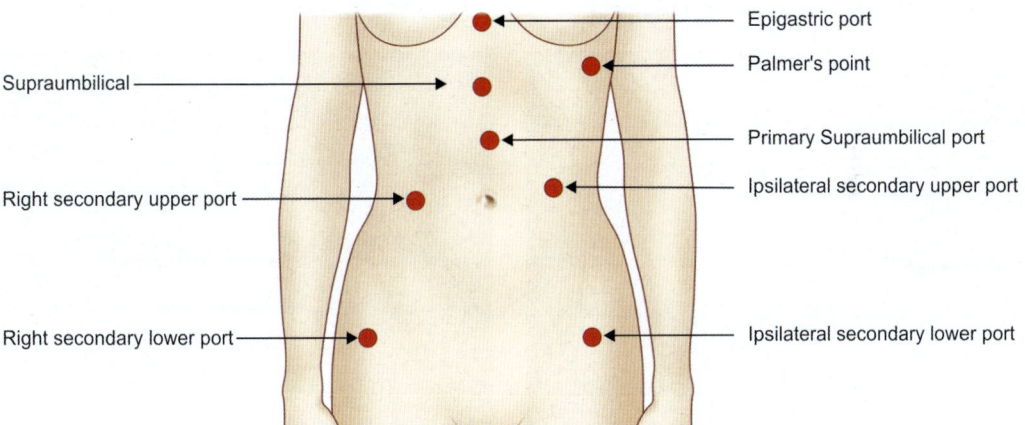

Fig. 7.1C: For larger myomas

is lacking. In cases of large and multiple myomas it is better to have a limited MRI of pelvis done as surgeon can decide preoperatively his incision sites, number of incisions, how many myomas can be removed via one incision and relation of myomas with uterine cavity. Though after putting a laparoscope one needs to re-evaluate his/her own preoperative decisions.

It is advised to perform hysteroscopy in all cases before proceeding for laparoscopic myomectomy[8] as smaller submucosal myomas can be missed out in presence of large and multiple myomas.

Procedure[9]

- Placement of primary and secondary trocars depends upon the size and site of myomas.
- Relation of myomas with the uterus and fallopian tube should be carefully assessed after inserting primary trocar and then site of secondary trocars to be decided.
- Vasopressin 1 in 100 dilution is injected into myomas at 3 to 4 sites to minimize bleeding (action will remain only for 20-30 min).
- Careful planning of incision is done.
- Incision can be taken with a monopolar hook/harmonic spatula **(Figs 7.2A and B)**.
- Most preferred incision is transverse incision, as it will cut fewer vessels.
- Incision should be of sufficient depth, so that capsule of myoma is visualized.
- With 2 non-traumatic forceps, cut edges are pulled apart so as to expose capsule of myoma well and make space for myoma screw insertion.
- Once the myoma screw is inserted, myoma is pulled outward and upward keeping counter traction on uterus downward with 2 allis forceps applied on the anterior lip the cervix.

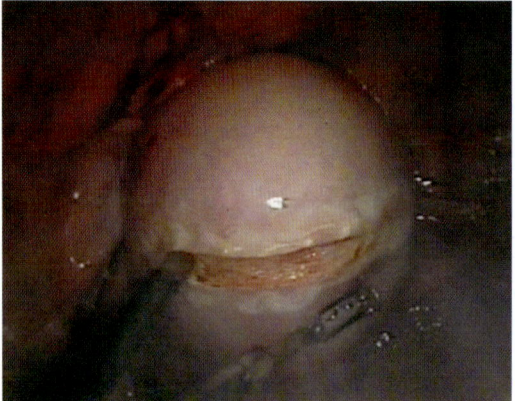

Fig. 7.2A: Incision with monopolar hook

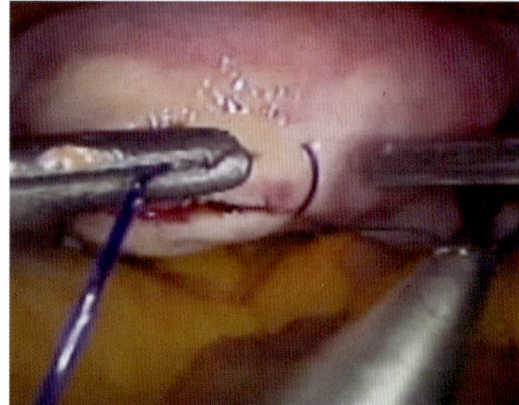

Fig. 7.3A: Placement of suture beyond the angle

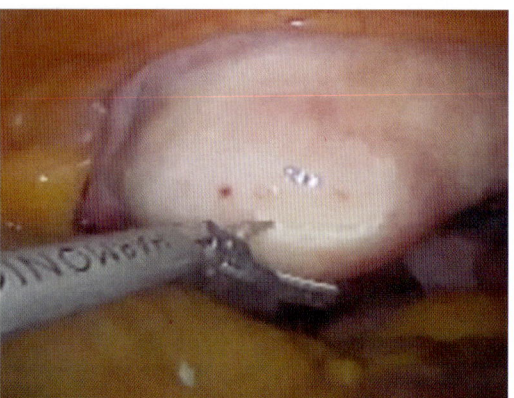

Fig. 7.2B: Incision with harmonic scalpel

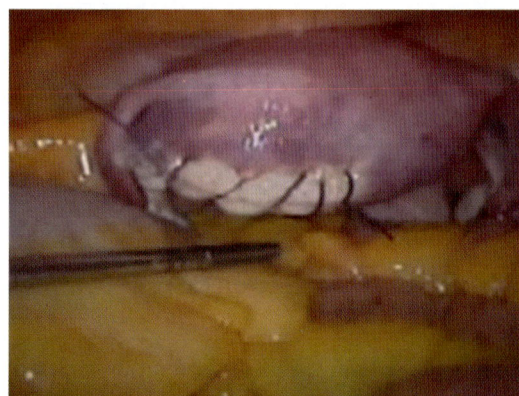

Fig. 7.3B: End result no migration of suture line tension all across the suture line

- If one is in the right plane, myoma is usually extracted easily and there is minimal bleeding.
- Position of myoma screw is changed from time to time so that traction is applied next to cleavage line.
- For a larger myoma, 10 mm myoma screw helps in better extraction and hence shortens operative time.
- Usually the base of myoma will have large feeding vessels, which should be cauterized and cut.
- Only active bleeders of the bed are cauterized which can be easily identified by underwater inspection.
- Undue cautery should be avoided, as it will give defective healing.
- Myoma after removal is parked at right paracolic gutter.

Closure of Uterine Flap

- Reconstruction of myoma bed can be performed with vicryl no. 1 suture **(Figs 7.3A and B)** or barbed suture **(Table 7.1)**/V loop **(Table 7.2)**.
- Whether single or multiple layer closure is individual's decision-but the ultimate aim is to obliterate the dead space completely so as to avoid hematoma formation, which is another cause of weakening of scar.
- Start from one angle, first stitch is placed beyond angle either with intracorporeal or extracorporeal suture and then rest of defect is closed by taking deep continuous locking sutures and the end suture should be again beyond the angle of opposite side.
- If it is a single layer closure, ensure that stitches are deep enough to obliterate the dead space.

- Studies have shown that three-layer closure with first layer, as endometrial layer doesn't compromise pregnancy or pregnancy outcome.

Extraction of Myoma

- Myomas are extracted by electronic morcellation **(Figs 7.4A to C)**. Smaller myomas can be extracted by colpotomy

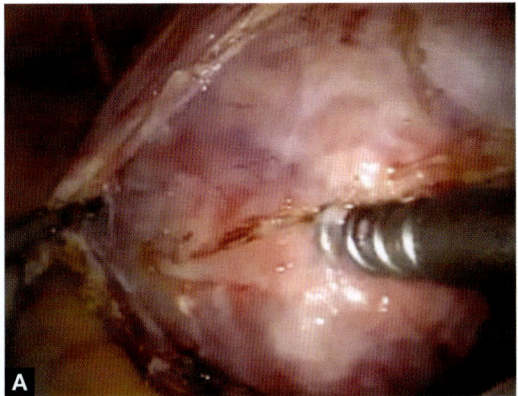

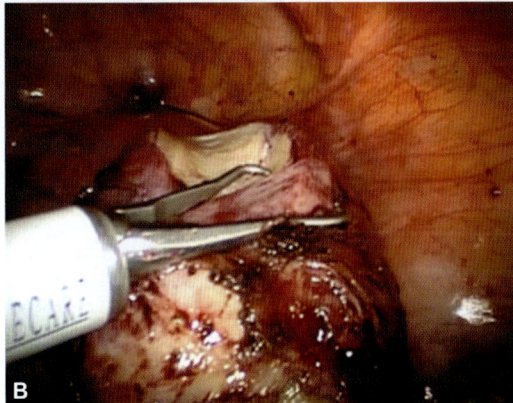

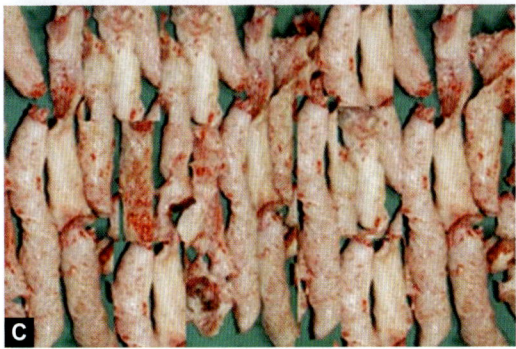

Figs 7.4A to C: (A) Morcellated pieces, (B) Extraction of myoma, (C) Morcellation in process

- A meticulous lavage is given and hemostasis is checked
- End result should be a clean pelvis
- To keep a drain in the postoperative period is again an individual's choice.

In difficult situations-

Pedunculated myomas with a broad base

- Instead of transverse incision, circular incision should be taken at the base of myoma in a circumferential manner
- With myoma screw, myoma is pulled up and enucleated after cauterizing base of the pedicle.

Table 7.1: Barbed suture[10] DemeTECH, MedSURGE, USA
• Newer silhouette type suture, got FDA approval in November 2006.
• Available in both absorbable and non-absorbable materials.
• Via micromachining techniques, the bidirectional suture is fabricated from monofilament fibers combined with etching of the filament in order to create barbs in a helical fashion.
• The barbs vary in lengths and oppose one another from the midpoint of the suture length.
• This configuration ultimately allows for a linear "drawstring" closure of the wound. This type of closure translates into a well-approximated wound at multiple tissue levels, with a decrease in tension in the X, Y, and Z-axis.
Advantages
• It self-anchors and is balanced by the countervailing barbs, no knots and third hand is not required.
• Yields more consistent wound opposition which gives a more 'watertight' seal.
• Dead space obliteration is excellent.
• Controls and distributes tension across the entire length of the wound.
• Enables use of running vs. interrupted sutures.
• Increases efficiency by saving time.
• Allows two individuals to close a wound at the same time.
• Eliminates the need of a third hand or an assistant.

Table 7.2: V Loc Suture TM 180 (Covidien, Mansfield, MA, USA)[11-13]

- Improvised unidirectional knotless barbed suture Won FDA approval in March 2009 for soft tissue approximation.
  Surgical needle at one end and loop at the other.

- Unidirectional, shallow barbs with circumferential distribution.
  Loop – used to secure the barbed suture
  Tension on the suture line causes the suture to resist migration.

- No change to standard wound closure technique

- Unique circular shape

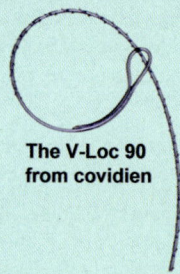

The V-Loc 90 from covidien

- Needle held securely in optimal position.

Advantages

Same as that of barbed suture.

In addition preloop enhances the security of the stitch at angle.

Tips

- In case of multiple myomas where the shape of the uterus is distorted, round ligaments help in identification.
- As far as possible, incision should be taken anteriorly than on posterior wall. Self pre-operation USG always helps to enhance surgical performance on table especially in cases of multiple myomas. One can decide the number of myomas that can be taken out through a single incision. There is no tactile sensation in laparoscopy so small myomas hidden under large myomas, if known before hand, can be removed successfully.
- We don't advocate use of pre-op GnRH analogues to reduce the size of myoma.

- Traction on uterus downwards with allis forceps applied to anterior lip of cervix and upward counter traction on myoma with myoma screw, next to cleavage line will facilitate dissection.
- Myomas up to 5-6 cm can be delivered with colpotomy
- Proper serosal approximation, hemostasis, clean pelvis at the end, early mobilization will help in prevention of postoperative adhesions.
- Instillation of vasopressin, speedy surgery, skillful and rapid suturing, good knot tying techniques will help to minimize bleeding.
- Occasionally one can encounter excessive bleeding from vasopressin injection site so one should keep in instilling vasopressin even while withdrawing the needle.

STRENGTHENING OF MYOMA SCAR

Laparoscopic myomectomy has received many controversies and debates for the obvious reason that strength of myomectomy scar gets tested in subsequent pregnancies and rupture of uterus can sometime lead to maternal morbidity and mortality apart from fetal mortality (Fig. 7.5).

To prevent the weakening of a scar one has to take care of following triad.

A. One can think of avoiding hematoma formation by –
1. Using excellent energy source for incision and extraction of myoma so that vessels get sealed before cutting.
2. Excellent closure: Barbed/V Lock/Vicryl no 1.

B. Avoiding tissue necrosis: By applying the above principles of closure one can think of

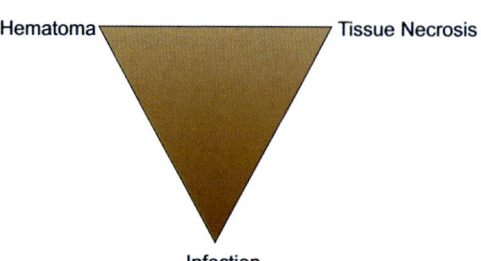

Fig. 7.5: Weakening of scar

avoiding cauterisation of myoma bed and hence tissue necrosis.

Cauterisation of myoma bed for sealing of vessels should be avoided unless it has a large bleeder. Immediate and excellent suturing will otherwise also achieve hemostasis. Needless to say good sterile precautions, shorter duration of surgery, and avoidance of hematoma formation will avoid infection automatically.

> Determination of surgeon, his/her operative skills, willingness to learn and use newer modalities of energy sources and suture materials, learning with his/her own mistakes will make an excellent laparoscopic surgeon.
>
> It is important for every surgeon to ask himself/herself at the end of the day, whether I would have done the same case in better way? And if yes what way? Adopt that technique or mind for the next case and needless to say he/she becomes better, faster and safer day by day.
>
> **Limitations of Laparoscopic Myomectomy:**
> - The size
> - Number and positions of myomas
> - Whether future fertility is desired
> - The experience of surgeon especially mastery over endosuturing
>
> **How big is big? and How many are too many?**
> *The answer varies from surgeon to surgeon depending upon which part of learning curve he/she is on. It is a relative term but -*
> *The easiest myomas to remove are those that are subserous than deep intramural and anterior and fundal than posterior and isthmic.*

REFERENCES

1. Laparoscopic Myomectomy: A Current View– Jean Bernard Dubuisson, Chapron C, Arnaud Fauconnier, et al. Human Reproduction Update 2002;6(6):588-94.
2. Endoscopic Management of Uterine Fibroids. Agdi M, Tulandi T. Best Pract Res Clin Obstet Gynecol. 2008; 22(4):707-16. Epub 2008 Mar 6.
3. Pregnancy Outcomes after Laparoscopic Myomectomy with Ultrasonic Energy and Laparoscopic Suturing of the Endometrial Cavity: Nelson H, et al. The Journal of the American Association of Gynecologic Laparoscopists. 2001;8(1):129-36.
4. Treatment of Myomas by Laparoscopic and Laparotomic Myomectomy and Laparoscopic Hysterectomy: L Mettler, T Schollmeyer, E Lehmann, Willenbrock, J Dowaji and A. Zavala, Informa Healthcare, Minimally Invasive Therapy and Allied Technologies 2004;13(1):58-64.
5. Factors Influencing Laparoconversions During The Learning Curve of Laparoscopic Myomectomy: H Marret, M Chevillot, B Giraudeau, K Lalitha, Acta Obstetricia Et Gynecologica Scandinavica, 2006;85(3):324–9.
6. Nezhat's Operative Gynecologic Laparoscopy and Hysteroscopy Camran Nezhat, Farr R. Nezhat, Ceana Nezhat, Page 155,316-22.
7. Uterine Leiomyoma (Fibroid) Imaging : Hilip Thomason, Director of Diagnostic Radiology, Department of Radiology, Beverly Hospital Contributor Information And Disclosures Emedicine WebMD Updated: May 6, 2008.
8. Laparoscopic Myomectomy : Feasibility and Safety—A Retrospective Study of 762 Cases: P G Paul, Aby Koshy And Tony Thomas, Gynecological Surgery. 2006;3:97-102.
9. Endoscopy Simplified : Practical Tips By Experts – Dr Sunita Tandulwadkar, Jaypee Publication, 2008.
10. The Power of The Barbed Suture: Michael S Kluska, Plastic Surgery Practice, Jan 2010.
11. Motion Study – Comparison of Wound Closure Time Using Conventional Techniques and Knotless, Self Anchoring Surgical Sutures In Ex-Vivo Porcine Model For Single Layer Closure With Barbed Devices Vs. Double Layer Closure With Traditional Suture. Royal College Of Surgeons, London, UK; Covidien, 2010.
12. Time Study - V-Loc™ 180 Absorbable Wound Closure Device, Robert T. Grant, MD, Msc, FACS, New York-Presbyterian Hospital, Argent Global Services, 2010.
13. Utilization of A Porcine Model to Demonstrate The Efficacy of An Absorbable Barbed Suture For Dermal Closure, UTSW, S Brown, 2010.

CHAPTER 8

Ectopic Pregnancy: How to Make it Safe for Patient, Tubes and Fertility

Pandit Palaskar

Chapter Outline

- Etiology of Ectopic Pregnancy
  - Sites of Ectopic Pregnancy
  - Diagnosis of Ectopic Pregnancy
  - Management of Tubal Ectopic Pregnancy
- Conservative Medical Therapy of Ectopic Pregnancy
- Surgical Management
  - Conservative Surgical Treatment
  - Segmental Resection
  - Radical Surgical Treatment
  - Indications for Salpingectomy
- Comparison of Surgical and Medical Therapy
  - Interstitial (Cornual) Pregnancy
  - Pregnancy in Rudimentary Horn
  - Cervical Ectopic Pregnancy
  - Ovarian Ectopic Pregnancy
  - Abdominal Ectopic Pregnancy
  - Heterotopic Pregnancy
  - Our Experience of Ectopic Pregnancy

INTRODUCTION

A pregnancy that develops following implantation anywhere other than the endometrial cavity is called ectopic pregnancy. The risk of ectopic pregnancy increases three to four times in women between the ages of 35 to 44 compared to those from 15 to 24 yrs. About 64 percent of ectopic pregnancies occur in the ampulla, where fertilization occurs. The recent increase in incidence of ectopic pregnancy has been attributed to a greater incidence of sexually transmitted disease (STD), Increased Infertility and ART, delayed childbearing, previous surgical interference and easy diagnosis.[1]

ETIOLOGY OF ECTOPIC PREGNANCY

1. **Tubal damage secondary to inflammation**
   Both increased incidence of STD resulting in salpingitis and the efficacy of antibiotic therapy in preventing total tubal occlusion after an episode of salpingitis are related to the increasing incidence of ectopic pregnancy. History of PID increases the incidence of ectopic pregnancy by six fold.

2. **Contraceptive devices**
   Subtle tubal epithelial damage or actual PID episodes are likely responsible for the observed association between IUDs and increases relative risk of ectopic pregnancy by 11.5 percent.[2]

3. **Infertility treatment and ART**
   Delayed pregnancy and treatment for conception has increased incidence of ectopic pregnancy due increased tubal factor.[3]

4. **Prior tubal surgery**
   Any operative procedure on the tube, whether a sterilization procedure or tubal reconstructive surgery, can cause an ectopic pregnancy. The incidence of ectopic pregnancies occurring after neosalpingostomy for distal tubal obstruction ranges from 2 to 18 percent. The rate of ectopic pregnancy after a microsurgical reversal of sterilization procedure is only about 4 percent, presumably because the tubes have not been

damaged by prior infection. If sterilization is by coagulation and cutting the tubes, 67 percent of failures are ectopic pregnancies.

5. **Assisted reproductive technologies**
   Ectopic pregnancies are known to occur with increased frequency after *in vitro* fertilization and related techniques. Incidence of ectopic pregnancies after ART techniques is 2.1 percent. Potential factors include, the possibility of direct injection of embryos into the fallopian tube, uterine contractions provoked by the transfer catheter that propel the embryos retrograde, position or depth of the transfer catheter in the uterine cavity, and the volume of transfer medium. Verhulst and colleagues reported that tubal damage was a major risk factor. They found that the ectopic pregnancy rate after IVF was significantly greater in patients with tubal disease (3.65% vs 1.19%). History of previous ectopic pregnancy also appears to be risk factors for ectopic pregnancies following IVF. Also there is 2 percent risk of heterotopic pregnancy in women undergoing IVF who had distorted tubal anatomy and this risk increase proportionately with the number of embryos transferred.[4]

6. **Infertility**
   Risk of ectopic pregnancy is more in infertile woman as compared to general population of same age. This may be due associated tubal factor infertility due to PID and use of ART techniques.

7. **Other causal factors**
   Cigarette smoking, multiple sex partners, early age at first intercourse and vaginal douching are associated with an increased risk of ectopic pregnancies.

Sites of Ectopic Pregnancy

Tubal ectopic pregnancy (most common) 95 to 97 percent.

Interstitial (cornual) ectopic pregnancy 2 to 4 percent.

Cervical ectopic pregnancy 0.1 percent.

Ovarian ectopic pregnancy 0.5 percent.

Abdominal ectopic pregnancy 0.03 percent.

Diagnosis of Ectopic Pregnancy

For a successful outcome, an ectopic pregnancy must be diagnosed early, preferably before rupture.

Serum β-hCG assay: Serum β-hCG levels are useful in determining the viability of pregnancy, levels increase in an exponential fashion in early pregnancy.[5] During the early gestation, β-hCG mean doubling time is 2 days. The β-hCG doubling time can differentiate an ectopic pregnancy from intrauterine pregnancy, a 66 percent rise in the β-hCG over 48 hours represents the lower limit of normal values for viable intrauterine pregnancies. About 15 percent patients with viable intrauterine pregnancies have less than 66 percent rise in β-hCG levels 48 hours, and a similar percentage with ectopic pregnancy have more than 66 percent rise. Serum β-hCG pattern that is most predictive of ectopic pregnancy is one that has reached a plateau (a doubling time of more than 7 days).

Transvaginal ultrasonography: Pelvic ultrasound has revolutionized the diagnostic process of ectopic pregnancy. Transvaginal ultrasonography in particular can identify masses in adnexa as small as 10 mm in diameter and can provide more detail about the character of the mass than clinical examination. At the same time, TVS can evaluate the contents of the endometrial cavity and can document the presence of a viable pregnancy with great accuracy. In addition, TVS allows for the simultaneous assessment for the presence of free peritoneal fluid.[6]

Dilatation and curettage: In tubal pregnancies, uterine curettage showed atypical epithelial changes of the gestational endometrium, which was first described by Polak and Wolfe and further expanded by Arias-Stella. These endometrial criteria, seems to have limited value in the specific diagnosis of extrauterine pregnancy today.

Culdocentesis: It is a diagnostic tool for identifying the presence of intraperitoneal bleeding. Culdocentesis provides immediate clinical information when unclotted blood is aspirated from the cul-de-sac. It cannot be used for a definitive diagnosis, because a tubal pregnancy may not have ruptured or leaked into the peritoneal cavity.

Laparoscopy: It remains the gold standard in the detection of ectopic pregnancy. In addition to permitting the diagnosis of an ectopic pregnancy, it enables surgical treatment. Laparoscopy also provides an opportunity to visualize the entire pelvis and other peritoneal organs. In particular, the condition of the unaffected fallopian tube can be assessed as well as the presence of pelvic adhesions and endometriosis. This information may be particularly valuable for those patients interested in future fertility. Laparoscopy may be useful when an ectopic pregnancy is suspected but no signs of an ultrasonographically visualized extrauterine gestational sac are evident. This includes situations in which there is an inability to visualize an intrauterine gestational sac and serial β-hCG levels are rising inappropriately.

Management of Tubal Ectopic Pregnancy

Ectopic pregnancy can be treated either medically or surgically. Both methods are effective and the choice depends on the clinical circumstances, the site of the ectopic pregnancy and the available resources.

CONSERVATIVE MEDICAL THERAPY OF ECTOPIC PREGNANCY

- Pharmacological therapy using methotrexate was introduced by Tanaka (1982)
- It is proven to be successful in 90 percent of selected cases
- American College of Obstetrician and Gynecologists recommend methotrexate for patients who desire future fertility and have an ectopic mass less than 3 cm in diameter, with β-hCG levels less than 1500 mIu/ml and no evidence of fetal heart on ultrasonography
- Methotrexate can be given as single dose (1 mg/kg) or multiple dose therapy[7]
- Follow-up is by monitoring β-hCG
- Even though for a patient who is thought to be a candidate for conservative therapy, access to the peritoneal cavity is essential to determine the most appropriate procedure
- Tubal patency is 80 percent in both conservative surgical and pharmacological therapy
- Comparison of laparoscopically treated patients with methotrexate treated patients suggest that the two methods have similar reproductive outcomes.

SURGICAL MANAGEMENT

The classical surgical approach for an ectopic pregnancy was by open laparotomy. Lawson Tait first described the life saving procedure of salpingectomy by laparotomy in 1884. It was not until some 70 years later that less radical operations with conservation of the involved tube during laparotomy were performed. In 1973, Stromme first reported the successful use of salpingetomy to treat tubal ectopic pregnancy. Laparoscopy has been used in the diagnosis of ectopic pregnancy for many years. Since the first excision of a tubal pregnancy through a laparoscope by Manhes and Bruhat in 1980, it has been used with increasing frequency in the surgical treatment of ectopic pregnancies. Laparoscopy permits diagnosis and treatment to be combined in the same procedure and ectopic pregnancies can be diagnosed and treated at an early stage. In fact, laparoscopy is not only suitable for early ectopic pregnancies but it is also safe and feasible in instances where there is tubal rupture and hemoperitoneum, provided the patient is not severely compromised hemodynamically.

Indications for surgery in ectopic pregnancy include women with the following criteria:
- Not suitable candidate for medical therapy
- Failed medical therapy
- Heterotopic pregnancy with a viable intrauterine pregnancy
- Hemodynamically unstable and need immediate treatment.

Conservative Surgical Treatment

Conservative surgical management of an unruptured ectopic pregnancy usually consists of one of two possible procedures, linear salpingostomy or segmental resection. A conservative surgical approach is possible when the diagnosis of ectopic pregnancy is made sufficiently early so that rupture of the tube has not yet occurred. Currently, most ectopic pregnancies are treated by laparoscopic surgery. In fact, most studies have suggested that laparoscopic surgery is superior to laparotomy in hemodynamically stable patients.

Linear salpingostomy (Figs 8.1A to E): In women, who wish to preserve their fertility, linear salpingostomy is considered the gold standard for the management of a distal tubal pregnancy. After conservative and radical surgery for ectopic pregnancy, most of the available information suggests that the subsequent intrauterine pregnancy rate is higher after conservative surgery (linear salpingotomy).[8]

If laparoscopy is planned, the location, the size, and the nature of the tubal pregnancy are

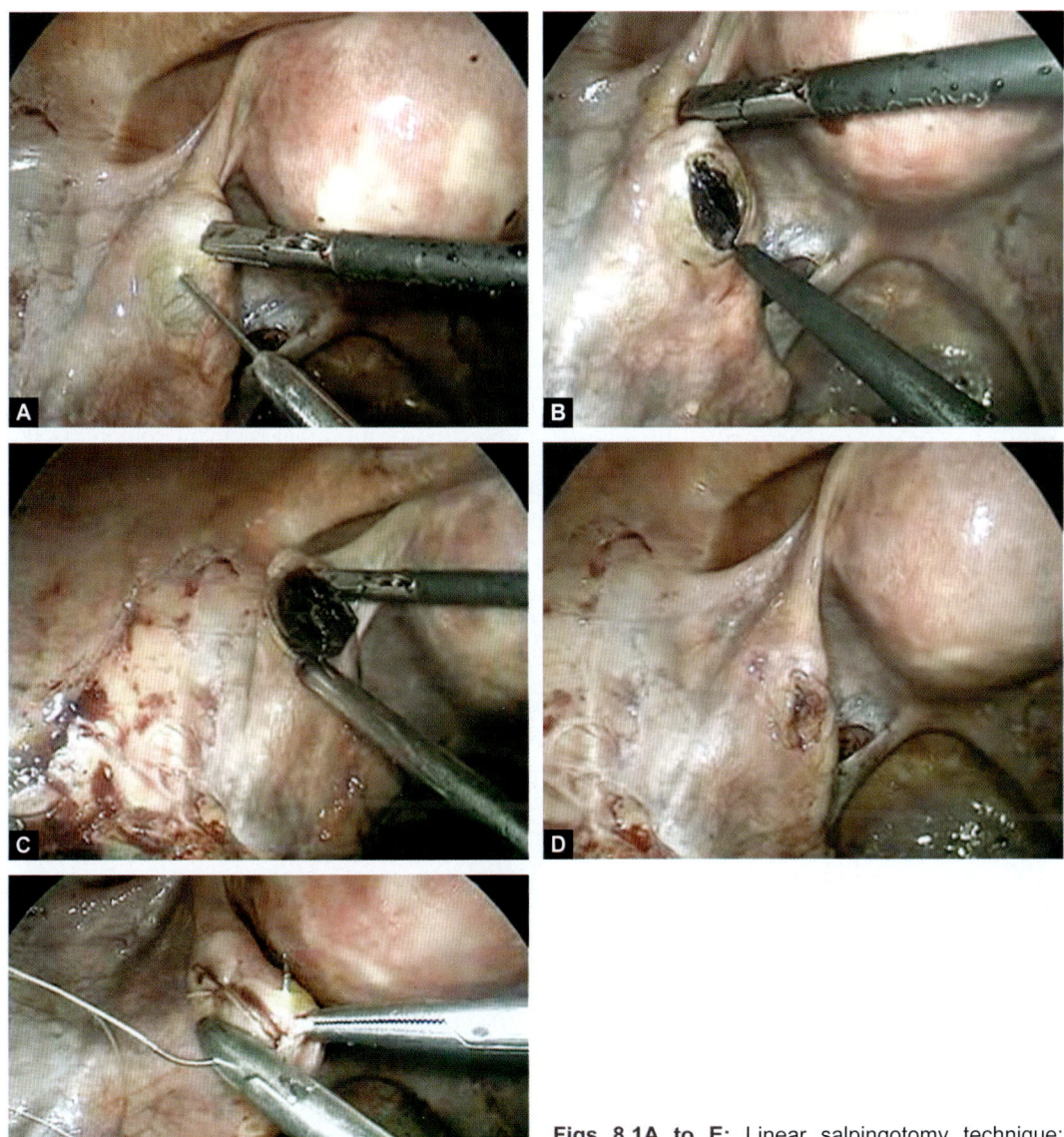

Figs 8.1A to E: Linear salpingotomy technique; (A) Left tubal ectopic, (B) Salpingotomy, (C) Removal of ectopic, (D) Salpingotomy complete, (E) Suturing tubal incision

ascertained. If the bleeding has ceased or can be arrested adequately, ruptured tubal pregnancies can be treated endoscopically. Once bleeding is controlled, the products of conception and blood clots are removed. Heparinized saline should be used in cases of large hematoma. A 10 mm suction instrument is used to clean the abdominal cavity. Forced irrigation with normal saline should dislodge the clot and trophoblastic tissue from the serosa of the peritoneal organs with minimal injury to these structures.

For unruptured tubal pregnancy, the fallopian tube is identified and mobilized to minimize bleeding, a 5 to 8 ml diluted solution containing 20 unit vasopressin in 100 ml of saline is injected with a 20 gauge spinal or laparoscopic needle. It should be injected in the mesosalpinx just below the ectopic sac and over the antimesentric surface of the tubal segment containing gestational sac. After stabilizing the tube by grasper in one hand and microelectrode in other, a linear incision is made on the antimesenteric surface extending one to two cm over the thinnest portion of tube. The fine needle tip should be used in the cutting mode and should barely touch the tissue surface. With electrosurgery, thermal damage may spread if large tips are used on large surface areas in contact with tissue. The pregnancy usually should protrude through the incision and slowly slips out of tube. It may be teased gently out using hydrodissection or atraumatic forceps. Sometimes, forceful irrigation in the tubal opening can dislodge the gestation from implantation. As pregnancy is pulled out or extrudes from the tube, some of the products of conception can remain adhered to the implantation site by a ligamentous structure containing blood vessels. Using bipolar this structure should be coagulated before removing the tissue. The tube is then left to heal by secondary intention or sutured, with secondary intention being appropriate for most cases. Depending upon the size of the product of conception ectopic is removed usually though a 10 mm trocar sleeve. Intraperitoneal drain can be kept in cases of large hemoperitoneum.

Persistent ectopic pregnancy (Follow-up after linear salpingotomy): About 5 to 10 percent patients who undergo linear salpingotomy are at risk of persistent ectopic pregnancy due to residual live ectopic tissue remaining at the ectopic site.[9] The incidence can be minimized by removing all the chorionic tissue using thorough lavage. Serial β-hCG estimations are performed in the postoperative period. It may take several weeks for the titer to become negative. In patients at risk, the titers plateau or rise after an initial fall.

Risk factors for persistent ectopic: Ectopic in proximal portion of tube, small ectopic pregnancies (< 2 cm diameter), early therapy (<42 days from last menstrual period), and high concentrations of β-hCG (> 3000 IU/L) preoperatively.

Treatment includes expectant medical therapy (methotrexate) or salpingectomy. In high-risk cases, a single dose of methotrexate 1 mg/kg can be administered postoperatively for prophylaxis.

Segmental Resection

Resection of the tubal segment containing the gestation is preferable to salpingotomy for an isthmic pregnancy or a ruptured tube or if hemostasis is difficult to obtain. The optimal surgical approach to isthmic ectopic pregnancy remains controversial. Three conservative approaches have been described: segmental resection of the involved portion of the tube with primary microsurgical reanastomosis, segmental resection with reanastomosis at a later operation and linear salpingotomy. In the isthmus the tubal lumen is narrower and muscularis is thicker than the ampulla. Thus, the isthmus is more predisposed to severe postoperative damage, and the rate of proximal tubal obstruction seems to be higher following linear salpingotomy.

Technique of segmental resection: The tube grasped proximal and distal to the ectopic sac with atraumatic graspers. Bloodless resection is accomplished by using bipolar forceps or harmonic scalpel. The tube is cut using scissors. Mesosalpinx is coagulated and cut serially till the segment is excised. The mesosalpinx if bleed should also be cauterized by using bipolar forceps, particular attention given to the arcuate anatomizing branches of the ovarian and uterine arteries. The tube may be reanastomosed at a later date if desired. Primary tubal reanastomosis is a time consuming process requiring special expertise and extensive microsurgical experience; it should not be undertaken by an inexperienced hand.

Radical Surgical Treatment

Total salpingectomy is required when a tubal pregnancy has ruptured and a substantial hemoperitoneum has occurred.

Indications for Salpingectomy

- Ruptured ectopic pregnancy with hemoperitoneum
- A recurrent ectopic pregnancy in the same fallopian tube
- An ectopic pregnancy in a severely damaged tube
- Size of ectopic mass more than 5 cm
- Uncontrolled bleeding during linear salpingotomy
- An ectopic pregnancy in a women who has completed her family.

Total salpingectomy is performed by coagulating and cutting the mesosalpinx, beginning with the proximal portion of the tube to the fimbrial end **(Figs 8.2A to D)**. The tube is separated from the uterus using bipolar coagulation and scissors or harmonic scalpel. Care should be taken to completely remove the tube from cornual end; otherwise, it can be a site for repeat ectopic pregnancy. The mesosalpinx should be cut close to the tube, avoiding damage to blood vessels in mesosalpinx, to preserve the blood supply to the ovary. The isolated segment containing the tubal pregnancy is removed intact or in sectioned part, through the 10 mm trocar sleeve. If the tissue is bulky and cannot be accommodated through cannula, endobag can be used for retrieval of tissue. Lavage the upper

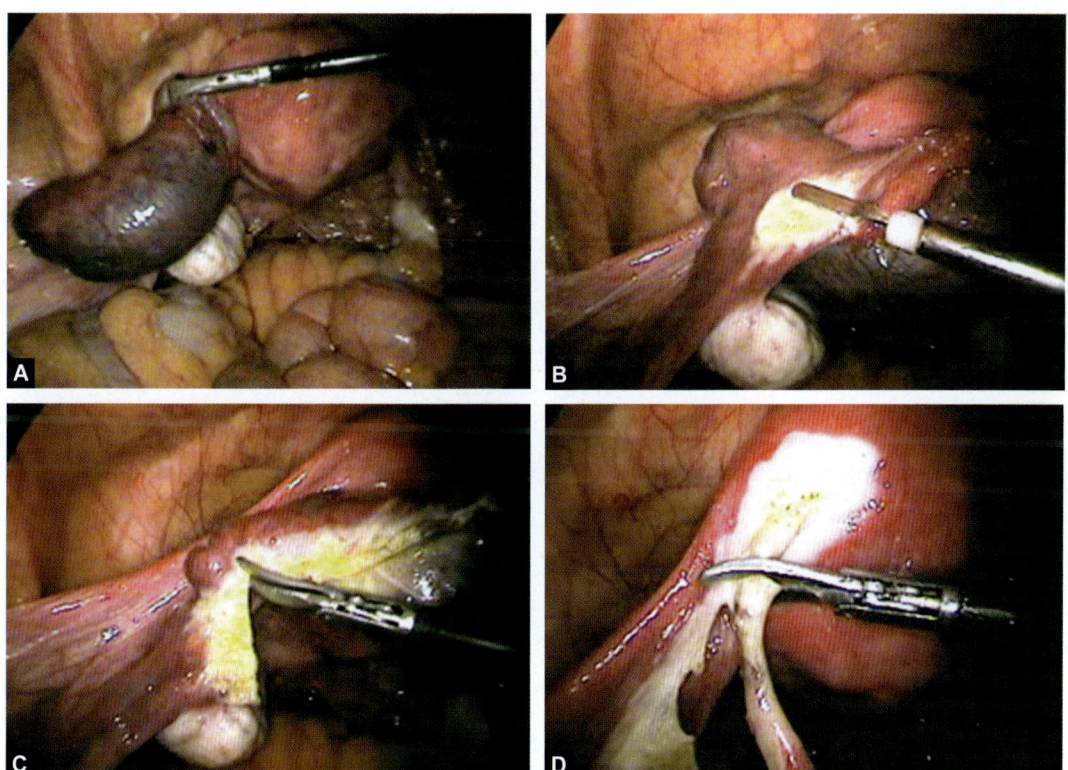

Figs 8.2A to D: Technique of salpingectomy; (A) Left tubal ectopic, (B) Mesosalpinx coagulated, (C) Mesosalpinx cut, (D) Tube transected

abdomen in reverse Trendelenburg position to remove blood collected in the subdiaphragmatic space. Adhesion can be treated simultaneously without significantly prolonging the operation. In one week the β-hCG should return to baseline.[10]

What is the Benefit of Laparoscopic Management of Tubal Pregnancy?

Laparoscopic management provides less postoperative morbidity. Most cases of ruptured as well as unruptured tubal pregnancy can be treated laparoscopically. Laparoscopic management is a useful method for reducing hospital stay, complications and return to normal activity.

The main advantages are:
1. Less postoperative pain.
2. Faster recovery.
3. Short hospital stay.
4. Less postoperative complications like wound infection and adhesion.
5. Cost-effective in working group.

COMPARISON OF SURGICAL AND MEDICAL THERAPY

Several studies have compared conservative laparoscopic treatment with systemic methotrexate in the management of ectopic pregnancy. Hemodynamically stable patients who meet strict criteria, without excessively large or advanced ectopic pregnancies, may therefore be offered either medical or conservative surgical therapy. The immediate clinical and long-term outcomes in these selected patients appear to be similar. Saraj et al reported a randomized trial comparing single dose methotrexate with laparoscopic salpingotomy. They reported similar immediate treatment success rates: 94.7 percent for methotrexate and 91.4 percent for laparoscopic salpingotomy. Additional methotrexate injections were required in 15.8 percent of patients in single dose methotrexate group.

Interstitial (Cornual) Pregnancy

Interstitial (cornual) pregnancy is a rare condition that accounts for no more than 2 to 4 percent of all tubal pregnancies. Timor-Tritsch and colleagues established transvaginal ultrasonographic criteria for interstitial pregnancy. These criteria include:
- An empty uterine cavity
- A chorionic sac seen separately and more than 1 cm from the most lateral edge of the uterine cavity
- A thick myometrial layer surrounding the chorionic sac.

Treatment of interstitial pregnancy: The choice of treatment depends on the extent of trauma that has occurred in the uterine wall and on the interest of the patient in preserving her childbearing function. Systemic methotrexate has been used in a limited number of patients with unruptured interstitial pregnancies. If an interstitial pregnancy is observed when it is still small, it might be excised using conservative laparoscopic techniques.[11] For many surgeons cornual resection and repair of the defect by laparotomy remains the standard conservative surgical procedure. In cases when uterine rupture has occurred or a very large interstitial pregnancy is present, a hysterectomy may be required.

Cornual resection and salpingectomy technique (Figs 8.3A to D): Whenever possible, the ovary should be saved. Myometrium is infiltrated with diluted vasopressin (20 units in 100 ml saline) to optimize intraoperative hemostasis. The interstitial pregnancy sac is incised in V-shaped manner. Care should be taken to excise minimal myometrium as the tissue retracts once sac is excised and remove all the chorionic tissue by thorough lavage. Myometrial walls are approximated with intracorporeal suturing like myomectomy.

Pregnancy in Rudimentary Horn

Pregnancy can occur in a rudimentary horn of the uterus, which may be attached to the uterus. At times, it may be difficult to differentiate tubal ectopic pregnancy from pregnancy in rudimentary horn. In such situations, laparoscopy is useful, both for diagnosis and treatment. Laparoscopically, the rudimentary horn is excised completely, preserving the ovary.

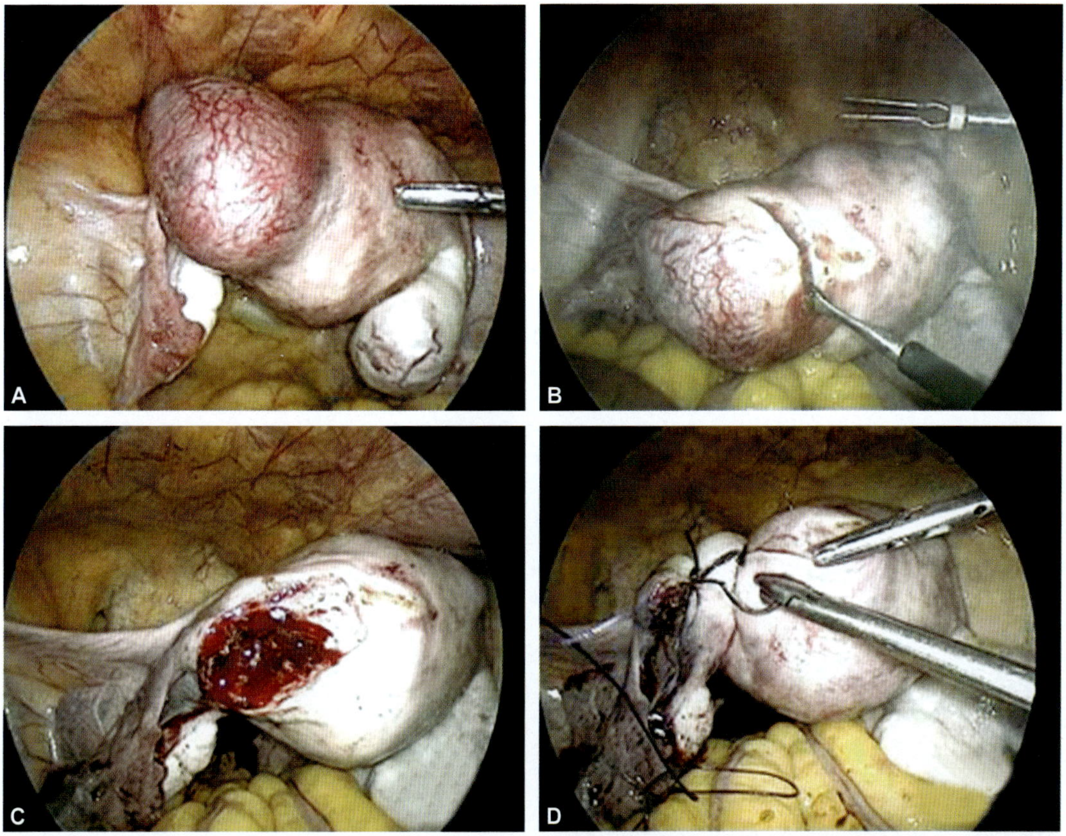

Ectopic Pregnancy: How to Make it Safe for Patient, Tubes and Fertility

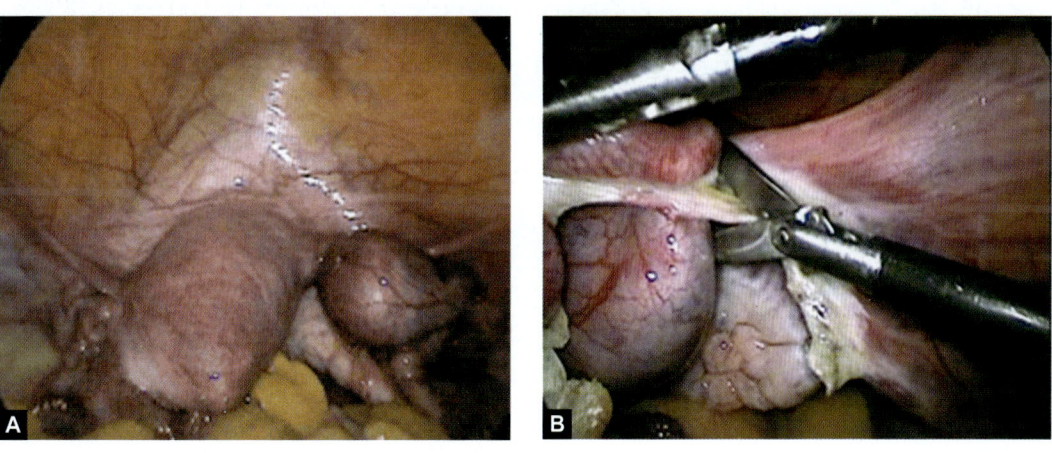

Figs 8.3A to D: Cornual resection and suturing; (A) Left cornual ectopic, (B) Cornual resection, (C) Cornu resected, (D) Cornual suturing

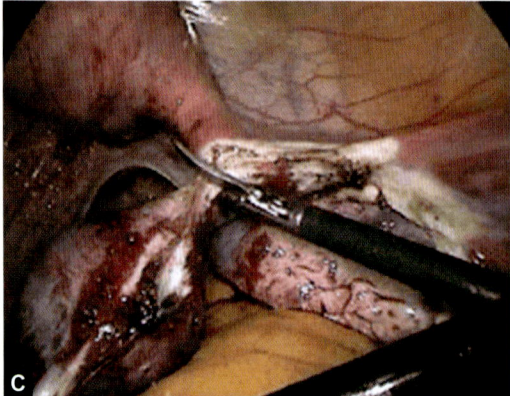

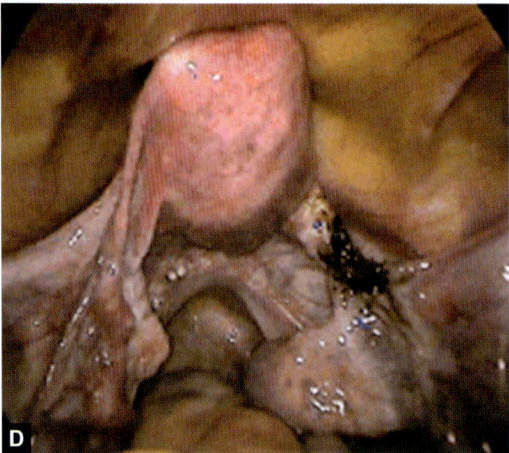

Fig. 8.4A to D: (A) Right rudimentary horn pregnancy; (B and C) Exicision of horn; (D) Excision of horn complete

Right rudimentary horn pregnancy and its excision are shown in **Figures 8.4A to D.**

Cervical Ectopic Pregnancy

The cervix is a rare but hazardous site for placental implantation because the trophoblast can penetrate through the cervical wall and into the uterine blood supply. The three anatomical and histological criteria for diagnosis of cervical pregnancy were established by Rubin in 1911.
- Cervical glands must be opposite the placental attachment
- Placental attachment to the cervix must be situated below the entrance of the uterine vessels or below the peritoneal reflection of the anterior and the posterior surfaces of the uterus
- Fetal elements must be absent from the corpus uteri.

Paalman and Mc Elin proposed five more clinically practical criteria for the diagnosis of this condition:
- Uterine bleeding without cramping pain following a period of amenorrhea
- A soft, enlarged cervix equal to or larger than the fundus (the hourglass uterus)
- Products of conception entirely confined within and firmly attached to the endocervix
- A closed internal cervical os
- A partially opened external cervical os.

Treatment of cervical ectopic pregnancy: The treatment for a cervical pregnancy is surgical, that is a skillful D and C, and the procedure has the potential to be complicated by profuse bleeding, which may require hysterectomy, which can be laparoscopic or abdominal. The preoperative preparations directed to reduce the vascularity of uterine cervix– such as transvaginal ligation of cervical branches of uterine arteries, a Shirodkar type cerclage, angiographic uterine artery embolization or intracervical vasopressine injection may reduce operative morbidity.[12,13]

Medical therapy can also be considered for the primary treatment of cervical pregnancy or as an adjunct to surgical therapy through decreased vascularization of the mass. Uterine artery ligation or embolization does reduce bleeding in treating with later D and C.

Ovarian Ectopic Pregnancy

The pregnancy confined to the ovary represents 0.5 percent to 1 percent of all ectopic pregnancies and is the most common type of nontubal ectopic pregnancy. The only risk factor associated with the development of an ovarian pregnancy is the current use of intrauterine device. The diagnostic criteria by Spiegelberg (1878) are:
- The fallopian tube on the affected side must be intact
- The fetal sac must occupy the position of the ovary

- The ovary must be connected to the uterus by ovarian ligament
- Ovarian tissue must be located in the sac wall
- A well preserved corpus luteum can be identified in the wall of the gestational sac.

Early diagnosis of an ovarian pregnancy, of all the diagnoses relating to extrauterine gestations, is perhaps most difficult. Persistent pelvic pain is the most frequent clinical manifestation of an ovarian gestation. Transvaginal ultrasound, β-hCG assay are helpful in confirming the diagnosis. Sometimes laparoscopy may be necessary to confirm or refute a diagnosis of suspected ovarian pregnancy.

Left ovarian pregnancy and their excision are shown in **Figures 8.5A to D**.

Treatment of ovarian ectopic pregnancy: An ovarian pregnancy is easily confused with a leaking corpus luteum hematoma. For this reason, a safe approach is to proceed with localized surgical resection of the bleeding mass with conservation of the ovary, if possible. It is possible to perform surgical resection by laparoscopic techniques. Unless the diagnosis is made late the ovary can usually be preserved. If the last trophoblastic villus cannot be removed in the ovarian resection, the ovary should be preserved. Any remaining trophoblastic tissue will usually degenerate rapidly or respond to postoperative methotrexate therapy and therefore should produce no long-standing clinical problem. Only rarely is the hemorrhage so profuse that oophorectomy is required to control the bleeding.

Abdominal Ectopic Pregnancy

An abdominal pregnancy is perhaps both the rarest and the most serious type of extrauterine

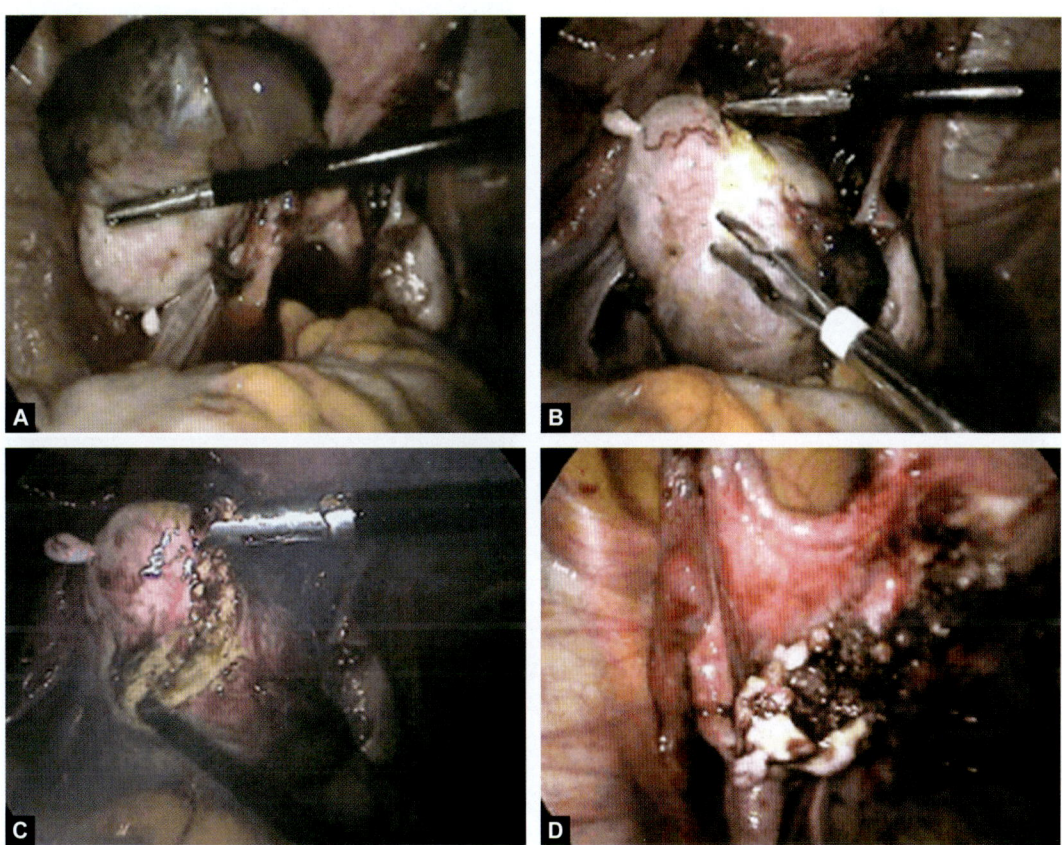

Figs 8.5A to D: Left ovarian pregnancy and its excision; (A) Left ovarian ectopic pregnancy, (B) Excision of ectopic mass, (C) Excision of ectopic mass, (D) Excision complete

gestation. Abdominal pregnancies are classified as primary or secondary. Most are secondary, the result of early tubal abortion or rupture with secondary implantation of the pregnancy into the peritoneal cavity. A primary abdominal pregnancy must meet the three criteria defined by Studdiford in (1942). These are:
- Both tubes and ovaries must be in normal condition with no evidence of recent or remote injury
- No evidence of uteroperitoneal fistula should be found
- The pregnancy must be related exclusively to the peritoneal surface and be early enough to eliminate the possibility that it is a secondary implantation following a primary implantation in the tube.

Management of abdominal pregnancy: Because the pregnancy can continue to term, the potential maternal morbidity and mortality are very high. As a result, early surgical intervention is recommended when an abdominal pregnancy is diagnosed. Early abdominal pregnancy can be managed by laparoscopy. Advanced abdominal pregnancy is usually managed by laparotomy. At surgery, if the vascular supply of the placenta is identified, it can be ligated and removed. If the vascular supply cannot be identified the cord is ligated near the placental base, and the placenta is left in place. Placental involution can be monitored using serial ultrasonography and assessment of β-hCG levels. Methotrexate is not recommended in this clinical setting because it can hasten trophoblastic degeneration, leading to accumulation of necrotic placental tissue, which may become infected.[14,15]

Heterotopic Pregnancy

Combined intrauterine and tubal ectopic pregnancies are rare (1:30,000). The incidence is on the rise due to IVF-ET. Five percent of ectopic pregnancies in IVF-ET are heterotopic.

Treatment of heterotopic pregnancy: Laparoscopy has been employed with reasonable success for the treatment of heterotopic pregnancy. Expectant management has no role, methotrexate therapy is contraindicated. During laparoscopic procedure uterine manipulator is not used. Three accessory ports may be used. Salpingectomy is performed using endoloop technique; electrocoagulation is avoided if possible.[16,17]

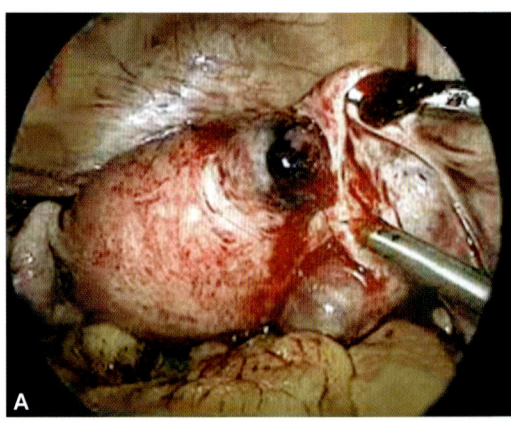
A

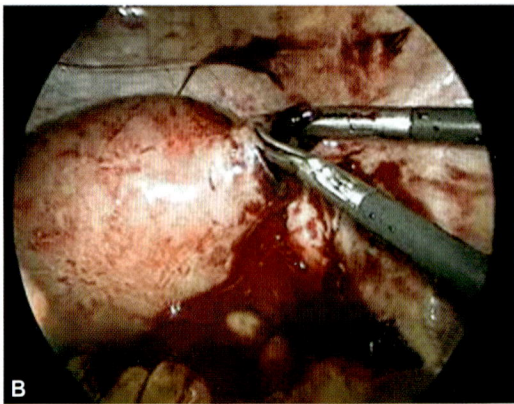
B

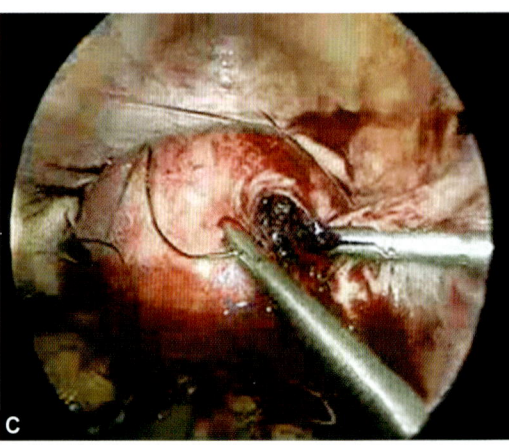
C

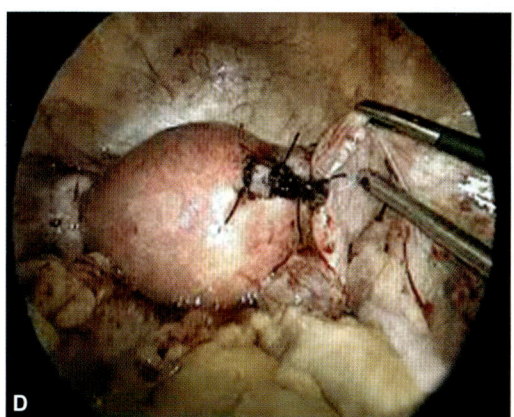

Figs 8.6A to D: (A) Intrauterine and cornual pregnancy; (B) Cornual resection; (C) Cornual suturing; (D) Cornual suturing complete

Intrauterine and cornual pregnancy and resection of corneal pregnancy are shown in **Figures 8.6A to D**.

Our Experience of Ectopic Pregnancy

In last ten years, we have managed 370 cases of ectopic pregnancies at various sites and size. Tubal ectopic were 363, ovarian ectopic were 3, cornual were 2 and heterotopic were 2. All were managed either with medical therapy (methotrexate, 32 cases) or laparoscopy (348 cases). None of the patients required laparotomy. Even patients with massive hemoperitoneum and hemodynamically unstable patients (22 cases) were also managed by laparoscopy.

REFERENCES

1. Bouyer J, Coste J, et al. Risk factors for ectopic pregnancy: A comprehensive analysis based on large case control, population based study in France. Am J Epidemiol. 2003;157:185-94.
2. Rachou E, Germain E, et al. Risk factor for extra uterine pregnancy in women using an intra uterine device. Fertil Steril. 2000;74;899-908.
3. Fernandes H, Gerviase A. Ectopic preg after infertility treatment; Modern diagnosis and therapeutic strategy. Hum. Repro, 2004;10:503-13.
4. Strandell A, Hamberger L, Risk factor for ectopic pregnancy in assisted reproduction., Fertil Steril. 1999;71:282.
5. Barnhart K, Jacobson S, et al. Prompt diagnosis of ectopic pregnancy in emergency dept. setting. Obstet Gynecol. 1994;84:1010-5.
6. Shalev E, Yarom I, et al. TVS as the ultimate diagnostic tool for the management of ectopic pregnancy, Experience with 840 cases. Fertil Steril. 1998;69:62.
7. Stovall TG, Ling FW, et al. Single dose methotrexate for tratment of ectopic pregnancy. Obstet Gynecol. 1991;77:754.
8. Dcherney AH, Kase N. The conservative surgical management of unruptured ectopic pregnancy. Obstet Gynecol.1979;54-451.
9. Farquhar CM. Ectopic pregnancy. Lancet. 2005;366(9485);583:91.
10. Nezhat F, Winer W, et al. Salpingectomy via laparoscopy. A new surgical approach. J Laproendo Surg. 1991;1:91.
11. Ostrzenski A. A new laparoscopic technique for interstitial pregnancy resection; A case report. J Repro Med. 1997;42-363.
12. Pasqual MA, Ruiz J, Tresserra F, Sanuy C, Graces JP, Tur R, et al. Cervical ectopic pregnancy: diagnosis and conservative treatment. Hum Reprod 2001;16:584-6.
13. Kung, FT, Chang, SY, Tsai, YC et al. Subsequent reproduction and obstetric outcome after methotrexate treatment of cervical pregnancy: a review of original literature and international collaborative follow-up. Hum. Reprod. 1997;12:591-95.
14. Varma R, Mascarenhas R, Jame D. Successful outcome of advanced abdominal pregnancy with exclusive omental insertion. Ultrasound Obstet Gynecol. 2003;21:192-4.
15. Onan MA. Turp AB, Saltik A, Akyurek N, Taskiran C, Himmetoglu O. Primary omental pregnancy: case report. Hum Reprod. 2005; 20(3):807-09.
16. Cheng PJ, Chueh HY, Qiu JT. Heterotopic pregnancy in a natural conception cycle presenting as hematometra. Obstet Gynecol. 2004, 104:1195.
17. Ludwig M, Kaisi M, Bauer O, Diedrich K. The forgotten child—a case of heterotopic, intraabdominal and intrauterine pregnancy carried to term. Hum Reprod. 1999;14(5):1372-4.

CHAPTER 9

How to Make Laparoscopic Surgery Safe for Advanced Endometriosis

PG Paul

Chapter Outline

- Preoperative Assessment
- Technique
- Mild Endometriosis
- Moderate to Severe Endometriosis
- Correction of Retroflexion of Uterus
- Salpingo-Ovariolysis
- Cystectomy

Endometriosis is a leading cause of pelvic pain and infertility in women. The gold standard for diagnosis of endometriosis is by direct visualization or histological findings or both.[1] Endometriosis has a variety of appearances and forms including the classic 'powder burn' lesions, red lesions, white lesions, peritoneal retractions, and endometriotic cysts or 'chocolate cysts'.[2] Endometriosis is usually associated with scar tissue and adhesions. The severity of endometriosis is usually expressed by the classification system developed by the American Society for Reproductive Medicine that incorporates implant scores and adhesion scores.

In planning treatment many variables must be considered, such as age of patient, extent of disease, degree of symptoms and desire for fertility.[3] Current evidence based data suggests that laparoscopic excision of endometriosis offers good long-term results with regard to infertility results and regression of pain symptoms.[4]

PREOPERATIVE ASSESSMENT

Good preoperative evaluation is necessary to plan the surgery and for counseling. Importance should be given to patient's severity of symptoms. Patients, whose main complaint is pain and completed family may be treated more aggressively like salpingectomy or adnexectomy. Additional procedures like presaral neurectomy can be performed for patients with severe dysmenorrhea.[5] In infertile patients, ovarian conservation is given prime importance. Transvaginal sonography can help to identify whether the endometrioma is single or multiloculated. Cystectomy for a multiloculated endometrioma is very difficult and ovarian tissue loss can be more. It is important to assess the involvement of rectovaginal septum to plan for a difficult dissection or a probable rectal repair.

TECHNIQUE

Patient should be positioned with the buttocks well beyond the edge of the table to allow free movement of the uterine manipulator. We use a spackman cannula with a tenaculam to antevert the uterus which also allows chromopertubation. Good antevertsion is essential for treating Pouch of Douglas obliteration. Use of uterine sound or dilator is very inconvenient and should be avoided. Legs are properly strapped in an Allen stirrup **(Fig. 9.1)**. Primary trocar is placed infraumbilically. Two accessory 6 mm trocar are placed in either quadrant, lateral to inferior epigastric arteries. Third trocar is placed in midline 4 to 5 cm suprapubically.

Very few special instruments are necessary for endometriosis surgery. A good suction irrigation system is very essential to suck and wash the thick chocolate material. A pair of sharp scissors and bipolar instruments is essential. A pair of graspers with fine teeth (Like Allis's forceps) as well as traumatic teeth (Like Kocher's forceps) is needed for cyst enucleation. A bowel grasper is useful for reconstruction of the ovary. A rectal probe may be needed during dissection of the rectovaginal septum.

MILD ENDOMETRIOSIS

Superficial implants can be easily coagulated with bipolar forceps. Washing and rubbing the implants with suction irrigation cannula and simultaneously coagulation of the implants avoids charring **(Fig. 9.2)**. Deeper implants are excised with scissors. Any active bleeders can be coagulated.

MODERATE TO SEVERE ENDOMETRIOSIS

In severe endometriosis, there will be adhesions, endometriomas and or obliteration of Pouch of Douglas (POD). Adhesions can involve bowel, bladder, tubes, ovaries and uterus. The severity of adhesions depends on the number and type of previous surgeries, duration of endometriosis and previous medical treatment. Rupture of endometrioma or previous pelvic infections can make the adehesions dense. Ovarian endometriosis can be in the form of surface implants with adhesions or endometriomas. Endometriomas can be small, large or multiloculated.

Severe endometriosis surgery needs a very systematic approach, patience and perseverance. Surgeon and the team should be mentally prepared for a prolonged surgery. The results of the surgery depend on the restoration of anatomy and completeness of the removal of the disease.

The aims of laparoscopic conservative surgery are:

- Complete adhesiolysis with restoration of normal tubo-ovarian relationship to enhance fertility potential
- Removal of both typical and atypical endometriotic implants
- Complete removal of endometriotic cyst.

The steps of a typical case of severe endometriosis are illustrated in the following figures:

General inspection of the pelvis and abdomen is done first. Uterus and adnexa is examined for extent of adhesions and size of endometrioma **(Fig. 9.3)**.

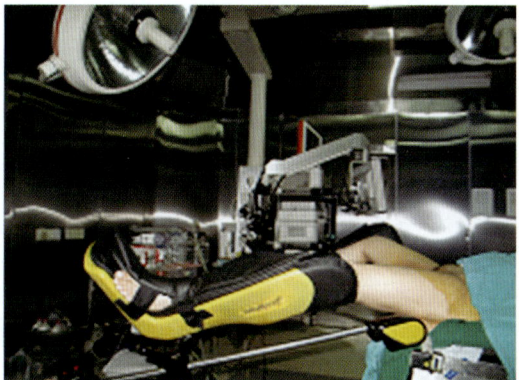

Fig. 9.1: Patient's legs are placed in allen stirrups

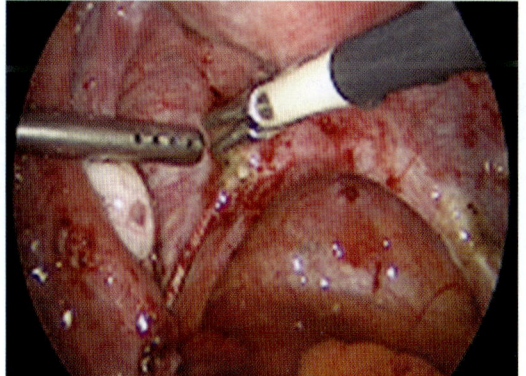

Fig. 9.2: Superficial endometrial implants are coagulated with bipolar forceps

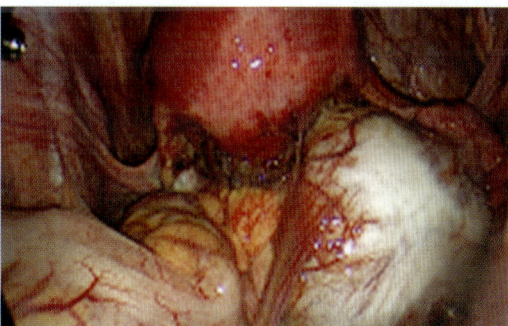

Fig. 9.3: Severe endometriosis - bilateral endometrioma with adhesions

CORRECTION OF RETROFLEXION OF UTERUS

The fleshy broad adhesions over the uterus and adnexa are excised with scissors or any energy source **(Fig. 9.4)**.

The bleeding normally stops without coagulation. The uterus is anteverted with the Spackman cannula, simultaneously assisted by suction irrigation cannula. The endometriomas and uterosacral adhesions to uterus get released spontaneously. Sometime chocolate material gets partially drained during this process **(Fig. 9.5)**.

The spilled chocolate material is sucked out immediately to reduce contamination. This spillage is inevitable in most situations. Large chocolate cyst can be aspirated with direct trocar puncture and lavaged as an initial step to reduce the spillage. The retroflexion of uterus is further corrected by applying pressure with an open grasper to release the uterosacral adhesions and expose the fleshy endometrial tissue **(Fig. 9.6)**.

This step sometimes drains chocolate material. Sharp dissection is needed when this adhesions is fibrosed especially, in previously operated case.

SALPINGO-OVARIOLYSIS

Usually, ovary will contain chocolate cysts of varying size with pelvic side wall adhesions. If the cyst is more than 5 cm, it is drained before ovariolysis as already mentioned. Smaller chocolate cyst is held with an atraumatic grasper with Ally's forceps like teeth and start releasing from the pelvic side wall with a suction irrigator **(Fig. 9.7)**.

The separation of cyst from the pelvic peritoneum is started from normal site and pressure is applied more on the cyst rather the pelvic side wall to avoid injury to pelvic peritoneum and underlying structures like ureter and veins. The contents of the chocolate cyst gets drained during this step as most of these cysts are extraovarian in origin **(Fig. 9.7)**. Spilled chocolate contents

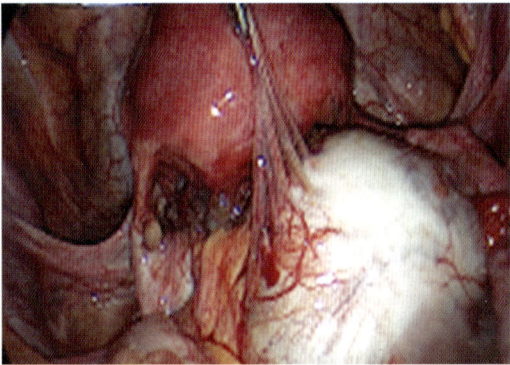

Fig. 9.4: The fleshy broad adhesions are excised

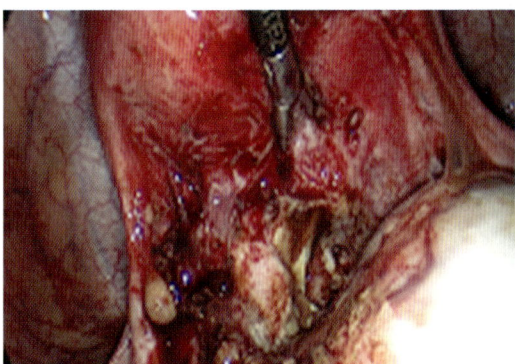

Fig. 9.6: Further correction of retroflexion exposing the fleshy endometrial tissue

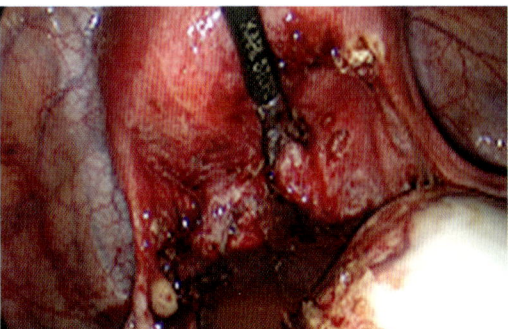

Fig. 9.5: Correction of retroflexion of uterus with spill of chocolate material

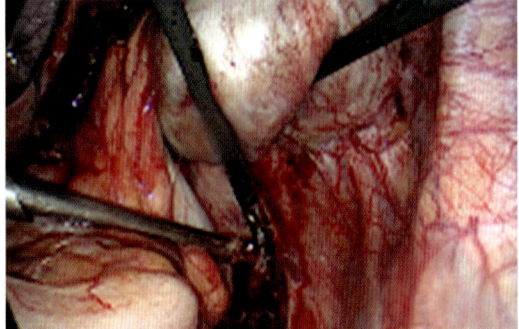

Fig. 9.7: Releasing the right endometrioma from pelvic side wall

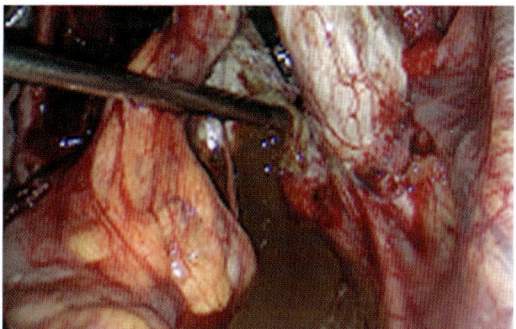

Fig. 9.8: Drainage of chocolate material during the dissection

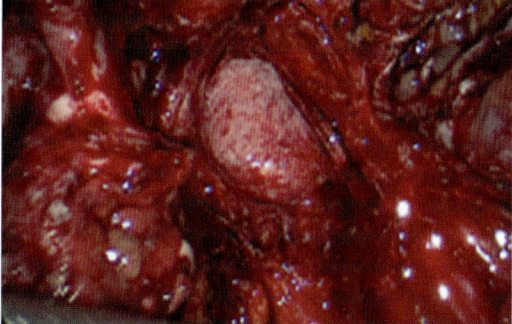

Fig. 9.11: Part of normal peritoneum is seen in the POD after adhesiolysis

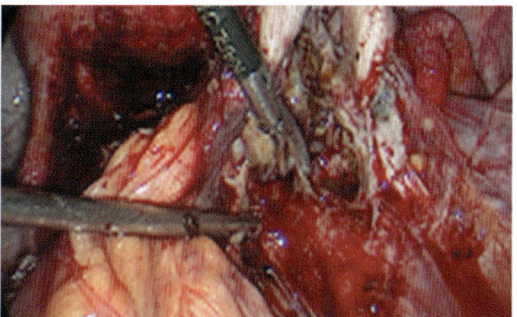

Fig. 9.9: Ovariolysis assisted with a third grasper

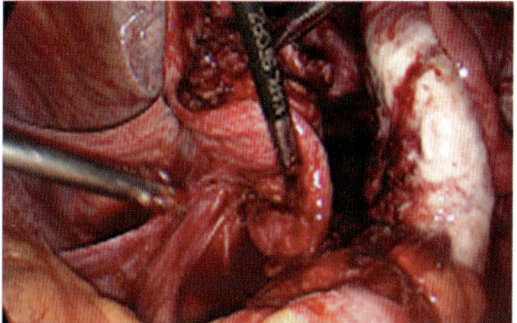

Fig. 9.12: Left adnexa already released from pelvic side wall

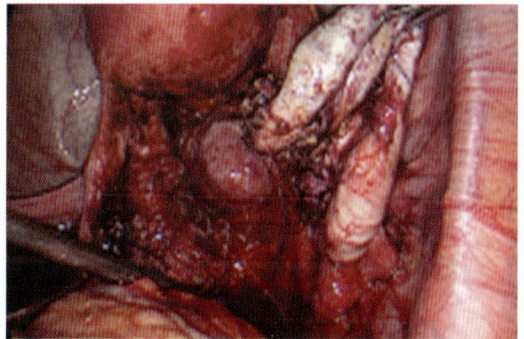

Fig. 9.10: Right adnexa completely released from the pelvic side wall

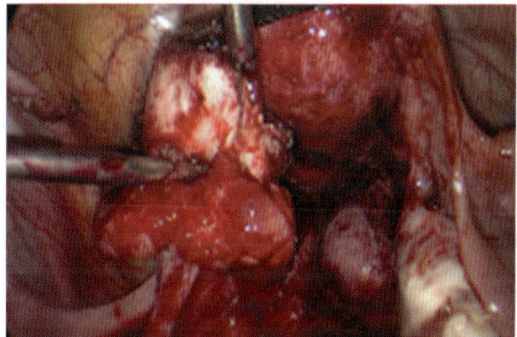

Fig. 9.13: Left salpingolysis

are immediately sucked and washed with saline **(Fig. 9.8)**. The ovariolysis is continued with help of a third atrumatic grasper from suprapubic port **(Fig. 9.9)**. The adnexa is completely released from the pelvic side wall **(Fig. 9.10)**.

Over enthusiastic adhesiolysis can result in damage to the hilum of ovary with profuse bleeding. If the dissection plane is proper, there is no need for any energy use for hemostasis. Once the adnexal and uterosacral adhesions are corrected, POD anatomy will be clear. Although the initial appearance was suggestive of complete obliteration of POD, after adhesiolysis, part of normal peritoneum could be identified **(Fig. 9.11)**. Left adnexa is also released from the pelvic side wall in a similar fashion **(Fig. 9.12)**.

Usually, the sigmoid covers the left adnexa and it has to be released before this step can be undertaken. Left tube is then gently released from the ovary with blunt dissection with suction irrigation **(Figs 9.13 to 9.15)**.

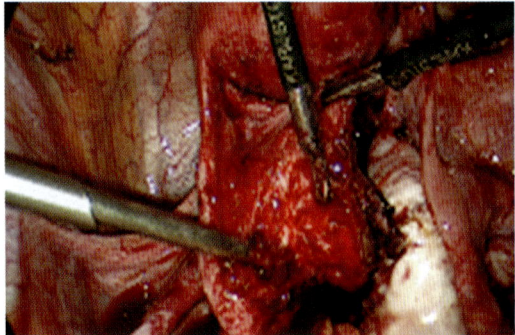

Fig. 9.14: Salpingo-ovariolysis continued

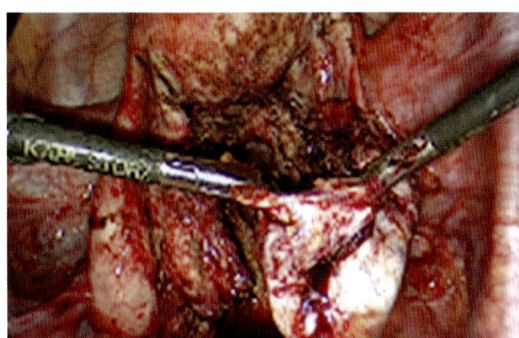

Fig. 9.16: Right cyst enucleation–tearing the edges for identification of layers

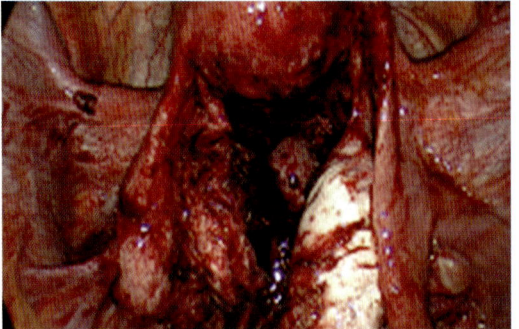

Fig. 9.15: Salpingo-ovariolysis completed

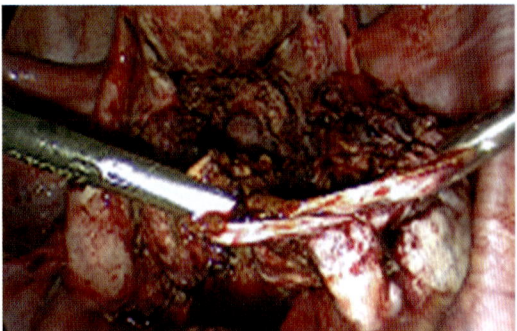

Fig. 9.17: The cyst layer is seen separately from the ovarian tissue

This step may need sharp dissection in long standing endometriosis or previously operated cases. Gentle handling is needed for releasing the fimbrial end. Energy source is avoided as far as possible as bleeding from vascular fimbriae stop spontaneously.

CYSTECTOMY

Current evidence suggests that cystectomy is a better treatment for endometrioma as far as the disease recurrence and pregnancy results are concerned.[6] Endometriotic cyst enucleation is different from usual cystectomy as there is no true cyst lining. The pseudocyst lining of endometrioma has to be peeled off without compromising the ovarian tissue. Different techniques can be used for identifying the layers for peeling. We hold the edge of the cyst with 2 graspers and try to tear by pulling the graspers apart till the cyst lining is seen separately **(Figs 9.16 and 9.17)**.

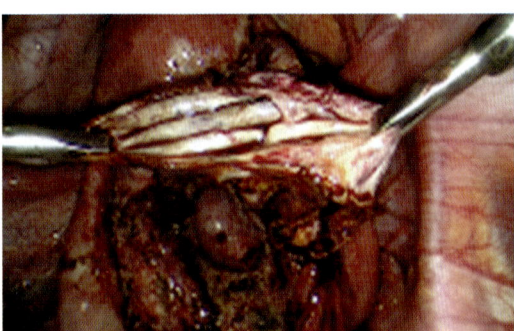

Fig. 9.18: Enucleation of the cyst in progress

Once the cyst lining is identified, it is peeled from the ovarian tissue holding with a Kocher's like toothed grasper **(Fig. 9.18)**. A third atraumatic grasper is useful for precise enucleation while other two graspers keeps the layers wide apart **(Fig. 9.19)**.

Always make sure there is no ovarian tissue (usually reddish in color) on the cyst side **(Fig. 9.20)**. During the final stages of separation take

How to Make Laparoscopic Surgery Safe for Advanced Endometriosis

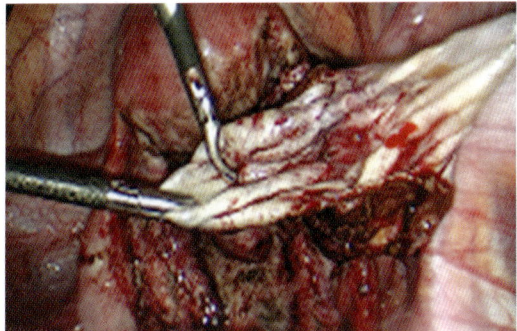

Fig. 9.19: Enucleation of the cyst—cyst and ovarian tissue are pulled apart and third grasper assisting

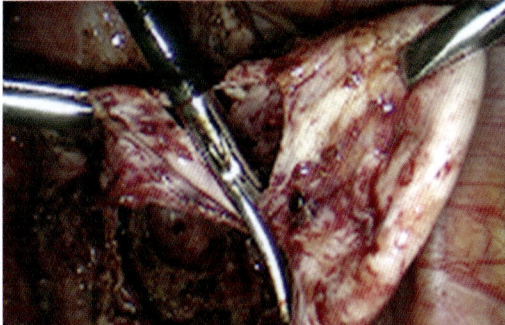

Fig. 9.22: Thinned-out edges of the ovarian tissue is excised with a sharp scissors

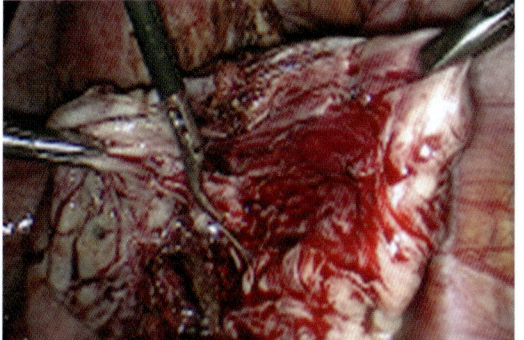

Fig. 9.20: Enucleation of the cyst – avoiding ovarian tissue getting enucleated with the cyst

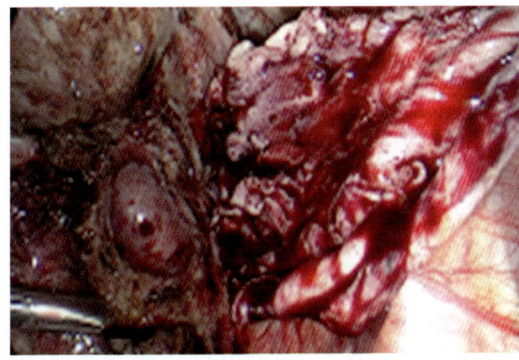

Fig. 9.23: Inspection of ovary to look for hemostasis

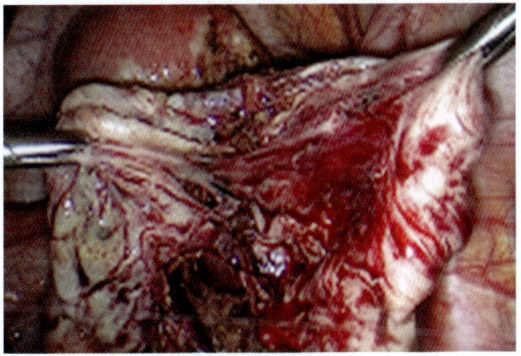

Fig. 9.21: Enucleation of the cyst – final stages separation of cyst

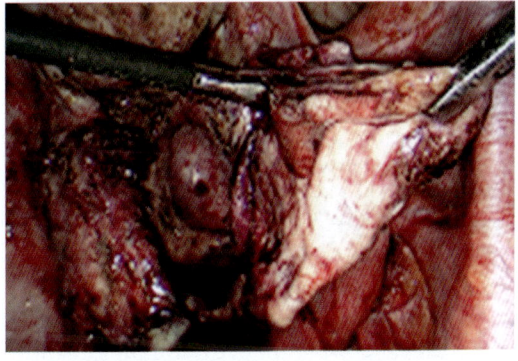

Fig. 9.24: Ovarian reconstruction

care to avoid injury to ovarian ligament **(Fig. 9.21)**. Sharp dissection may be needed during this step. The edges of the remaining ovarian tissue may be either thinned out or may contain remnants of endometrial implants which can be excised with a sharp scissors **(Fig. 9.22)**. Inside of the ovary is then inspected for any active bleeders **(Fig. 9.23)**. Minimal oozing is ignored as coagulation can further damage the ovarian tissue. Minimal blood and fibrin is useful for reconstruction of ovary without suturing. The reconstruction is done by holding the edges with graspers to make a near normal ovarian shape **(Fig. 9.24)**. Ovary is then compressed

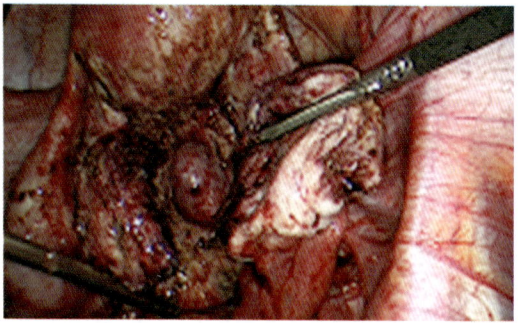

Fig. 9.25: Ovarian reconstruction without suturing—bowel grasper keep the ovary compressed

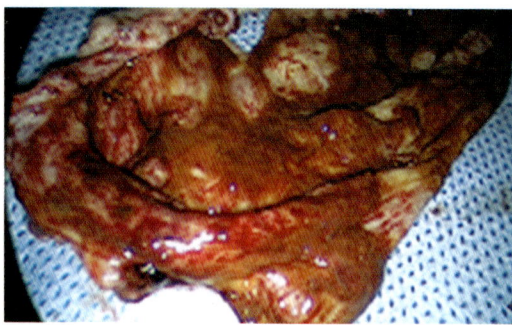

Fig. 9.28: Specimen – cyst side

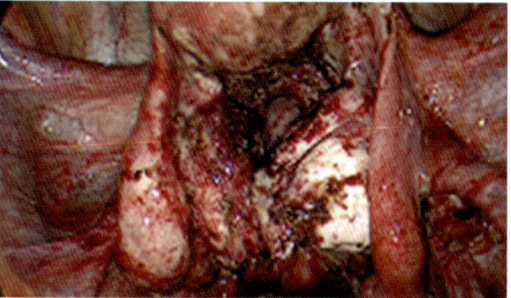

Fig. 9.26: Appearance of ovaries after reconstruction

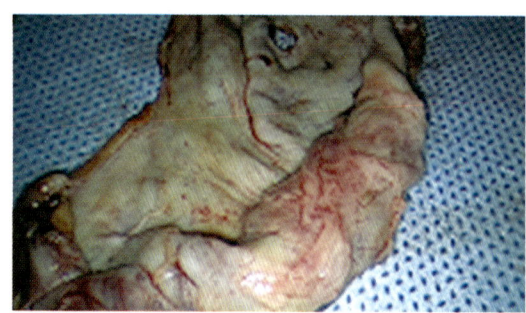

Fig. 9.29: Specimen – ovarian side

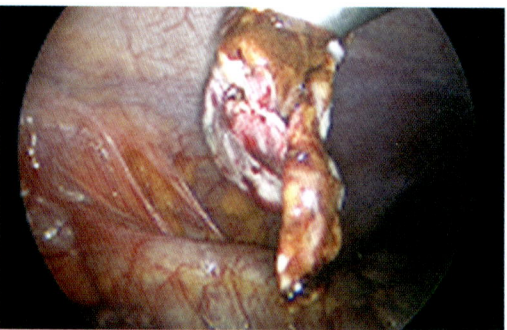

Fig. 9.27: Specimen removal through the primary port

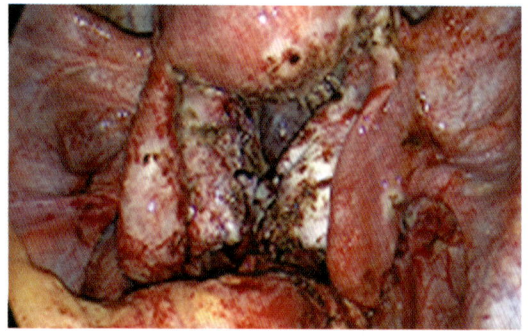

Fig. 9.30: Final picture of pelvis after conservative surgery

with a bowel grasper for 3 to 4 minutes to allow the natural fibrin to act as glue **(Fig. 9.25)**. Thus ovarian suturing is avoided to reduce adhesions formation. The reconstructed ovary looks near normal shape **(Fig. 9.26)**. Specimen is removed through the primary 10 mm trocar by visualizing through a 5 mm telescope introduced thorough one of the secondary port to avoid enlarging the 6 mm secondary port **(Fig. 9.27)**.

The specimen inspected on both sides to check for the presence of any inadvertent ovarian tissue removal **(Figs 9.28 and 9.29)**. To perfect your cystectomy technique, it is a good practice to ask the pathologist for presence of ovarian tissue on the specimen. Peritoneal cavity is lavaged with normal saline to wash off any spilled chocolate material and blood. Finally, pelvis is inspected for complete hemostasis **(Fig. 9.30)**.

SUMMARY

Laparoscopic surgery for severe endometriosis is a demanding surgery. Patient should be thoroughly evaluated both, clinically and sonographically. This helps in planning the surgery as well as counseling the patient about the potential complications. Laparoscopic surgery for severe endometriosis should be done in a systematic manner. Every effort should be taken to restore the anatomy and to remove all visible endometriosis. Potential complications are high, unless extreme care is taken during surgery.

REFERENCES

1. Brosens I, Puttemans P, Campo R, Gordts S, Kinkel K. Diagnosis of endometriosis: pelvic endoscopy and imaging techniques. Best Pract Res Clin Obstet Gynaecol. 2004;18:285-303.
2. Donnez J, Van Langendonckt A. Typical and subtle atypical presentations of endometriosis. Curr Opin Obstet Gynecol. 2004;16:431-7.
3. American Fertility Society. Revised American Fertility Society classification of endometriosis. Fertil Steril. 1985;43:351-2.
4. Adamson GD, Pasta DJ. Surgical treatment of endometriosis associated infertility: meta-analysis compared with survival analysis. Am J Obstet Gynecol 1994;171:1488-504.
5. Zullo F, Palomba S, Zupi Eetal. Effectiveness of presacral neurectomy in women with severe dysmenorrhoea caused by endometriosis who were treated with laparoscopic conservative surgery. Am J Obstet Gynecol .2003;189;720-1.
6. Hart R, Hickey M, Maouris P, Buckett W, Garry R. Excisional surgery versus ablative surgery for ovarian endometriomata: a Cochrane Review. Hum Reprod. 2005 Nov; 20(11):3000-7. Review.

CHAPTER 10

How to Make Total Laparoscopic Hysterectomy Safe?

Prakash H Trivedi, Shaily Jain

Chapter Outline

- Indications of Laparoscopic Hysterectomy
- Philosophy of Patient's Safety in Laparoscopic Hysterectomy
- Contraindication for Laparoscopic Hysterectomy
  - Key Points in Laparoscopic Hysterectomy Till 14 Weeks Size Uterus
- Debulking of Uterus
  - The Key Areas for Effective TLH
  - Special Situations and Difficulties

INTRODUCTION

During the last two decades, Gynecological Endoscopic and Minimal Access Surgery have revolutionized approach to various pathology of different organs; removal of uterus was no exception. In many countries and particularly in India there are expert vaginal surgeons in every corner. They made removal of uterus vaginally, a truly natural orifice minimal access surgery. However, still there were many hysterectomies done abdominally which was justifiable for malignancy, very large uterus or previous abdominal surgery with bowel adhesions close to scar or uterus,[1] but in remaining situation an expert laparoscopic surgeon replaced it with ease and expertise an efficient outcome for patient. At no stage laparoscopic approach is thought, if the desired outcome is achieved vaginally. It is imperative for every gynecologist to be a good vaginal surgeon before becoming a good laparoscopic surgeon.

Laparoscopic hysterectomy is totally a patient plus consumer and industry driven advance, which has sealed a place in modern gynecology.

INDICATIONS OF LAPAROSCOPIC HYSTERECTOMY

A new surgical skill and techniques do not wait but it creates opportunities to deliver with adequate safety to patients. The indications vary from centers and operating surgeons specially the line of demarcation to do abdominal or laparoscopic hysterectomy.

In our armamentarium the following are the indications of laparoscopic hysterectomy:

1. Patient with excessive menstrual bleeding not responding to medical therapy with a uterus which is more than 14 weeks in size or vaginal space is restricted like in a nulliparous case and in unmarried women with advanced age.
2. Patient with multiple or large fibroids symptomatic and has finished child bearing.
3. Patient for hysterectomy with pain in abdomen, possibility of associated pathology like pelvic adhesions, inflammatory disease, endometriosis or endometriomas, suspected appendicitis rarely with cholecystectomy for gall stones- symptomatic.

4. Patient with 2-3 cesarean sections and the gynecologist is not comfortable to do a safe vaginal hysterectomy.
5. Patient with vault laxity and removal of uterus is also indicated, wherein vault can be suspended by a mesh anchored from sacral promontory to vault.

PHILOSOPHY OF PATIENT'S SAFETY IN LAPAROSCOPIC HYSTERECTOMY

Proper care has to be taken by the operating surgeon to achieve sufficient experience and skill to have safe use of energy sources, suturing, bipolar and tissue dissection for removal of uterus. Also, removal of large uterus by good morcellator, if it is likely to cause laceration in the vagina, which is narrow for a very big uterus.

Indications of doing a laparoscopic hysterectomy should be defined and it should not be like 'me-too'. phenomena or peer pressure to do or for longer survival or due to glamor of laparoscopic surgery. Full conscious attempt is made to justify the skill, infrastructure, set up and safety to do laparoscopic hysterectomy.

Further as laparoscopic surgery promises minimal invasion, more safety and patient expect a miracle, then complications tarnish image of both laparoscopic surgery and the center. Thus, safety is of utmost importance.

In any case of laparoscopic hysterectomy, a detailed counseling explaining the procedure by a short film or photographs to patients and relatives with limitations, rare complications and your own data has to be given. Further an elaborate exhaustive yet simplified consent form and in certain cases, special high-risk consent is mandatory, explaining the patient in a language in which they understand.

General surgeon doing laparoscopic hysterectomy with gynecologist assisting is not preventable at all. But it is necessary for us to enhance there team skills in vaginal hysterectomy and the better steps which a gynecologist will do in comparison to a general surgeon for the safety for our women patient.

There cannot be a standard technique for laparoscopic hysterectomy as in the last 17 years it has changed from LAVH, supracervical hysterectomy to total laparoscopic hysterectomy first with bipolar, scissors and monopolar for colpotomy on a nonconducting tube, then it was dominated by addition of harmonic scalpel. In the 21st century, there was a brigade of new vessel sealing device like Martin maxi with Robi grasper, Gyrus Plasma Kinetic transector 10 and 5 mm, Ligasure from Valley lab 10 mm and recently 5 mm Atlas, the Erbes Biclamp, now a 5 mm Enseal is preferred due to lesser lateral spread. However, many Laparoscopist are still feeling that for suturing of uterine arteries, bipolar for coagulation (dedicated Wolf or Erbe) and scissors for dissection are still more satisfying and tension free. The vessel sealing device reduces change of instruments but if used improperly can lead to injury to surrounding structures.

CONTRAINDICATION FOR LAPAROSCOPIC HYSTERECTOMY

1. Medical conditions do not permit Pneumoperitoneum like hiatus or umbilical hernia or poor respiratory or cardiac reserve.
2. Surgeon is not groomed for the technique or center is not well equipped.
3. Very large uterine masses >26–28 weeks in size.
4. Previous abdominal surgery with likelihood of bad bowel adhesions.
5. Gross obesity (relative).
6. Ovarian malignancy or advanced cervical or endometrial carcinoma.

Operative technique for a total laparoscopic hysterectomy in mild to moderately difficult cases

The operation theater facilities, consent, etc. with the team is ready as described in Chapter Step By Step Laparoscopic Surgery.

Key Points in Laparoscopic Hysterectomy Till 14 Weeks Size Uterus

Patient is under general anaesthesia with endotracheal intubation or laryngeal mask apparatus with multiparameter monitoring observing pulse rate, $ETCO_2$, DO_2, ECG Plethysmograph and temperature. Patient is in modified lithotomy position with leg rest at 45° to have free movement of lower port instrument.[2] Verres needle, CO_2 Insufflation, primary and 3 ancillary trocars are introduced. (as mentioned in Chapter Step by Step Laparoscopic Surgery). Next a head low position is given to take bowels away from operative field. An epidural anaesthesia can lead to contracted bowels and avoiding N_2O which is excreted in intestines gives a good field. Foley's catheter is kept in the bladder; uterine manipulator like a simple Hulka's or thicker longer version of the same is used initially. Use of laparoscopic myoma screw **(Fig. 10.1)** is good for manipulation but may block one port, this, however, is best to manipulate big uterus, as other manipulators do not work.

Hysterectomy starts with cutting the round ligaments with harmonic ace[3,4] or monopolar spatula **(Fig. 10.2)**.

Once a free plane is seen on cutting the round ligament, peritoneum is dissected to push the bladder and also the ureter more lateral **(Figs 10.3A to C)**.

The vessels are skeletonized and the ascending, descending and the knuckle of the uterine artery with uterine vein also visible clearly. The cornu or infundibulopelvic ligament is dissected with Enseal or bipolar and cut **(Fig. 10.4)**.

The posterior peritoneum is dissected with harmonic scalpel till uterosacral ligaments, which are also detached from the uterus **(Fig. 10.5)**. This makes the uterine vessels very prominent for dissection or suturing. On both sides skeletonization of the vessel is done meticulously **(Figs 10.6A to C)**. Now we can coagulate, suture or dessicate and cut with vessel sealing devices.[5,6]

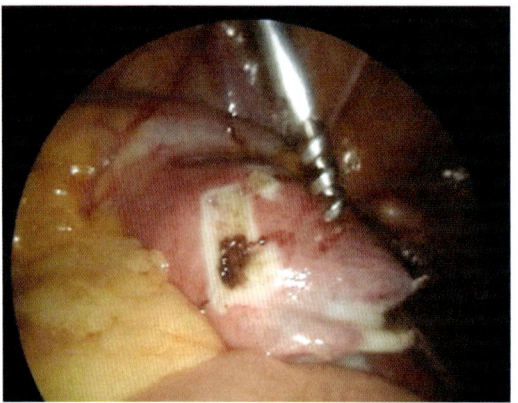

Fig. 10.1: Myoma screw used for manipulation, introduced through left port and fixed on right side and uterus manipulated towards the left side for right sided dissection and vice versa

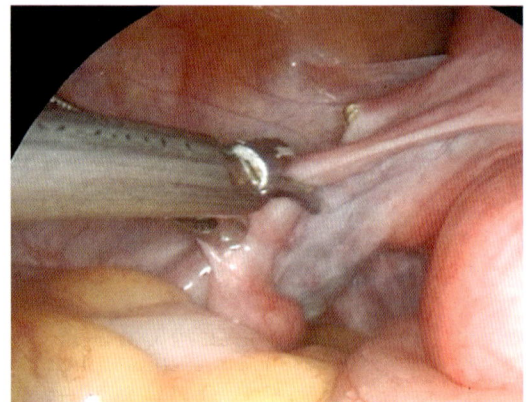

Fig. 10.2: Round ligament being cut with harmonic ace

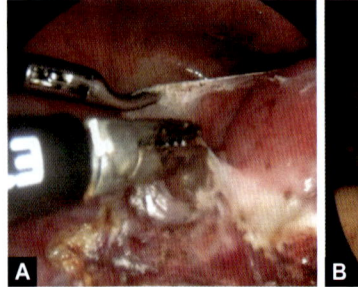
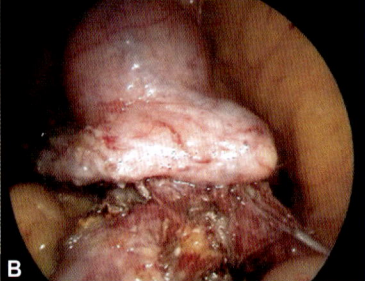
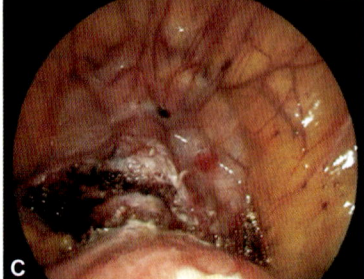

Figs 10.3A to C: Peritoneum dissected to push bladder down; (A) Bladder dissected with enseal, (B) Dissected bladder with Foley's bulge seen, (C) Bladder pushed down

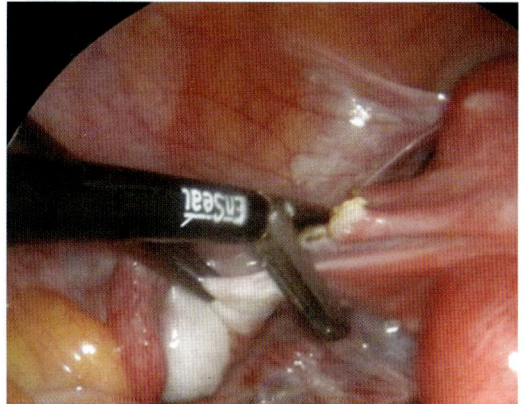
Fig. 10.4: Cornu dissected with enseal

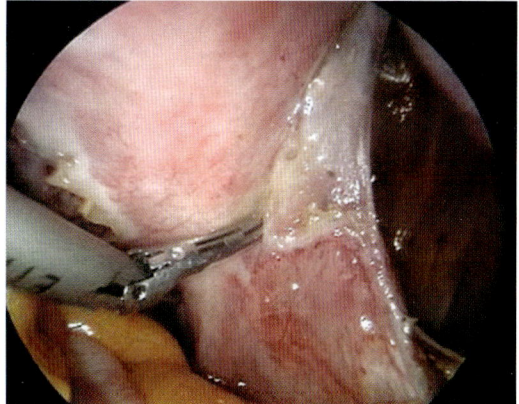
Fig. 10.5: Uterosacral dissected with harmonic

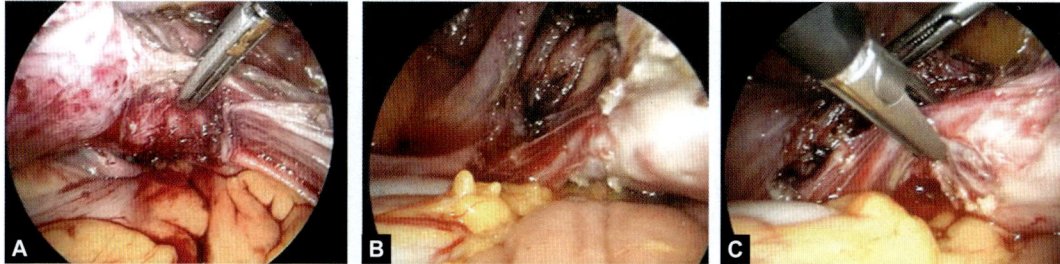
Figs 10.6A to C: After skeletonisation, coagulate uterine with 5 mm vessel sealing device; (A) Skeletonising uterines, (B) Skeletonised uterines vessel, (C) Coagulate with enseal

After tissue dissection, both sides are sealed to avoid back flow bleeding **(Fig. 10.7)**. The next very important step is to separate the medial attachment of tissues engulfing uterine vessels, which are already coagulated or sutured. This prevents avulsion bleeding of uterine vessels due to a pull from below while delivering the uterus.

As the uterosacral was already divided before this tissue separation, uterus is only attached to the vagina which is made prominent by a colpotomizer tube introduced vaginally enhancing it over the cervix **(Fig. 10.8)**.

With a harmonic scalpel or a hook, the vagina is opened and a circumferential incision is completed with cervix held by a single hooked grasper in the left upper port and the left lower port having the harmonic scalpel **(Fig. 10.9)**. The assistant should safeguard the surrounding structures.

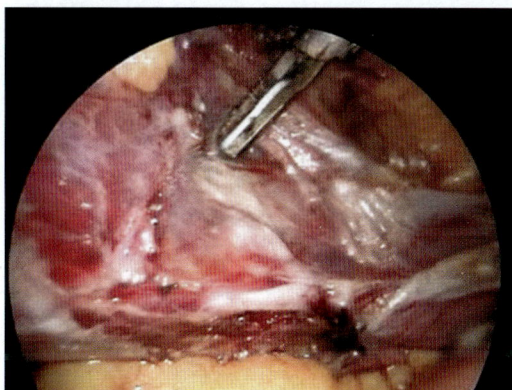
Fig. 10.7: Dissection of tissue around vessels with coagulation

The uterus, depending on the size, is removed vaginally or morcellated by introducing a morcellator from the left lower port.

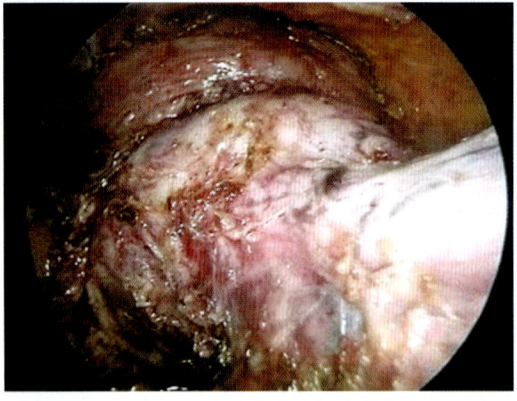
Fig. 10.8: Vagina made prominent by colpotomiser

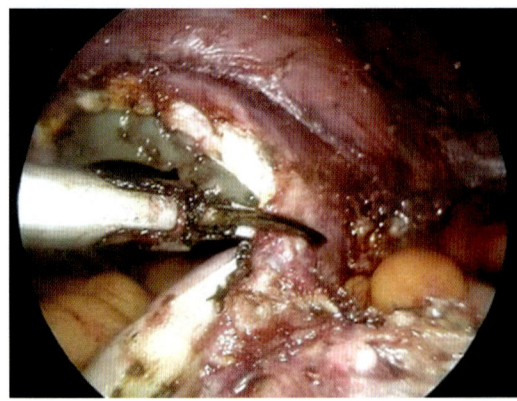
Fig. 10.9: Circumferential incision around cervix

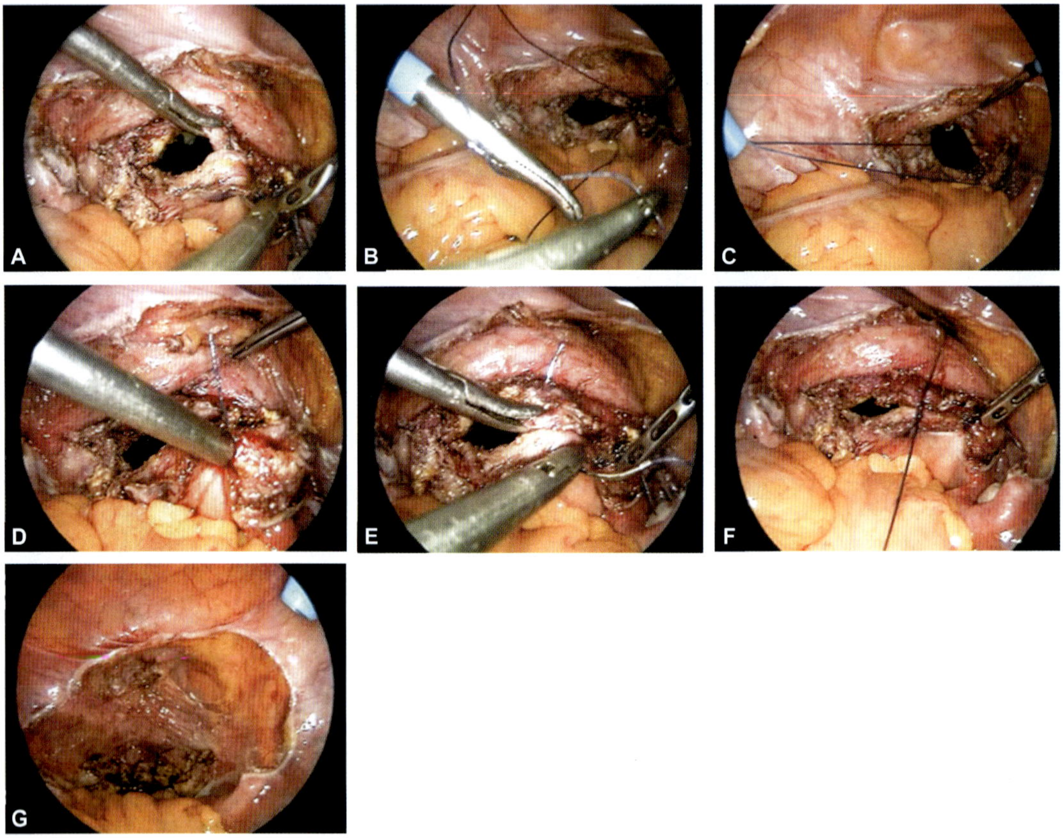

Figs 10.10A to G: Vaginal vault sutured with interrupted stitches

Then the vaginal vault is closed by interrupted sutures laparoscopically or vaginally **(Figs 10.10A to G)**.

Foley's catheter is removed in 24 hours. Patient can be discharged within 24-36 hours and moderate rest is advised for a week. She can resume work within 10 days. Sexual relations should be avoided for 6–8 weeks.

DEBULKING OF UTERUS

In case of bulky uterus with multiple fibroids, uterus can be removed vaginally by debulking. This may be done after cauterizing all three pedicles of the uterus on both sides and cutting the vagina circumferentially and then bisecting the uterus and enucleating the fibroid vaginally **(Figs 10.11A to F)**. Alternatively, myomectomy may be done laparoscopically thereby debulking the uterus **(Figs 10.12A to K)**. Following the hysterectomy is done by the standard laparoscopic technique and uterus is delivered through the vagina along with the enucleated fibroid.[7,8]

Irrespective of the size of the uterus the recovery duration is the same.

The Key Areas for Effective TLH

1. Specially designed uterine manipulator to antevert or retrovert, with side movements, a bulging colpotomizer with prevention of gas leak or a myoma screw as the sole manipulator, blocking vagina with gauze to prevent gas leak.
2. 30° 10 mm telescope gives better visualization of lateral dissection, uterine arteries and anterior or posterior colpotomy.
3. Standardize a bipolar, scissors and endosuturing **(Fig. 10.13A)** or harmonic and a bipolar or 5 mm good vessel sealing device like Enseal, 5 mm gyrus transector **(Fig. 10.13B)** or 5 mm Atlas of Valley labs or Robi grasper and Martin Maxim.
4. Assistant and nurses have their destined role. Main responsibility of the 1st assistant is to hold the camera and instrument on his/her side, one OT expert nurse to give instruments and a standby on right side of the surgeon to hold camera to relive the 1st assistant.
5. Each machine has a standardized setting for hysterectomy viz. Bipolar 30 watts, harmonic at 2 and 5 marks, monopolar if used-100 watts cutting, coagulation 60 watts, rest vessel sealers are automatically set on plugging in the machine.

Special Situations and Difficulties

- Case of previous cesarean section.
- Infraumbilical scar of any surgery.
- Uterus more than 20 weeks size.

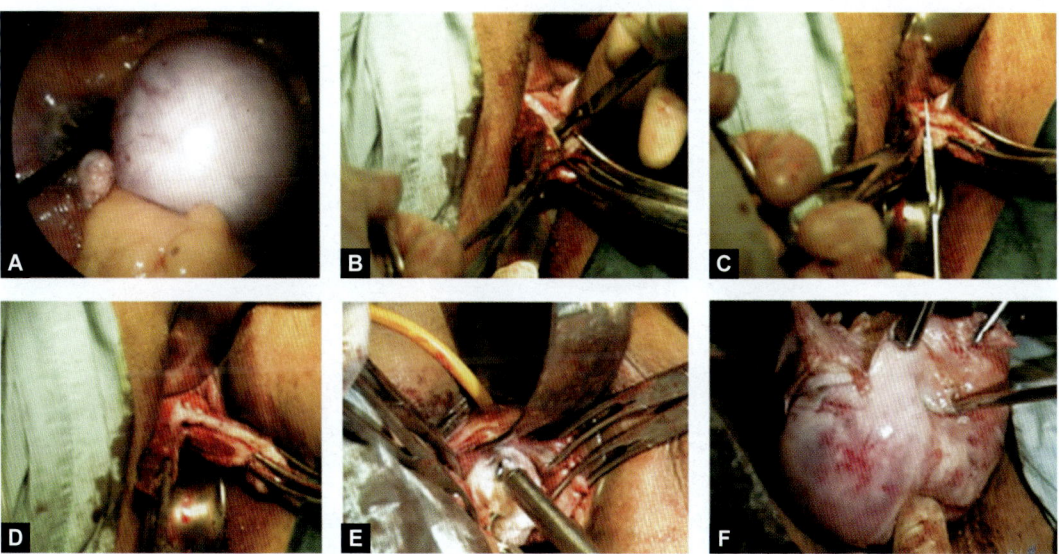

Figs 10.11A to F: Debulking uterus vaginally by enucleating fibroid

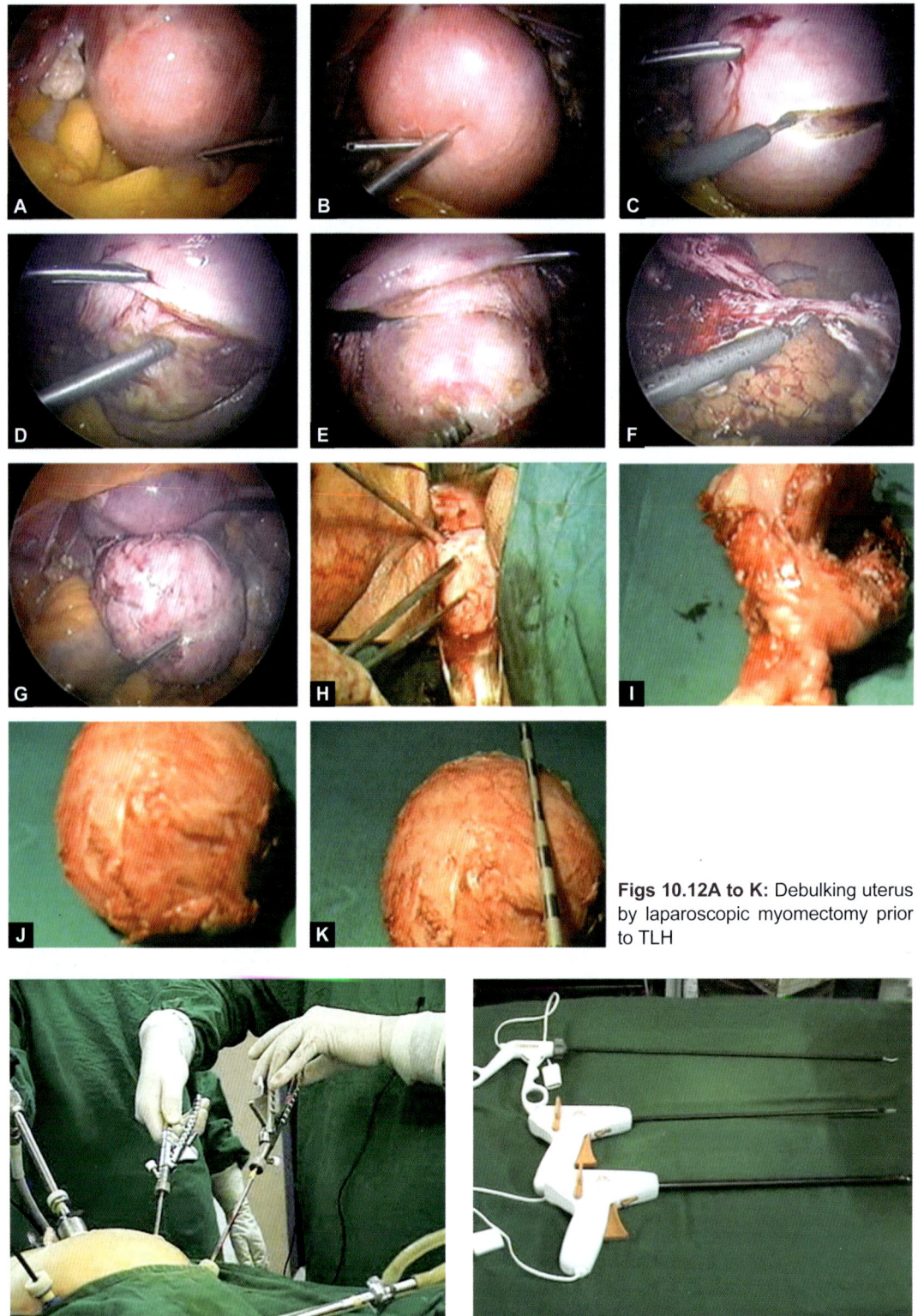

Figs 10.12A to K: Debulking uterus by laparoscopic myomectomy prior to TLH

Fig. 10.13A: Endosuturing

Fig. 10.13B: 5 mm Gyrus

How to Make Total Laparoscopic Hysterectomy Safe?

- Very obese patient
- Supracervical hysterectomy.

1. **Case of previous cesarean section**
   In this case care is taken to insert verres and trocar avoiding bowel injury. Occasionally, primary trocar is 2 inches above the upper limit of umbilical scar with nasogastric tube to deflate stomach. Palmer's point below the rib cage can be used with a long verres needle for insufflation and also to pass needle scope to see presence or absence of adhesion **(Figs 10.14A to D)**. The adhesion with the abdominal wall is dealt with harmonic ace or scissors and bipolar on the same side. Special care is taken for dissection of the uterovesical peritoneum from the lateral aspect giving a window access to the plane to push bladder with blunt dissection or best with harmonic scalpel **(Figs 10.14E to G)**. Rarely in bad case, supracervical hysterectomy is also acceptable (given ahead).

2. In infraumbilical scars due to other surgeries. In this case the management is similar to that of previous cesarean except that bladder may not be adherent and bowel can be dangerously close.

3. Very obese patient. In this case the management is same, except veress and trocars are

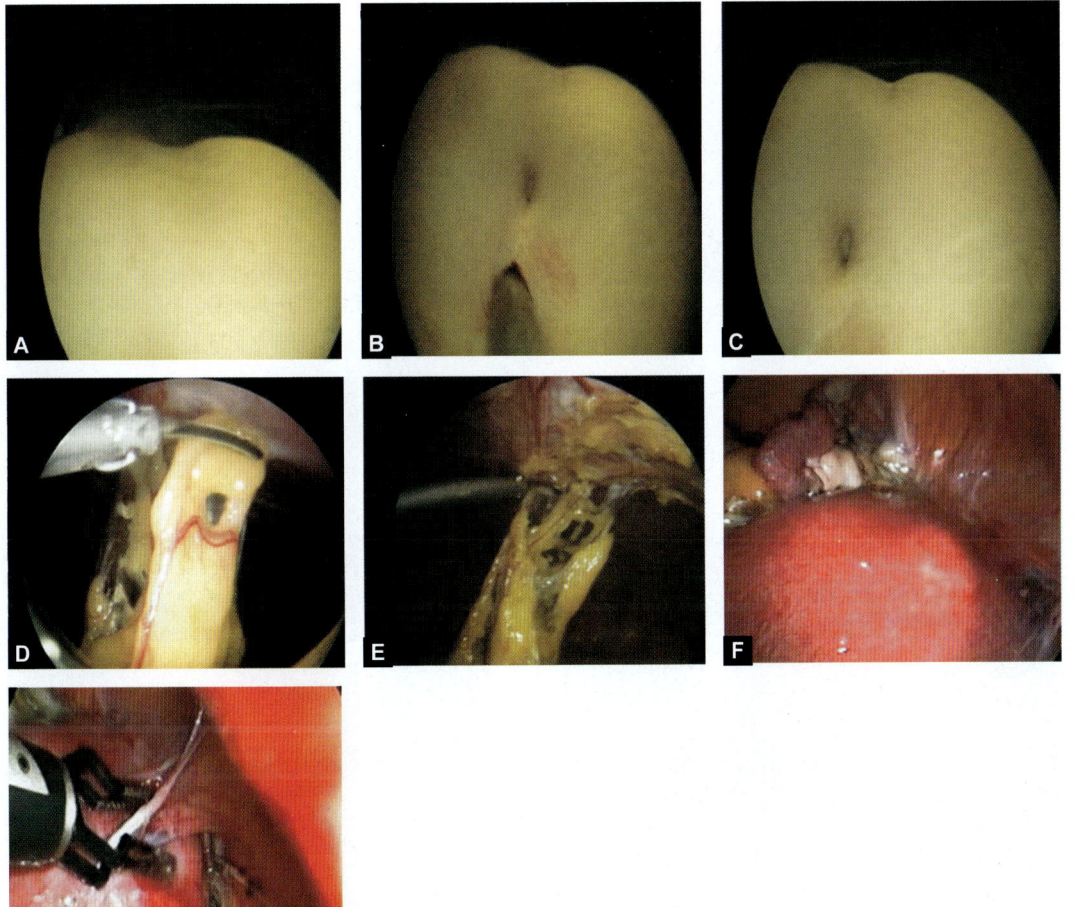

Figs 10.14A to G: Previous 2 LSCS with adhesions; (A and B) Scar of previous surgery, (C) Dip in skin due to scar of previous surgery, (D and E) Dissection of abdominal wall adhesions (cauterized with harmonic), (F) Bladder adhesions (G) Dissection with Gyrus, (F and G) Adherent bladder being dissected

long. Once inside the peritoneal cavity, it is like any other hysterectomy **(Fig. 10.15)**.

4. i. **Uterine size of more than 20 weeks**

The veress and ports are at least 3 inches above the upper most part of the uterus. 10 mm myoma screw and a vessel sealing device can be used through the supraumbilical midline port and a 30° telescope and vessel sealing instrument can be used through the right side 10 mm port, e.g. right sided dissection is done from the right sided ports, but for left sided dissection, 30° telescope is inserted through the right 10 mm port and vessel sealing device is inserted through the supraumbilical port with uterus pulled towards right side.

ii. **Bulky uterus with endometriosis**

In case of endometriosis found in association with bulky uterus, there are likely to be adhesions around the uterus **(Figs 10.16A and B)**. These adhesions require meticulous adhesiolysis and carry the risk of bowel injury, especially sigmoid colon and rectum in posterior wall adhesions. Such cases require expertise in dissection. Harmonic is commonly used for the dissection **(Figs 10.16C to F)**. Adequate head low and good bowel preparation preoperatively is mandatory. Also, postoperatively, adequate monitoring of abdominal girth and starting oral intake after confirming peristalsis is a must.

A risk of selecting a right vessel sealer or bipolar, scissors or harmonic ace is made depending on case-to-case variation.

Big specimens are removed by morcellator to avoid lacerations in the vagina **(Figs 10.17A and B)**. Further idea of lateral spread

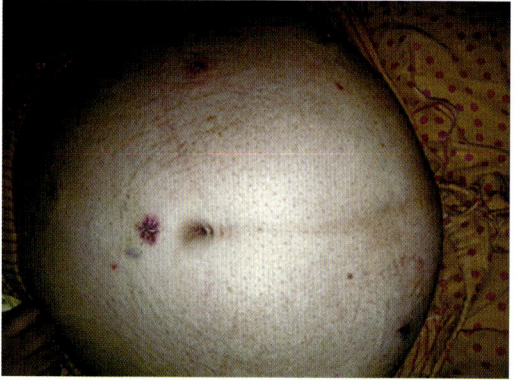

Fig. 10.15: TLH in an obese patient

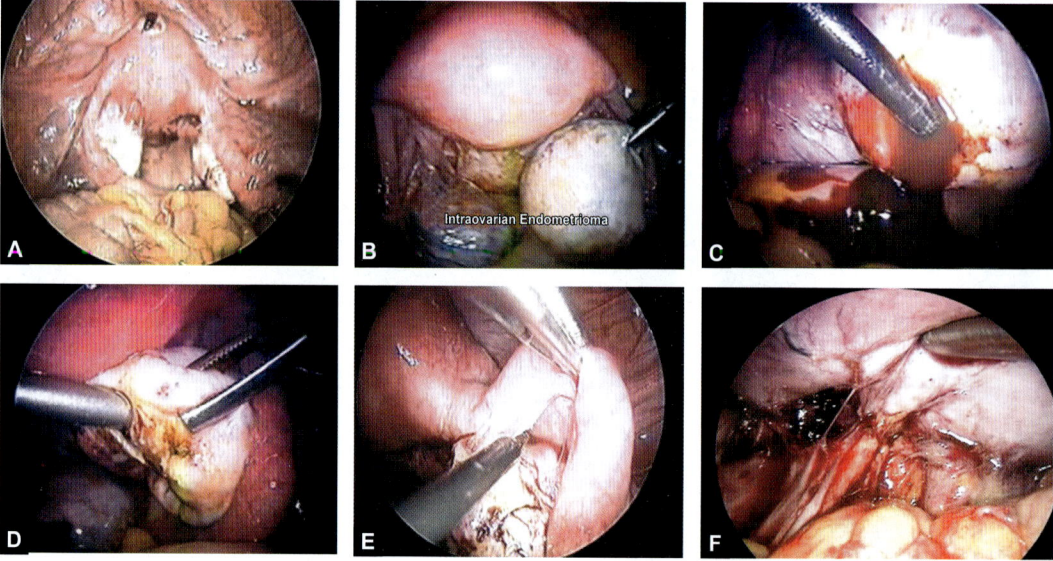

Figs 10.16A to F: Endometriosis ~ Endometriomas; (A and B) Endometriomas with adhesions, (C and D) Endometriotic cyst punctured, chocolate colored fluid drained, (E) Adhesiolysis to separate cyst from surrounding structures, (F) Posterior wall adhesions

How to Make Total Laparoscopic Hysterectomy Safe?

of any energy source is clear to avoid ureteric or bladder injury.

5. **Supracervical hysterectomy**

In cases of previous two or three LSCS, adhesions may be encountered, like adherent bladder anteriorly, adherent rectum posteriorly, omental adhesions, etc. In order to avoid deliberate injury to the bladder or rectum, one can opt for supracervical hysterectomy after confirming a normal pap smear. The body of the uterus is removed and cervix is retained thereby bypassing dissection involving the bladder and rectum **(Figs 10.18A and B)**. The cervical stump is closed with simple interrupted stitches **(Figs 10.18C and D)**. The uterus is then removed by morcellation **(Fig. 10.18E)**

Our experience of laparoscopic hysterectomy over 17 years – count of 25000 cases of laparoscopic surgery are:

Types of Hysterectomy	Cases
1. LAVH (earlier phase)	586
2. LH (with bipolar and scissor dissection, endosuturing)	729
3. TLH (with vessel sealing device and harmonic scalpel)	1026

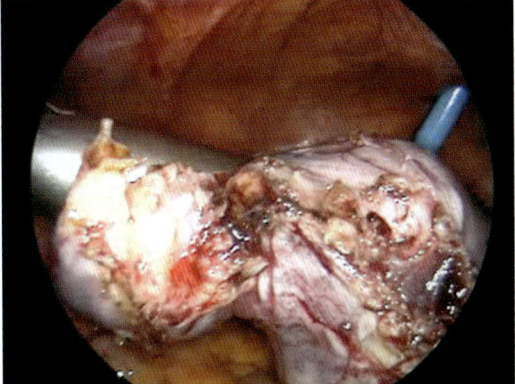

Fig. 10.17A: Uterus removed by morcellation

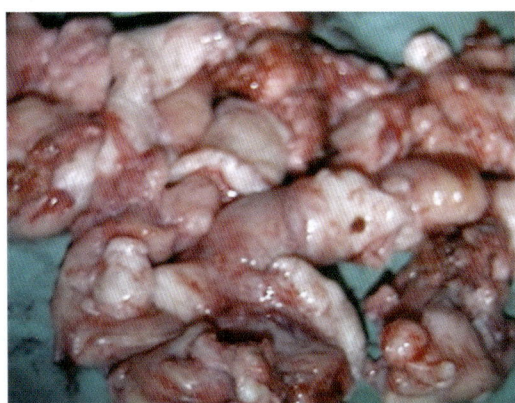

Fig. 10.17B: Morcellated pieces of uterus

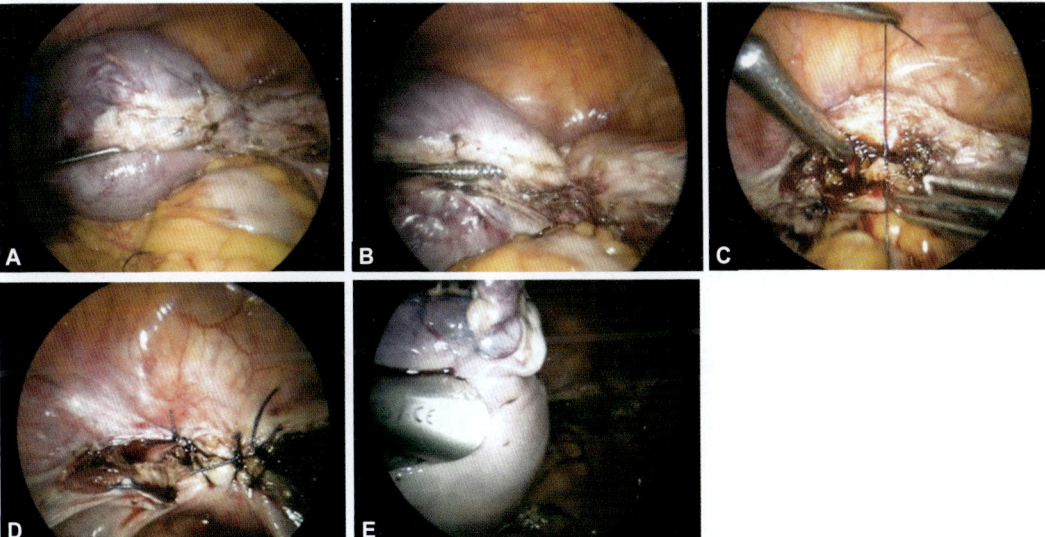

Figs 10.18A to E: Steps of supracervical hysterectomy; (A and B) Dissection till the level of the cervix, (C and D) cervical stump being sutured, (E) Uterus removed by morcellation

4. LASH- Supracervical Hysterectomy 18
   - Total no. of cases 2359
   - Conversion to open- 28
   - Bladder injury. 9
   - Bowel injury. 1
   - Ureteric injury. 5
   - Mortality. 1

Total laparoscopic hysterectomy from a consumer driven advance has established its place in modern Gynecology with excellent benefits in the hand of expert to avoid open abdominal surgery. Complications in learning phase are to be avoided as an excuse till you achieve mastery.

The new single port hysterectomy or single incision multiple port hysterectomy is in the phase of trial with iatrogenic difficulties to be mastered over a period of time.

Complications of TLH are covered in Chapter Complications of Laparoscopic Surgery.

The uterine vessels are very important and many endoscopist first deal with uterine vessel by creating a window in the broad ligament peritoneum after dissection and pushing the bladder peritoneum. The uterine vessels are sutured or coagulated or sealed on both sides with medial coagulation to avoid back flow. This technique may occasionally invite bleeding and ureteric injury. A better approach can be directly the anterior division of internal iliac artery after it gives out its first branch. This can be done by Qadar's technique between round ligament and infundibulo pelvic ligament following the uterine branch by pulling the obliterated umbilical ligament which is in continuity with the vessel. After skeletonizing one can suture, coagulate or seal the anterior division of internal iliac artery or uterine artery.

REFERENCES

1. Garry R, Reich H, Liu CY. Laparoscopic hysterectomy. Definition and indications. *Gynecol Endosc* 1994:1-3.
2. Koh C. A new technique of simplifying a total laparoscopic hysterectomy. *J Am Assoc Gynecol Lapros* 1998:5(2)186-7.
3. McCarus S. Physiologic mechanism of ultrasonically activated scalpel. *J Am Assoc Gynecol Loprosc* 1996:3(4):601-9.
4. Winter M, Mendelsohn S. TLH using the harmonic scalpel. J Soc Lapros Surg. 1999;3(3):185-6.
5. Kohler C, Hasenbein K, Klemm P, et al. LAVH with lateral transection of uterine vessels: *Surg Endos* 2003 Mar; 17(3):485-90.
6. Kovac SR, Curikshank SH, Retto HF. LAVH. J Gynceol Surg 1990; 6:185.
7. O'Shea RT, Cook JR , Seman EI. Total Laparoscopic Hysterectomy: A new option for removal of large myomatous uterus: *Aust NZ J Obstat Gynecol* 2002 Aug; 42 (3) :282-4
8. Wattiez A, Soriano D et al. TLH for very enlarge uteri : *J Am Assoc Gynecol Loprosc* 2002 May;9(2):125-30.

CHAPTER 11

Safe Laparoscopic Surgery for Prolapse in Young Patient and Vault Prolapse

Pravin Patel

Chapter Outline

- Preoperative Preparations
- Surgical Technique
  - Basic Surgical Techniques
- Anterior
- Uterine Prolapse
- Sacrocervicopexy
- Vaginal Vault Prolapse
- Sacrocolpopexy
- Enterocele
  - Rectocele (Posterior Vaginal Wall Repair)
  - Levator Ani Muscle Plication Repair
  - Robotic Sacrocolpopexy
- Complications

Pelvic organ prolapse is an increasingly common condition seen in women. Variety of treatment options are available depending on the degree and type of prolapse in conjugation with other circumstances of patient including age, parity and previous treatments taken.

Surgical reconstruction of pelvic organ prolapse may be performed by a variety of techniques.[1] One of the preferred options is vaginal approach because of its advantages in terms of reduced length of hospitalization and postoperative pain, as well as a faster return to normal activities and a better cosmetic result. However, some data suggest that anatomic outcomes are less than optimal.

Initially by laparoscopic reconstruction proven abdominal techniques were reproduced, but in a minimally invasive fashion. As more information was gained about the pathogenesis of prolapse, and as device innovations are introduced that improved surgical techniques have emerged.

Compared with open abdominal surgery, laparoscopic surgery[1,2] is associated with a number of advantages, including:

- Shorter hospital stay
- Decreased postoperative pain
- Smaller scars
- Potentially reduced time before resumption of work and other normal activities.

Technical advances include rapid carbon dioxide insufflators, three-chip and high definition cameras that improve picture clarity, ultra-bright light sources, safer energy sources, and changes in laparoscopic needle drivers and automated suturing devices.

PREOPERATIVE PREPARATIONS

Careful preoperative assessment should include anatomic and functional aspects of the pelvic floor. Establishing and understanding individual patient's prolapsed defect to achieve an optimal anatomic outcome.

Urinary incontinence is an area of concern as it can develop *de novo* or worsen following prolapse repair. The urethra may be anatomically kinked in patients with huge prolapse. Following prolapse repair, insufficient urethral sphincter function may result in new onset stress urinary incontinence.

Patients may not volunteer so to perform a preoperative cough stress test with a full bladder after manual reduction of any is recommended to decide whether to proceed with complex urodynamic testing of urethral function.

SURGICAL TECHNIQUE

Factors that should be considered include the overall health of the patient (including her ability to undergo general anesthesia and abdominal insufflation), body habitus, and previous approaches to prolapse surgery, such as retropubic procedures.

Informed consent should include the possibility of having to change the surgical approach intraoperatively to an open laparotomy in the event that adhesions or other factors. A mechanical bowel preparation often improves laparoscopic visualization by decompressing the bowel.

In absence of any previous surgery umbilical placement of 0° telescope is preferred. In a previous vertical abdominal incision consider either an open laparoscopic approach, or an alternative location for Veress needle and initial trocar placement, such as the left upper quadrant in the ninth intercostal space **(Fig. 11.1)**. The operating field is then carefully organized by fixing the sigmoid to the abdominal wall and clearing the pouch of Douglas.

Basic Surgical Techniques

The surgeon should be well verse and properly trained for extensive suturing and should use enough accessory trocars to allow for both retraction of tissues and transfer of needles from one needle driver or grasper to another.

Surgery can be divided into the anterior, posterior, or apical vaginal compartments correction. Several procedures are usually required for any individual case since multiple defects in the pelvic floor often occur, resulting in symptomatic and clinically evident prolapse of more than one organ.

ANTERIOR

The most common defect leading to cystocele or anterior vaginal wall prolapse is secondary to primary apical descent.

Paravaginal repair of cystocele may be performed after gaining access to the space of Retzius, or retropubic space. Most commonly, transperitoneal laparoscopy is performed and the retropubic space is entered using sharp dissection with electrocautery. Backfilling the bladder with 200 to 300 mL of stained fluid may be helpful in selected cases.[3]

After dissection, Cooper's ligaments are identified **(Fig. 11.2)**. Paravaginal repair involves placing a series of interrupted permanent sutures between the arcus tendineus fascia pelvis and the detached pubocervical fascia, starting near the ischial spine and working distally towards the pubic bone.

If a laparoscopic Burch procedure is performed for stress incontinence, the final paravaginal sutures are placed at the bladder neck, whereas if no Burch procedure is performed, the paravaginal repair is continued up to the insertion of the ATFP on the posterior-inferior surface of the pubis.[4-6]

There are no studies documenting equivalence of open abdominal versus laparoscopic paravaginal repair.

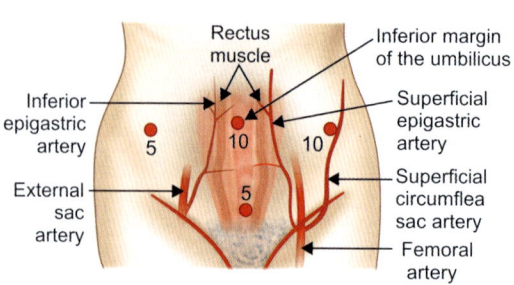

Fig. 11.1: Trocar placement

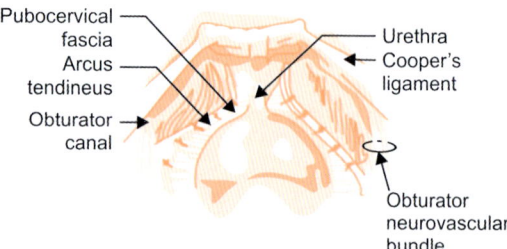

Fig. 11.2: Anterior compartment

UTERINE PROLAPSE

Uterine suspension should be considered as an option for women who either are considering future childbearing or who would prefer to avoid hysterectomy for other reasons.

Uterosacral ligament uterine suspension (Fig. 11): Mild to moderate degrees of uterine prolapse may be approached with uterosacral ligament uterine suspension.[7] Although techniques such as round ligament suspension were used, their long term beneficial effects and efficacy are doubtful. Uncontrolled case series have suggested the procedure may improve uterine prolapse. Further studies are necessary to confirm these reports.

The proximal portion of the uterosacral ligament, at the level of the ischial spine is identified and use permanent sutures to bind distal aspect of the ligament, near its insertion into the lower uterine segment and cervix **(Fig. 11.3)**.

The use of a uterine manipulator may assist with identification of the uterosacral ligaments. While working on uterosacrals, identification and proper retraction of pelvic ureters is mandatory to avoid complications.

SACROCERVICOPEXY (FIG. 11.4)

It is an alternative procedure for uterine suspension that involves suturing the posterior vagina and cervix to the sacrum using an intervening graft, which may be either synthetic (e.g. polypropylene, polyester) or biologic (e.g. fascia, dermis).[8] This procedure may be appropriate for specific patient populations including young women with Stages III or IV uterovaginal prolapse.

To perform this procedure with uterine conservation, the peritoneum and rectum are dissected off of the posterior vaginal wall, followed by placement of a series of sutures in the rectovaginal fascia, distal uterosacral ligaments, and cervix. A solid plastic rectal probe may help identify and avoid injury to the rectum during dissection in the rectovaginal space.

The presacral space, the peritoneum is opened over the sacral promontory and dissection is carried down until the anterior longitudinal ligament of the sacrum is exposed. The peritoneal incision is continued inferiorly, medial to the right uterosacral ligament and lateral to the rectum, until it meets the peritoneal incision over the posterior vaginal wall. The graft is then sutured, without tension, to the sacrum with several permanent sutures and buried underneath the peritoneum alternatively, some titanium coils or stainless steel tacks for affixing the graft to the sacrum can be used **(Figs 11.5A to H)**.

Many surgeons prefer to dissect para rectal space till the levator plate is exposed and performing addition fixing of distal end of mesh with levator ani to complete three point fixations.

VAGINAL VAULT PROLAPSE

Vaginal vault prolapse may occur after any hysterectomy **(Fig. 11.6)**, although it appears to

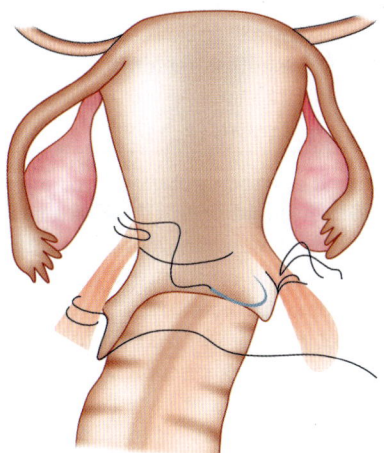

Fig. 11.3: Uterosacral ligament suspension

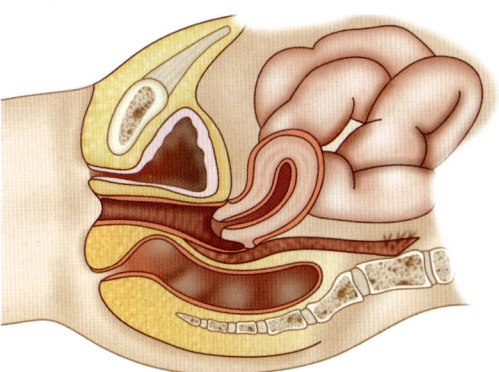

Fig. 11.4: Sacrocervicopexy

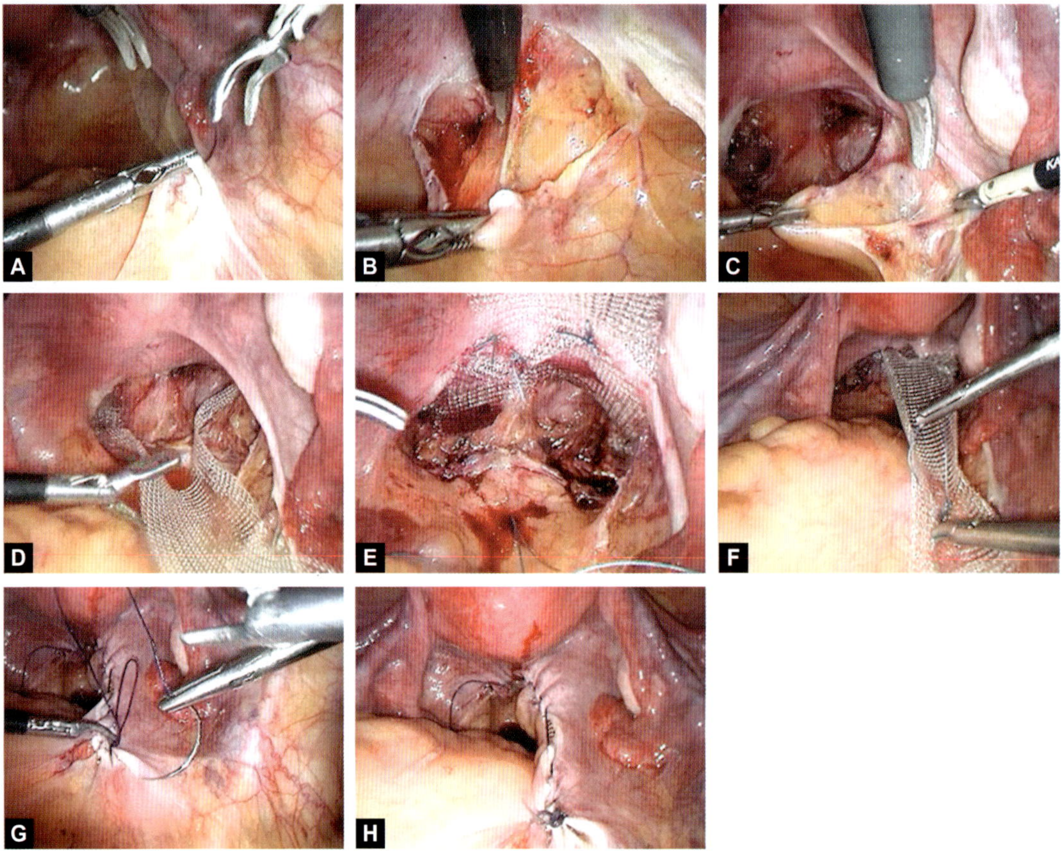

Figs 11.5A to H: Laparoscopic sacrocervicopexy; (A) Presacral space dissection, (B) Promontory, (C) Lateral peritoneal dissection, (D) Mesh placement, (E) Cervicoisthmic mesh fixation, (F) Promonto fixation, (G) Peritonization

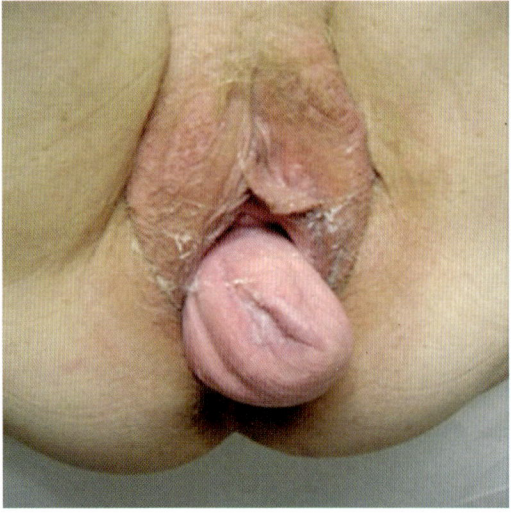

Fig. 11.6: Vault prolapse

occur more frequently in women whose hysterectomy was performed for prolapse, perhaps because the vaginal apex is insufficiently suspended following hysterectomy.

SACROCOLPOPEXY (FIG. 11.7)

Laparoscopic sacrocolpopexy[9-11] is an option when POP-Q stages II to IV vault prolapse is present. In these patients, it is often difficult to identify any useful remnants of the uterosacral ligaments for suspension.

In small nonrandomized studies, objective cure rates for the laparoscopic approach procedure of 93 to 100 percent have been reported at six months to five years follow-up. To perform laparoscopic sacrocolpopexy, after the bladder and rectum are dissected off the anterior and posterior vaginal walls, respectively, a Y-shaped synthetic graft is sutured to the anterior and posterior endopelvic fascia with a series of permanent sutures.[12-15] The graft is fixed to the anterior longitudinal ligament of the sacral promontory, after dissection is performed in the presacral space (as described for sacrocervicopexy). The procedure is typically completed by burying the graft under the peritoneum.

The goal of this laparoscopic procedure, is to duplicate the steps performed in the open procedure, as closely as possible, so that the results reported with the traditional surgery may be reproduced with minimally-invasive techniques. A retrospective chart review compared the outcome of laparoscopic versus abdominal sacrocolpopexy.[16-19] Surgical time was significantly increased in the laparoscopic group, blood loss was decreased. Rates of perioperative complications and subsequent procedures for pelvic floor defects were similar between the two approaches.

ENTEROCELE (FIG. 11.8)

Enterocele refers to herniation of bowel and the lining of the peritoneal cavity through the cul-de-sac of Douglas, without an intervening fascial layer.[20-22]

This most often occurs at the vaginal apex after hysterectomy, due to either a failure to properly reapproximate the anterior and posterior endopelvic fascia or breakdown of this repair.

Standard sacrocolpopexy technique does not require additional enterocele repair.[22] Some authors recommend resection of the enterocele sac (redundant vaginal epithelium) whereas others simply plicate fascia over the redundant tissue.

Rectocele (Posterior Vaginal Wall Repair)

Due to the ease of access via the vaginal route, there is no role for laparoscopic rectocele repair.

Levator Ani Muscle Plication Repair

Due to the risk of postoperative dyspareunia, it is not recommended as part of a laparoscopic reconstruction.

Robotic Sacrocolpopexy

The introduction of robotic surgery[23,24] to gynecologists has fueled a renewed interest in minimally invasive sacrocolpopexy and other procedures for prolapse that require endoscopic suturing. A number of small series have been published that appear to demonstrate the feasibility and short-term success rate of this approach to sacrocolpopexy.

COMPLICATIONS

Vascular and bowel injuries are the most common complications encountered during access in any laparoscopic procedure.

- *Urinary tract injury:* Injury to the bladder and ureters occurs more frequently in laparoscopic reconstruction procedures than in general gynecologic laparoscopy. Due to these risks, intraoperative cystoscopy can be considered as a part of these procedures.
- *Urinary retention:* Although more commonly associated with suburethral sling procedures, any anti-incontinence[25] surgery

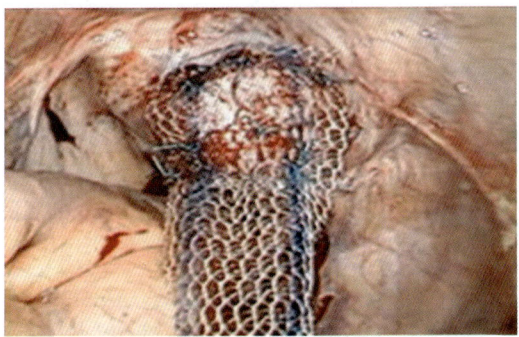

Fig. 11.7: Sacrocolpopexy

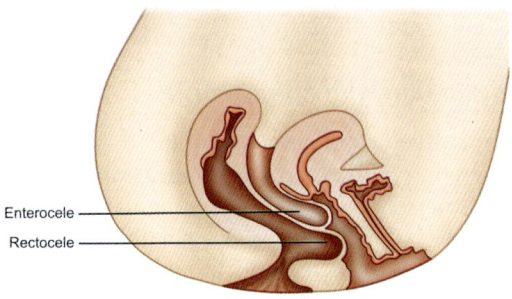

Fig. 11.8: Enterocele

(including Burch colposuspension) or vault suspension procedure may result in voiding dysfunction and/or urinary retention.[26] Continuous bladder drainage or intermittent self catheterization may be used as a part of treatment.
Prophylactic oral antibiotics, are given to reduce the risk of lower urinary tract infections.

- *Mesh Infection, mesh erosion:* Erosion of graft material or suture material, which may be caused by graft or suture infection usually secondary to vaginal wall penetration, performing the procedure adjacent to a vaginal incision, or securing the graft to an attenuated avascular wall with inadequate fibromuscular tissue.
Risks such as mesh infection or rejection are very rare with the newer mesh used, which is a macroporous soft polypropylene mesh.

Other common causes for mesh infection include:

- Intraoperative hemorrhage (especially in the presacral space)
- Postoperative ileus
- Wound complications, such as seromas and infections
- Early resumption of intercourse with vaginal wall penetration of sutures during repair.

Postoperative care: Patients undergoing laparoscopic pelvic floor reconstruction are usually discharged on the same day or the day after surgery.[27,28] A prescription for oral analgesics (e.g. ibuprofen or oxycodone) is given and stool softeners are recommended until normal bowel habits resume. Heavy lifting for eight weeks and intercourse for six weeks postoperatively should be avoided.

SUMMARY AND CONCLUSION

Laparoscopic promontofixation[29] is a feasible operation with a good anatomical success rate for young patients with utero-vaginal prolapse. This technique is applicable for the treatment of pelvic floor defects, including all the stages of prolapse. It would be desirable to improve the results concerning urinary incontinence by treatment with TVT-O, which could be systematic in women presenting considerable stress urinary incontinence preoperatively, while the use of the Burch procedure could correspond more to the repair of lateral cystocele, associated with paravaginal repair. Right use of patient selection, technique, material and equipment is essential for optimal outcome.

REFERENCES

1. Benson JT, Lucente V, McClellan E. Vaginal versus abdominal reconstructive surgery for the treatment of pelvic support defects: a prospective randomized study with long-term outcome evaluation. Am J Obstet Gynecol 1996;175:1418.
2. Maher C, Baessler K, Glazener CM, et al. Surgical management of pelvic organ prolapse in women. Cochrane Database Syst Rev 2004;CD004014.
3. Pulliam S, Chelmow D, Weld A, Rosenblatt P. Laparoscopic Paravaginal Repair: A Case Series 2005.
4. Kohli N, Jacobs PA, Sze EH, et al. Open compared with laparoscopic approach to Burch colposuspension: a cost analysis. Obstet Gynecol 1997;90:411.
5. Miklos JR, Kohli N. Laparoscopic paravaginal repair plus burch colposuspension: review and descriptive technique. Urology 2000;56:4.
6. Ferland RD, Rosenblatt P. Ureteral compromise after laparoscopic Burch colpopexy. J Am Assoc Gynecol Laparosc 1999;6:217.
7. Wattiez A, Goldchmit R, Canis M, Mage G, Pouly JL, Bruhat MA Laparoscopic treatment of uterine prolapse. In Tulandi T, Editor. Atlas of Laparoscopic and Hysteroscopic Techniques for Gynecologists, 2nd edition. London WB Saunders, 1999;153-8.
8. Rosenblatt PL, Chelmow D, Ferzandi TR. Laparoscopic sacrocervicopexy for the treatment of uterine prolapse: a retrospective case series report. J Minim Invasive Gynecol 2008;15:268.
9. Lo, TS, Wang, AC. Abdominal colposacropexy and sacrospinous ligament suspension for severe uterovaginal prolapse: a comparison. J Gynecol Surg 1998;14:59.
10. Nezhat CH, Nezhat F, Nezhat C. Laparoscopic sacral colpopexy for vaginal vault prolapse. Obstet Gynecol 1994;84:885.
11. Agarwala N, Hasiak N, Shade M. Laparoscopic sacral colpopexy with Gynemesh as graft material–experience and results. J Minim Invasive Gynecol 2007;14:577.

12. Higgs PJ, Chua HL, Smith AR. Long term review of laparoscopic sacrocolpopexy. BJOG 2005;112:1134.
13. Ross JW, Preston M. Laparoscopic sacrocolpopexy for severe vaginal vault prolapse: five-year outcome. J Minim Invasive Gynecol 2005; 12:221.
14. Paraiso MF, Walters MD, Rackley RR, et al. Laparoscopic and abdominal sacral colpopexies: a comparative cohort study. Am J Obstet Gynecol 2005;192:1752.
15. Yen CF, Wang CJ, Lin SL, et al. Combined laparoscopic uterosacral and round ligament procedures for treatment of symptomatic uterine retroversion and mild uterine decensus. J Am Assoc Gynecol Laparosc 2002;9:359.
16. Ross JW. Apical vault repair, the cornerstone or pelvic vault reconstruction. Int Urogynecol J Pelvic Floor Dysfunct 1997;8:146.
17. O'Brien PM, Ibrahim J. Failure of laparoscopic uterine suspension to provide a lasting cure for uterovaginal prolapse. Br J Obstet Gynaecol 1994;101:707.
18. Lin LL, Phelps JY, Liu CY. Laparoscopic vaginal vault suspension using uterosacral ligaments: a review of 133 cases. J Minim Invasive Gynecol 2005;12:216.
19. Schwartz M, Abbott KR, Glazerman L, et al. Positive symptom improvement with laparoscopic uterosacral ligament repair for uterine or vaginal vault prolapse: interim results from an active multicenter trial. J Minim Invasive Gynecol 2007; 14:570.
20. Miklos JR, Kohli N, Lucente V, Saye WB. Site-specific fascial defects in the diagnosis and surgical management of enterocele. Am J Obstet Gynecol 1998;179:1418.
21. Richardson, AC. The anatomic defects in rectocele and enterocele. J Pelv Surg 1995;1:214.
22. Paraiso MF, Falcone T, Walters MD. Laparoscopic surgery for enterocele, vaginal apex prolapse and rectocele. Int Urogynecol J Pelvic Floor Dysfunct 1999;10:223.
23. Daneshgari F, Kefer JC, Moore C, Kaouk J. Robotic abdominal sacrocolpopexy/sacrouteropexy repair of advanced female pelvic organ prolaspe (POP): utilizing POP-quantification-based staging and outcomes. BJU Int 2007;100:875.
24. Akl MN, Long JB, Giles DL, et al. Robotic-assisted sacrocolpopexy: technique and learning curve. Surg Endosc 2009;23:2390.
25. Nguyen JK. Diagnosis and treatment of voiding dysfunction caused by urethral obstruction after anti-incontinence surgery. Obstet Gynecol Surv 2002;57:468.
26. Kjerulff KH, Langenberg PW, Greenaway L, et al. Urinary incontinence and hysterectomy in a large prospective cohort study in American women. J Urol 2002;167:2088.
27. Gerten KA, Richter HE, Wheeler TL 2nd, et al. Intraabdominal pressure changes associated with lifting: implications for postoperative activity restrictions. Am J Obstet Gynecol 2008; 198:306.e1.
28. Weir LF, Nygaard IE, Wilken J, et al. Postoperative activity restrictions: any evidence? Obstet Gynecol 2006;107:305.
29. Wattiez A, Canis M, Mage G, Pouly JL, Bruhat MA Promontofixation for the treatment of prolapse. Urol Clin Nort Am 2001;28:151-7.

CHAPTER 12

Laparoscopic Adenomyomectomy

Sanjay Patel

Chapter Outline

- Transvaginal Ultrasonography
- Adenoma on Laparoscopy
- Adenoma on Hysteroscopy
- Coexisting Pathologies
- Preoperative Adenoma Mapping
- Aim of Adenoma Resection
- Technique of Adenomyoma Resection
- Technique of Endosuturing: Intracorporeal Slip Knot Technique

Definition: The heterotypic presence of the functioning endometrial glands and stroma within the myometrium at least 2.5 mm deeper to the basal layer is termed as Adenomyosis.[1]

It is common in patients with previous history of MTP, dilatation and curettage or any previous surgery on the uterus.

Classification: As per its morphological occurrence (1) Localized adenomyoma (2) Diffused Adenomyosis **Figs 12.1A and B**.

TRANSVAGINAL ULTRASONOGRAPHY

Adenoma is usually diagnosed on ultrasound. It appears as uncapsulated, heterogeneous, anechoic areas. All these changes will be more pronounced if seen during menstruation[2,3] **(Figs 12.2 and 12.3)**.

On color Doppler it may appear as diffuse, increased overall vascularity (PI >1.18 cm/s) **(Figs 12.4A and B)**.

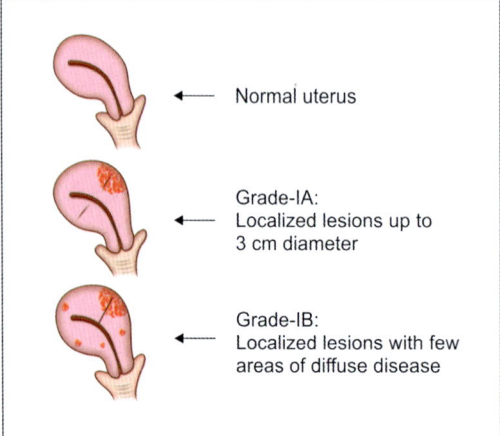

Fig. 12.1A: Classification of adenomyosis

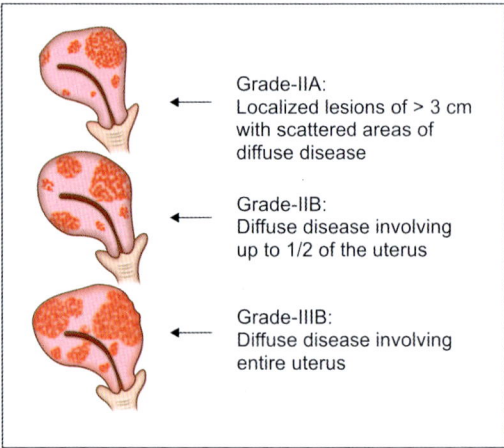

Fig. 12.1B: Classification of adenomyosis

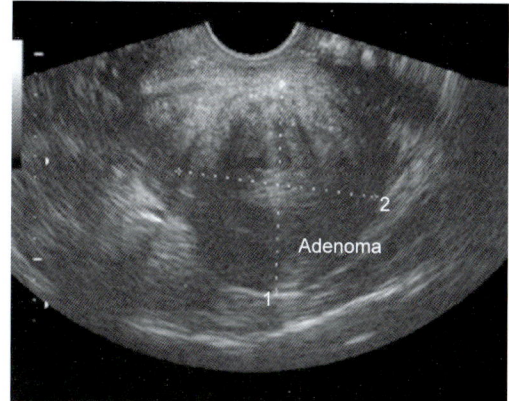

Fig. 12.2: USG findings of adenomyoma

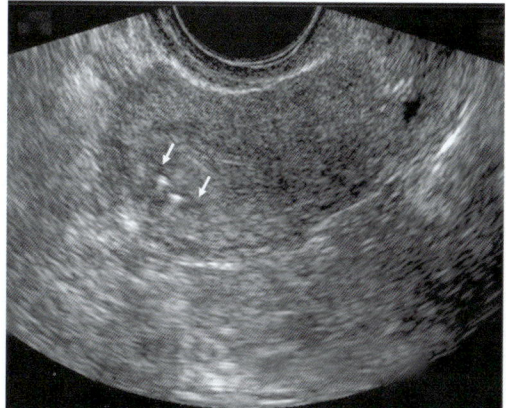

Fig. 12.3: Subendometrial adenoma on USG

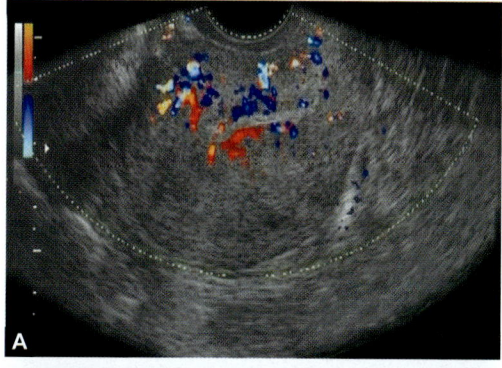

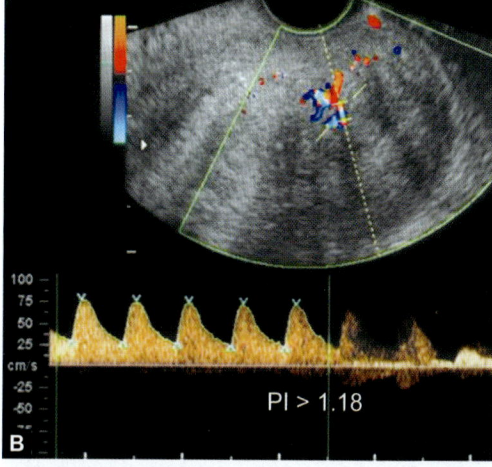

Figs 12.4A and B: Color Doppler showing vascular changes in adenomyoma

ADENOMA ON LAPAROSCOPY

Adenoma may be misdiagnosed as fibroid on ultrasound. If during surgery, one finds difficult to find the plane of cleavage then it is more likely to be adenoma[4] **(Fig. 12.5)**.

There may be chocolate colored fluid collection in the myometrium (intramyometrial cyst) **(Fig. 12.6)**.

ADENOMA ON HYSTEROSCOPY

Hysteroscopy shows increased endometrial vascularity[5] **(Fig. 12.7)**.

Subendometrial adenoma on hysteroscopy **(Fig. 12.8)**.

Endometrial puckering (looking like adhesions) due to adenomyosis **(Fig. 12.9)**.

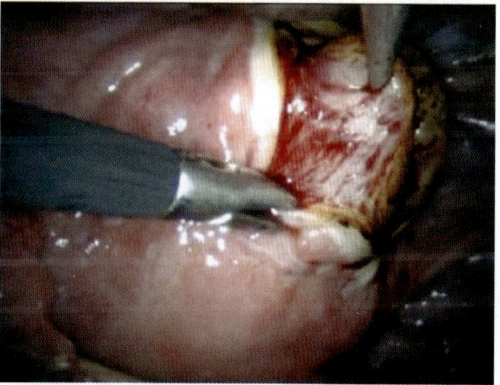

Fig. 12.5: Adenoma seen on laparoscopy

COEXISTING PATHOLOGIES

Adenomyosis/adenoma may coexist with endometriosis, fibroid **(Figs 12.10A and B)**,

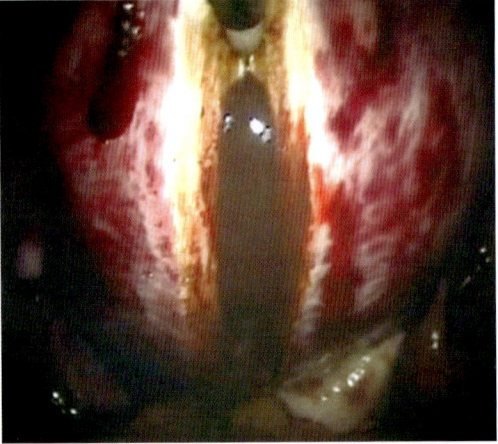

Fig. 12.6: Intramyometrial cyst containing chocolate color fluid

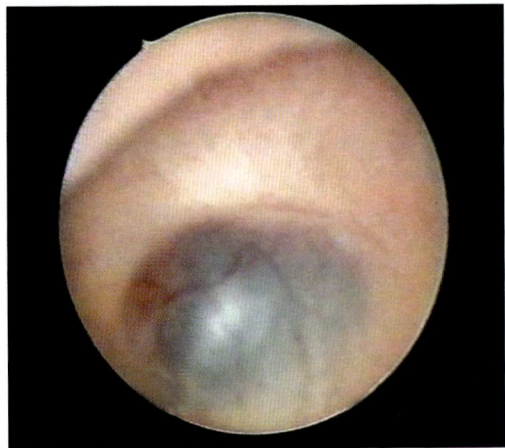

Fig. 12.8: Subendometrial adenoma on hysteroscopy

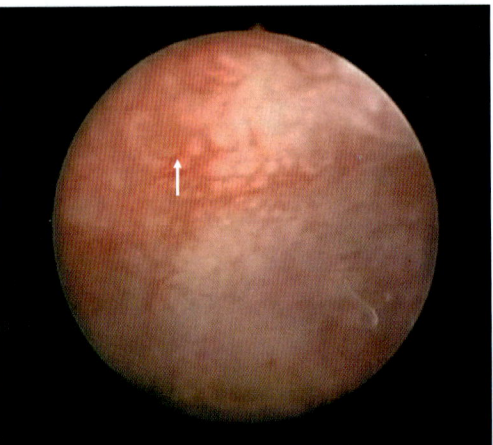

Fig. 12.7: Increased endometrial vascularity on hysteroscopy

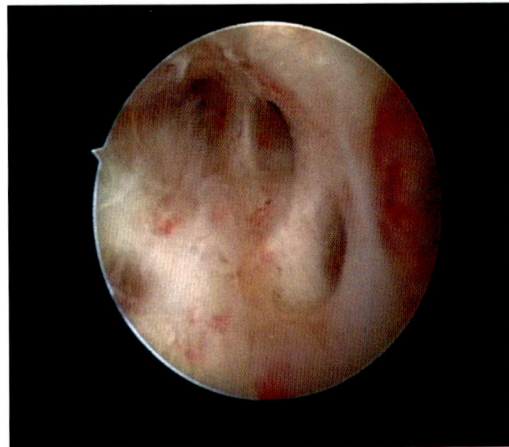

Fig. 12.9: Endometrial puckering visible on hysteroscopy

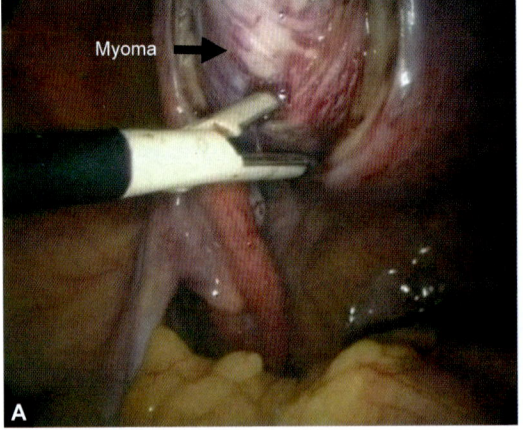

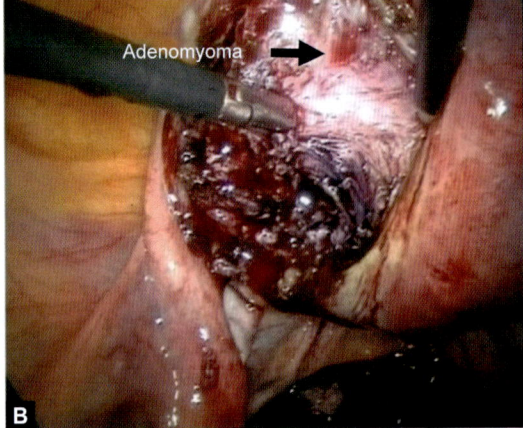

Figs 12.10A and B: Adenoma with fibroid

Laparoscopic Adenomyomectomy

endometrial polyp/hyperplasia, uterine adhesions and pelvic adhesions **(Figs 12.11, 12.12A and B)**.

PREOPERATIVE ADENOMA MAPPING

We routinely make a map depicting size, location of adenoma before starting the surgery **(Fig. 12.13)**.

Intraoperative transvaginal sonography is also done when needed.

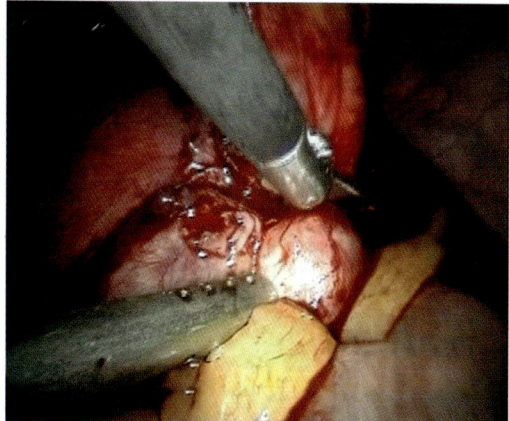

Fig. 12.11: Adenoma with anterior adhesions

AIM OF ADENOMA RESECTION

Resection helps in improving the symptoms by reducing the uterine vascularity, thus improving pain, menorrhagia and fertility. As adenoma/adenomyotic tissue is tough, it is better to use monopolar pure cutting current than scissor. Too much smoke generated during use of monopolar current should be evacuated periodically.

TECHNIQUE OF ADENOMYOMA RESECTION

It may not be possible to excise adenoma completely. Elliptical strip excision would be better for adenoma resection rather than attempting enucleation as in fibroid[6] **(Figs 12.14A and B)**.

It may be difficult to locate adenoma intraoperatively, for which intraoperative transvaginal sonography is useful.

Adenoma bleeds minimal. So if surgeon encounters more bleeding while resecting then he may have entered the healthy myometrium. The aim of resection is to reduce tension in

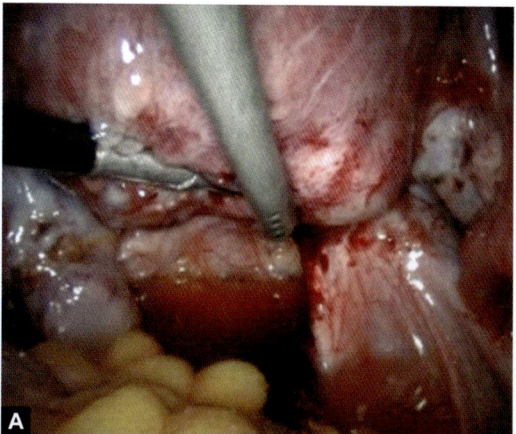

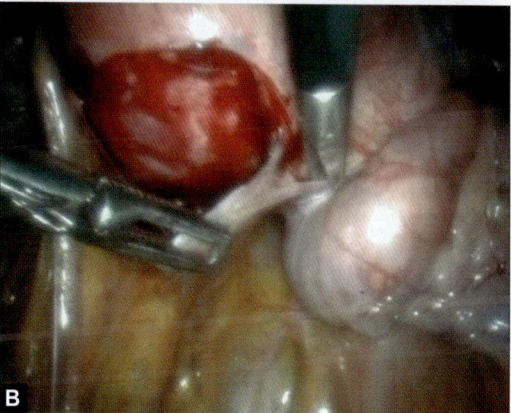

Figs 12.12A and B: Adenoma with posterior adhesions

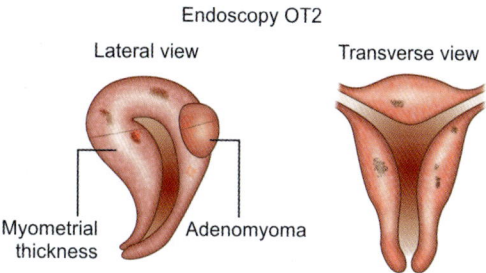

Fig. 12.13: Adenoma mapping

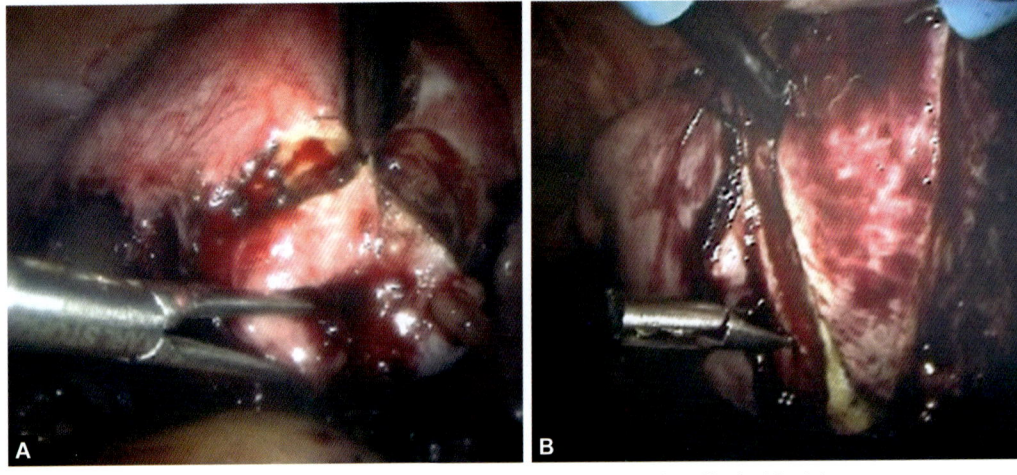

Figs 12.14A and B: Adenomyoma resection by elliptical incision

myometrium (similar to debulking surgery of benign SOL of brain without injuring vital areas of brain), which can be achieved by debulking the affected myometrium which is sometimes up to 50 percent leading to hemihysterectomy.

TECHNIQUE OF ENDOSUTURING: INTRA-CORPOREAL SLIP KNOT TECHNIQUE

Proper approximation should be done after resection. It can be achieved by intracorporeal slip knot technique.

First we take full thickness bite on right edge and then on left edge **(Fig. 12.15A)**. Then we place first half hitch and over that place second half hitch **(Fig. 12.15B)**. This makes it a square surgical knot **(Fig. 12.15C)**. This loose knot is then slipped as far as down as it goes. This knot is not tightened and is not complete and secured as yet. It is left half way through. First stitch acts as an assistant holding the edges together for us.

Then we go for second stitch 1 cm lower down in same manner as first stitch **(Fig. 12.15D)**. Then we go back to first stitch which is further tightened completely to secure it further approximating the myometrium **(Fig. 12.15E)**. This is how entire length of myometrium is approximated without leaving any residual dead space **(Fig. 12.15F)**.

Our Experience

Our series	Year 1996 – 2005
Localized adenoma	210 cases
Diffuse disease	46 cases
Total	256 cases

Symptomatic Improvements

Dysmenorrhea	92%	236 cases
Menstrual loss	84%	215 cases
Recurrence rate after 3 years	38%	97 cases
Note: Recurrence rate is higher in Grade II and Grade III.		

Pregnancy rates (Figs 12.16A to E)

Group	No. of cases
Localized adenoma	87 cases (37%)
Diffuse adenomyosis	20 cases (8%)

Adenomyomectomy may predisposes a pregnant uterus to rupture during labor. Therefore, such women should be offered elective cesarean delivery at term[7] **(Fig. 12.17)**.

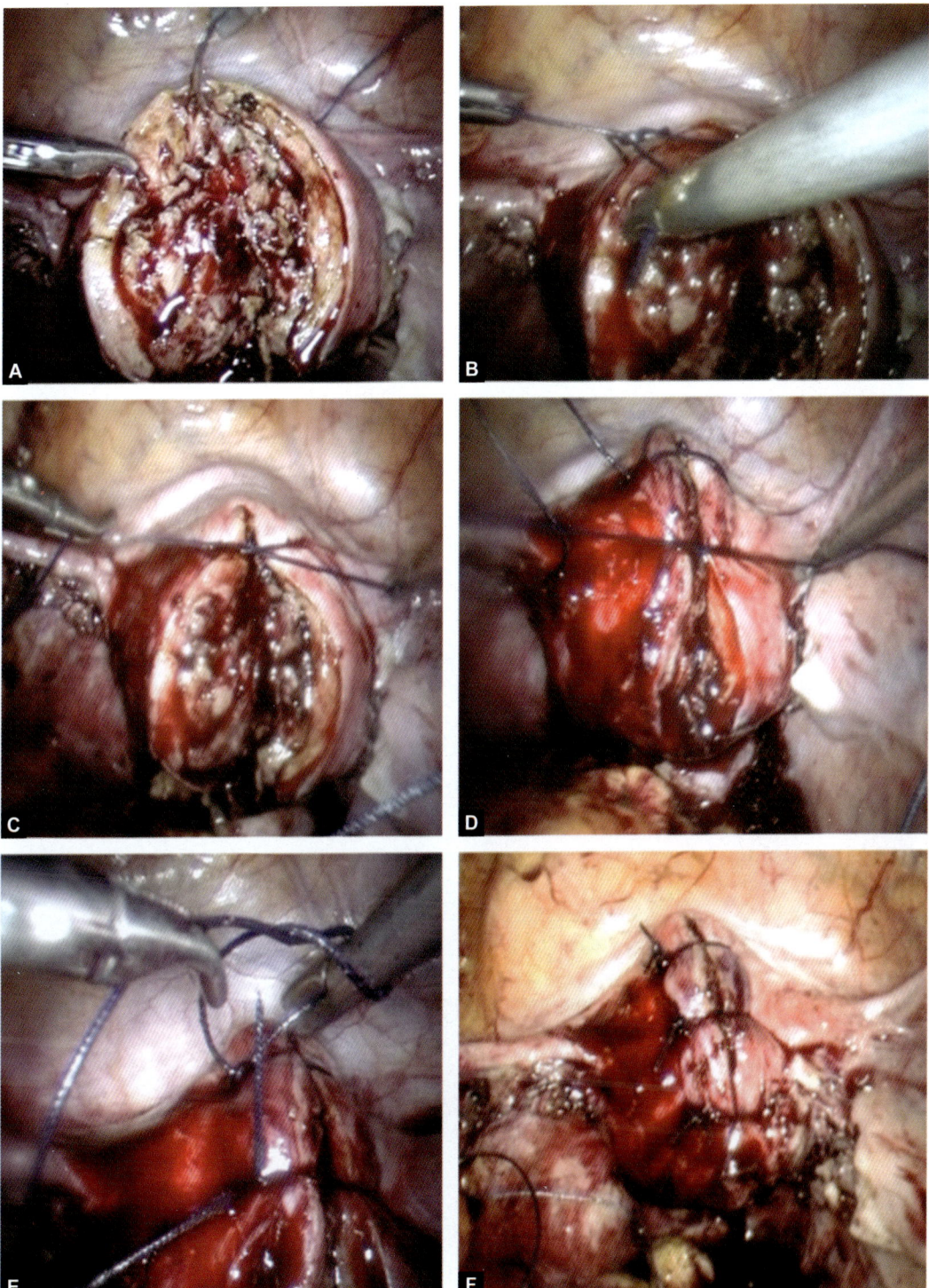

Figs 12.15A to F: Techniques of endosuturing: intracorporeal slip knot

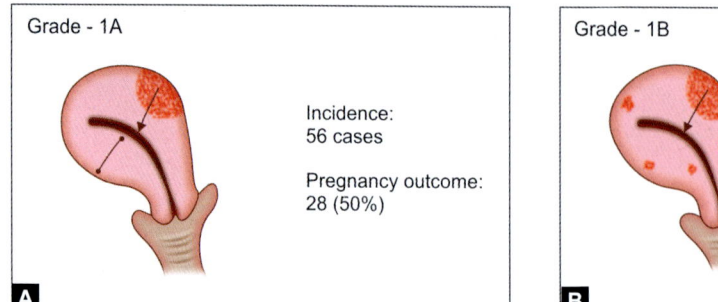
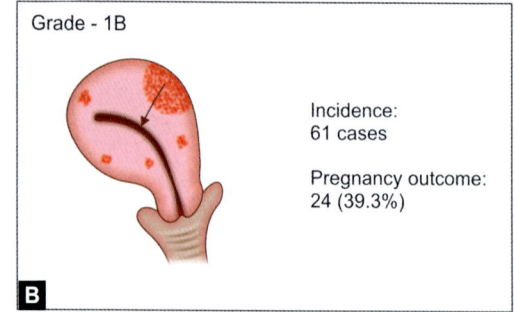
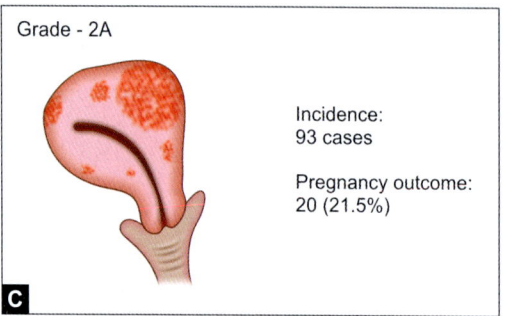
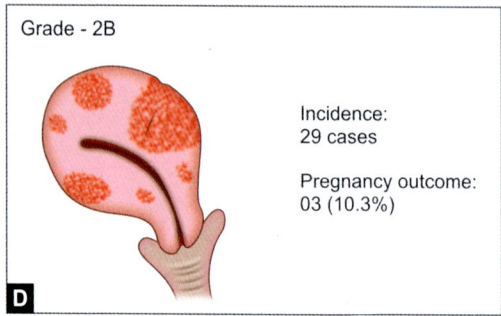
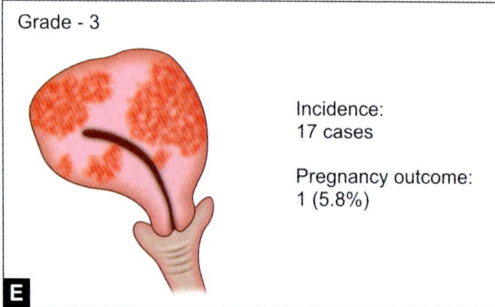

Figs 12.16A to E: Pregnancy outcome in different grades of adenomyosis

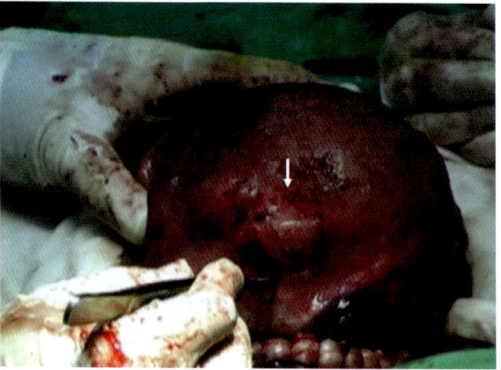

Fig. 12.17: Postadenomyomectomy cesarean section

CONCLUSION

Adenoma resection is technically more difficult but quite a rewarding surgery in early stage of the disease in terms of fertility and improvement in symptomatology in whom hysterectomy cannot be advised.

REFERENCES

1. Roland D, Thomas D, et al. Human Reproduction update, 2003;19(2):139-47.
2. Uterine adenomyosis: a need for uniform terminology and consensus classification. Reproductive BioMedicine Online 2008;17(2):244-8.
3. Karen L Reuter. Adenomyosis Imaging. Chief Editor: Eugene C Lin.
4. Wood C, Maher P, Woods R. Laparoscopic Surgical Techniques for Endometriosis and Adenomyosis. Diagn Ther Endosc. 2000;6(4):153–68.
5. Keckstein J. Hysteroscopy and adenomyosis. Contrib Gynecol Obstet. 2000;20:41-50.
6. Mineto M, Yasuyuki A. Laparoscopic Excision of Myometrial Adenomyomas in Patients with Adenomyosis Uteri and Main Symptoms of Severe Dysmenorrhea and Hypermenorrhea. Amer Assoc of Gynecol Laparoscop. 2004;11(1)86-9.
7. Cyril C Dim, Polycarp U, Agu, Ngozi R, Dim. Adenomyosis and uterine rupture during labour in a primigravida: an unusual obstetric emergency in Nigeria. Trop Doct. 2009;39:250-1.

CHAPTER 13

Safe and Efficient Laparoscopic Suturing

Mahendra Borse

Chapter Outline

- Patient's Position
- Instruments
- Port Placement
- Needle Insertion
- Ipsilateral Suturing
- Contralateral Suturing
- Needle Removal
- The Art of Camera Holding
- Needles
- Suture Material
- Barbed Suture
- Microsurgery
- Extracorporeal Knot

INTRODUCTION

Laparoscopic suturing has moved to a different level over the past few years. Earlier, the discussion was how laparoscopic suturing should be done; it was predominantly about convincing that it is possible. Now, we are trying to make it simple, efficient and safe so that there are no limitations regarding the location of the suturing sight and duration of surgery. It is possible to undertake suturing at any corner of pelvis, provided a few suggestions are followed meticulously. Talking about laparoscopic suturing today is different than what it was a few days ago. Learning curve was said to be long initially, which is not today. Suturing is the integral part of any surgery or procedure. It has to be easy and effortless to be safe and efficient.

Ipsilateral suturing is more physiological considering the surgeon's posture then contralateral suturing. It is possible to do using a long thread and do an extensive suturing. Contralateral suturing has advantage of being more logical regarding the handling of the thread inside the peritoneal cavity. One can follow any of the technique but principles of the surgical procedure should be sound and no variation from the most rewarding and time-tested technique should be allowed.

PATIENT'S POSITION

This starts from the proper positioning of the patient. Patient is placed in modified lithotomy position as shown in the photograph **(Fig. 13.1)**. Allen's stirrups are the ideal things to have but in absence of Allen's stirrups, tilting of the vertical stirrups by 45 degrees can serve the purpose. The principle is to avoid the thigh to obstruct the movements of the surgeon.

INSTRUMENTS

Manipulating the needle and thread in a limited space with limited range of mobility of instrument has been given so much importance as it takes time and demands good surgical sense to master this skill. Right and left, both the hands are to be used for manipulating the needle. Movements involved in laparoscopic suturing are manipulating the needle and the thread, holding the needle in the 'position of func-

Safe and Efficient Laparoscopic Suturing

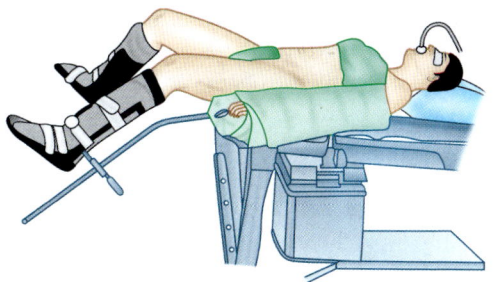

Fig. 13.1: Patient's position-modified lithotomy position

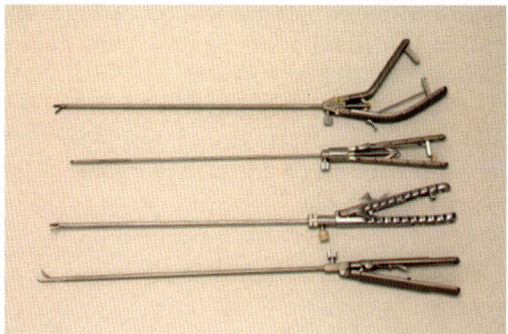

Fig. 13.2: Needle holders

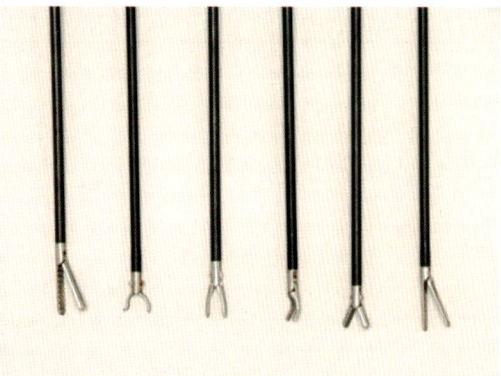

Fig. 13.3: Graspers

tion', holding the tissue, traversing the needle through the tissue and tying the knot.

The aim of choosing proper needle holder **(Fig. 13.2)** is to make sure that it grasps the curve needle securely. Inability to hold the needle securely makes inefficient passage of the needle through the tissue.

A light weight needle holder with a flat and titanium coated tip as a dominant needle holder and a parrot beak assisting needle holder are the ideal instruments for the laparoscopic suturing.

Handles made of titanium reduces the weight of needle holder significantly, which give a better feel for needle manipulation. It was very difficult to get an ideal needle holder few years ago, but now there is a wide range of instruments available to choose according to individual needs.

A needle holder with single tooth at the tip serves both the purposes as it can be used to hold and stabilize the tissue like tooth forceps. It has an added advantage that the needle does not slip out while holding in the desired position. The parrot beak needle holder with the tooth is an excellent instrument for handling the tough structures. A word of precaution–Never lock the needle holders with tooth in haste when the thread is close to the bowel loops.

Though a grasper **(Fig. 13.3)** can be used instead of assisting needle holder there are chances of the thread getting caught in the 'joints' which is a disaster at a critical moment. Out of variety of handles the one which is in line with the barrel of the needle holder is more versatile and useful at difficult sights of suturing. The curved handle (Coh's needle holder) is comfortable to use for prolong suturing.

PORT PLACEMENT

The distance between two suturing ports should be at least 10 cm **(Fig. 13.4)**, this is achieved naturally in contralateral technique, while it has to be achieved cautiously during ipsilateral suturing. Too close port placement makes the instruments to be parallel to each other and cause cluttering. Though it is not impossible to suture with closer ports it takes practice and good learning curve to execute it.

It is explained in terms of 'Triangle of success' **(Figs 13.5A and B)**. The line joining two ports forms the base of the triangle and the suturing sight forms the apex where the two instruments meet. What matters more is the angle between two instruments which should be more than 60 degrees, when we are trying to roll the thread on the instrument and secondly the quality of the fulcrum effect.

NEEDLE INSERTION

With Reich technique of needle insertion it is possible to introduce any type of needle into the peritoneal cavity for extracorporeal suturing. The needle holder pulls the tail of the thread through the cannula and again it is inserted through the cannula which holds the thread close to the swage point and the sequence of appearance in the peritoneal cavity is tip of the needle holder, small length of the thread, the needle and then the cannula which railroads over the needle holder, then the needle is left and the thread is pulled inside vertically down to drop the thread below the port side. When we do not want the push knot it is not necessary to pull the thread through the cannula and the needle can be inserted in the same way as described. During microsurgery the thread is coiled and pulled into the reducer and then the reducer is inserted in the cannula and suture is released inside the peritoneal cavity.

Once the needle is inside, it is manipulated by holding the thread close to the swage point with the grasper and a light grip of needle holder at the center of the needle. The thread can be pulled or pushed to get the desired position of the needle **(Figs 13.6A and B)**.

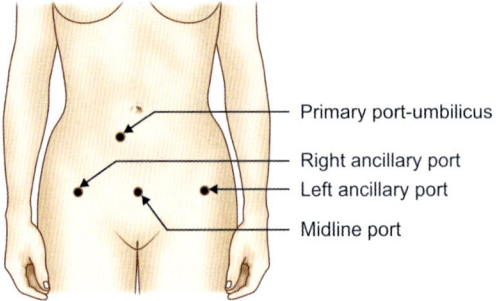

Fig. 13.4: Schematic presentation of the port placement

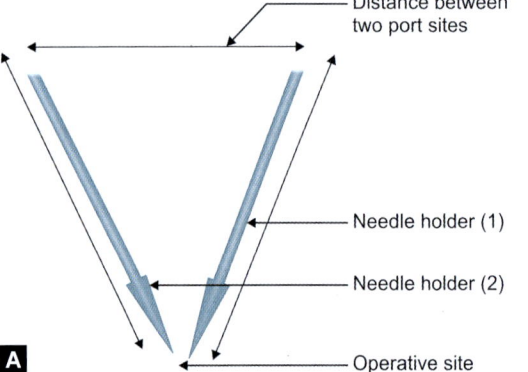

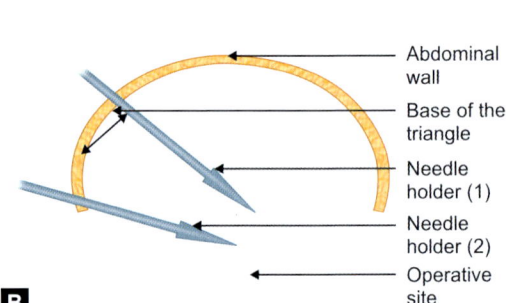

Figs 13.5A and B: (A) Triangle of success; (B) As seen through the laparoscope at the umbilical port

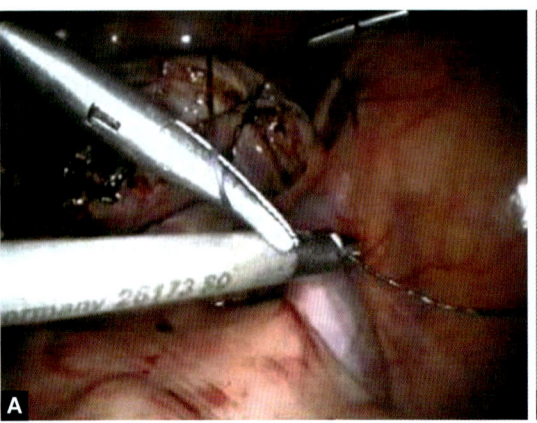
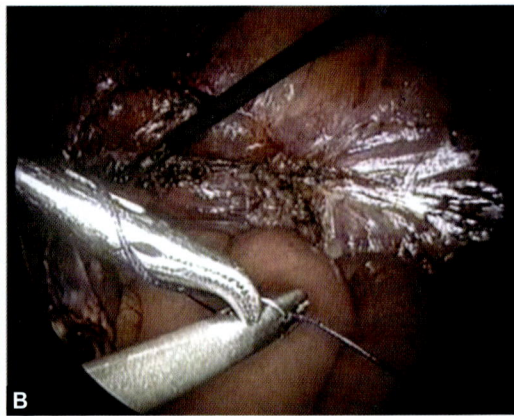

Figs 13.6A and B: Angle between two suturing instruments

IPSILATERAL SUTURING (FIGS 13.7A TO C)

The two instruments work from the same side of the patient out of which one is needle holder in the dominant hand and other can be assistant needle holder or a grasper which has tight grip on the thread like needle holder. Passage of the needle is an art where the depth of the tissue decides the position of the needle holder. If a deep bite through the tissue is required then the needle is held at the center and pierced perpendicular to the surface at adequate depth, the forearm is supinated to bring the needle tip out and the needle is pushed holding proximal to the previous grip similarly it is passed through the other half of the tissue and the knot is tide. We have to remember that the needle should be pushed through the tissue to get adequate length from the tip to grasp it and it is better to push rather than pull it by holding the tip. It is prudent to retain the original sharpness of the tip of the needle till the end of the suturing, it helps to get the anticipated passage of the needle through the tissue.

For all the purposes needle is held at the junction of proximal 1/3 and distal 2/3.

There are occasions when we have to change the direction of the needle after just insertion into the tissue, which is done by holding the needle with the needle holder and the thread with the grasper. The same manual, which is done to hold the needle in the desired position before suturing, can be done when the tip of the needle is inside the tissue.

The length of the thread is 12 to 20 cm for comfortable suturing but longer thread can be managed during ipsilateral suturing.

The standard technique of ipsilateral suturing is to make the 'C' on the surgeon's side and roll the thread above or below the assistant needle holder and pull the tail through the loops to tighten the knot. It is important to avoid 'strangulation' of the assistant needle holder while tightening the knot. It occurs if the loops are pulled and tightened prematurely before they come out of the tip of the assistant needle holder. Occasionally, the loop needs to be pushed if the strangulation occurs. The loops slide smoothly on the assistant needle holder as compared to the grasper, which have the joints bulging out when opened. The next loop is on the same side but the rolling of the thread is opposite to the previous one. It continues in the similar fashion, tightening in appropriate direction result in a proper surgical knot.

Longer length of the thread needs a patient handling in the peritoneal cavity. Once the needle comes out through the tissue it is pulled in upward direction then towards the left upper port (dominant needle holder) and then it is kept in the midline or towards the right side of the peritoneal cavity just below the liver, then the remaining thread is pulled in the same direction towards the left upper port and dropped down below it so the needle is most cranial and in the right half, then the loops of suture are caudal to it in the left half and both of them are not seen when ovary are focused on tying the knot.

For the next stitch the needle is picked up and passed through the tissue and kept again at the same point close to the liver, this time the remaining thread is pulled towards the right side and dropped caudal to the needle till the adequate length is available for tying the knot.

Though this sounds more cumbersome, with practice the required and adequate move-

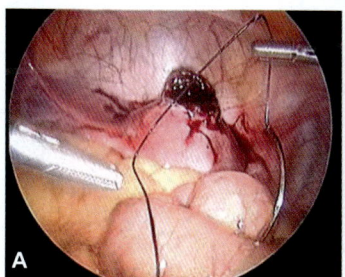
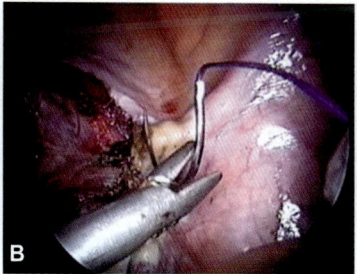
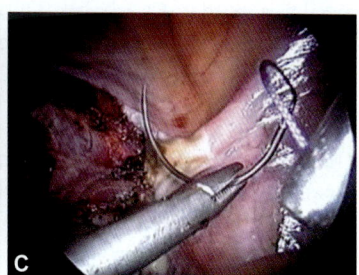

Figs 13.7A to C: Manipulation and positioning of needle, grasping and ready for suturing

ments of the needle holder can be mastered and performed without focusing the laparoscope for each movement the position of the bowels, the distance from the sight to the liver should be remembered and slightly conservative movements of the instruments are done to get a safe and required outcome.

CONTRALATERAL SUTURING

The laparoscope in the center and both suturing instruments from opposite sides make contralateral suturing resemble conventional suturing technique. Once the needle is passed through the tissue the 'C' is formed on one side for the first time, then the long thread is handed over to the other instruments. During this, the 'C' is automatically formed on the opposite side. The thread is rolled over the two instruments alternately. The direction of tightening the knot is such that it results in a proper surgical knot. There are less chances of "strangulation" of the instruments during contralateral suturing.

NEEDLE REMOVAL

Once the suturing is complete the needle is removed by holding the thread close to the swage point. First the cannula comes out followed by thread and then the needle.

THE ART OF CAMERA HOLDING

Good camera work can get a swift act of suturing out of a novice. Its importance cannot be expressed more than this. With the advent of high definition camera, monitors, laparoscope and excellent light source, we get an excellent picture which is illuminated in all the corners and does not need focusing repeatedly. Larger monitors with very sharp pictures avoid the necessity of repeated close-up view.

NEEDLES

Though, a cutting-edge needle can pass through the abdominal wall with ease, it can result into complications, which can go unnoticed. There are chances of laceration of blood vessels, especially vein, with the sharp tip and cutting edge.

The needle can be kept safely on a flat surface or it can be parked to the anterior abdominal wall. Depending on the length of the suture, the needle can be parked above the iliac fossa or more cranial to it, up to the liver. During this, one should always have the inferior epigastric vessels in vision and be aware about the vessels.

Minimum or optimum handling of the bowel loops is the best and safest strategy to avoid the complications arising from the needle prick.

Bowel retraction and packing should be complete and the suturing site should be well exposed before we grasp the needle and get ready to pierce the tissue. This helps to reduce the time required to suture as well as it becomes a pleasure as we can concentrate on the actual act of suturing.

Out of a variety of the needle sizes, most appropriate one should be chosen. Depending on the depth and consistency of the tissue, 35 mm or 40 mm needles are the most frequently used in gynecological surgeries.

Too thick needles or the cutting or reverse cutting edge needles are more prone for post suture oozing of blood through the stitch bite.

SUTURE MATERIAL

Performance of the surgeon varies depending on the suture material. Polyglycolic acid is the most commonly used suture material, which is suitable to all aspects of laparoscopic suturing. It does not retain its memory hence; the recoiling is not there, which is the property of prolene or nylon sutures. The suture material should really obey the surgeon's orders and act according to his wish. Besides, the knotting property of polyglycolic acid (Vicryl, Centicryl, Saffil etc.) is one of the best. Stiffness and knotting property of the polyglycolic acid varies according to the processing and coating on the suture. It is compared with prolene because prolene is the next commonly used suture material in gynecology. Properties of PDS are very much similar to prolene.

Catgut has better handling properties than prolene, but not as good as Vicryl. It has significantly less strength as compared to Vicryl or prolene. Catgut is easy to handle in laparoscopic suturing as it retains optimum stiffness once straightened. Silk is rarely used except in accidental bowel injury.

Vicryl is used for all the purposes, e.g. vault suturing, myomectomy, peritoneal closure, extracorporeal suturing for pedicles, uterine vessels, etc. Polyglycolic acid (Vicryl) really follows the orders of the surgeon and does not come repeatedly in front of the lens to obstruct the view.

Prolene is the next commonly used suture mainly used for the suspension procedures for uterine and vault prolapse. It is used where permanent fixation is desired. Handling prolene is significantly difficult because of its characteristic of retaining its memory. Stretching of the suture may help for a shorter thread or we should get a suture which is packed as straight one. Long thread can be used for extracorporeal suturing. When we have to deal with a long length of prolene following strategies can help:

1. Anchor the needle to the anterior abdominal wall peritoneum according to the length of the suture.
2. Anticipate the behavior of the suture. Anticipate how the loop of the suture is likely to lie after we pull it.
3. Never to leave the pulled thread off the needle holder. Never to leave the grip on the suture. This works as the guide for the next pull as well as it helps when we have many loops in front of the laparoscope.

Always remember the importance of the camera assistance in this procedure. These steps help while handling suture material of any type or length. 'Prolong focused attention' is required for laparoscopic suturing to become a pleasant act. Distraction makes us loose our grip on the movements as well as suture material. Maintaining a quiet temperament all throughout the procedure is the prerequisite of any laparoscopic surgery.

Perfect laparoscopic suturing is the pinnacle of laparoscopic surgery skill. It gives immense pleasure while performing and satisfaction at the end when it is complete with complete hemostasis and perfect approximation. It is one of the exercise for the mind which is difficult to focus anywhere for a longer time.

Handling properties of the prolene, PDS, PDO and barbed suture are the same.

There are occasions when we have to pass a blunt tip needle of the Mersilene tape through tough structures as anterior longitudinal ligament or pectineal ligament. In this case, the needle should be held close to the tip at the junction of 1/3rd and 2/3rd and inserted at the desired site. Then leave the needle and then rehold at the center of the needle. This makes it easy to change the direction and plane of driving the needle. Then push the needle until it emerges out from the tissue. Once the tip is pushed adequately, it can be pulled along its curvature, by holding proximal to the tip. The Mersilene tape should be pulled with two atraumatic instruments, as it needs strength without causing damage to the tape.

Gore-Tex is one of the best suture material to use for laparoscopic suturing as it glides very smoothly through the tissue and does not have stiffness (memory) as prolene. It is used for laparoscopic colposuspension.

BARBED SUTURE

It is similar to the fish scale or fence wire which has barbs. The barb does not allow the suture to slide back once it has passed through the tissue.

It is made of PDO, available in two types, one with a single needle and a loop at the other end. Bidirectional system is with needles at both the ends of the suture. It is divided at the center, where the barbs change the direction. Hence, if the suture is pulled through the tissue it meets resistance at the center of the suture. Each barb acts as a lock; as performed during conventional suturing, once passed through the tissue. It stays as it is and there is no need to keep it under traction. This property has eliminated the need of knotting at the end of the suturing. Knot tying is one of the aspects of laparoscopic surgery, which needs practice and consistency making it less amenable and more difficult. The apprehension about suturing is mainly because of the lack of opportunity or motivation to exercise it daily, at least initially during the learning phase.

Barbed sutures can be used at all the occasions, but myomectomy and vaginal vault suturing are best out of all. Adequate amount of firm tissue is required for the barbs to stay in the tissue. As it makes the laparoscopic suturing easy and convenient, the learning curve has shortened. It helps to reduce the duration of surgery and hemostasis is achieved very fast during myomectomy. Suturing in multiple layers to obliterate the dead space is no more a tedious and time consuming exercise.

Reducing the blood loss and duration of surgery reduces the anesthesia time and everything helps to improve the safety to a great level. Apposition of the tissue is excellent and very pleasant to perform if the stitches are placed at appropriate distance including adequate tissue.

Suturing pattern may vary according to personal choice. It can be either continuous from one angle to the other or we can start at the center and then proceed to the angles. The bidirectional system can be used in a crossing fashion to make it a shoe lace pattern. The exposed suture material is less as there are no knots and overall it results in less adhesion formation.

Barbed suture has made it possible to suture in reverse direction (backhand or anticlockwise) which is required for the fibroids at very odd and difficult locations. At such occasions the needle holder with the handle in line with the shaft (straight needle holder) is more convenient as supination and pronation can be directly transmitted to the needle.

Barbed suture is the need of time as we are progressing towards single port or single incision laparoscopic surgery (SILS). With the conventional sutures, though not impossible, but suturing is definitely very tiring and time consuming. It has its own learning curve, which starts when we master conventional laparoscopic suturing.

Though the invention of barbed suture seems to be inspired for SILS, it has really made a revolution in laparoscopic surgery.

MICROSURGERY

Laparoscopic microsurgical suturing is the most skillful and delicate activity, which needs very steady hand movements, appropriate instruments and an insight for the perfect port site selection.

The site of ancillary port entry should be decided after we enter the peritoneal cavity and it depends on where the suturing site is likely to be after anteversion of the uterus.

There is definitely a difference in handling the needle, suture material and the tissues as compared to the other gynecological surgeries. It has to be extremely gentle and smooth, with a very steady hand.

Instead of driving the needle through the tissue, in microsurgery the tissue is left on the needle tip so that the sharp tip pierces the tissue. The tip as it emerges out from the tissue, is held with the grasper and is allowed to fall down along the needle and the thread. Pulling the tissue is not wise in microsurgery. The thread is pulled and knot is tied by holding the required length of the thread only and the needle is never held, neither to tie the knot nor to tighten it.

As the tissues are so delicate and the tissue bite is very small, it is the approximation that is required and not tightening. If the needle gets detached from the thread, it becomes very difficult to find it out in the loops of intestines. When we are tying the knot, it is wise to keep the needle in front of the uterus (anterior pouch) where it is easy, safe and convenient to find for reholding purpose.

Unlike other suture materials (no 1, no O, 2-O), insertion and removal of the needle and thread should be done with the help of reducer and it should be confirmed every time that the needle is out. As a rule the entry and removal of the needle should be always under vision.

EXTRACORPOREAL KNOT

With the advances and improving skill of laparoscopic suturing, the occasions of extracorporeal knot tying have reduced. But it has its own place in suturing. Extracorporeal knot is designed mainly for tying the pedicles with larger vessels. The advantage of the knot is that once tied, it does not slip and get loosened. Apart from tying the pedicles like tubo - ovarian or infundibulopelvic ligament, it is used to approximate the uterine wall during myomectomy, during colposuspension or during the sling surgeries for prolapse, to fix Mersilene tape to the uterus or to the vault and to the anterior longitudinal ligament or pectineal ligament.

There two types of extracorporeal knots. In the first one, the knot is formed by half hitch and the thread is pushed inside to tighten the knot with the help of a variety of 'knot pusher'. It actually pushes the thread when we are holding both the ends outside.

Other type is actually a 'push knot'. The knot is formed outside with the lock and then pushed with the knot pusher. To avoid the pedicle getting pulled, the long thread should be held steady (without pulling it) and the knot is pushed until it reaches the site. Only then, the long arm should be pulled slightly to tighten the knot. Premature pulling of the long arm may result into avulsion of the pedicle.

Practically, extracorporeal suturing helps the surgeon in difficult situation, may it be inappropriate assistance or inadequate picture quality or bowel preparation.

Sometimes when we complete the suturing, there can be ooze from the needle prick site. Here it is wise to wait for sometime as the body's natural coagulation system can take care of it. If we interfere, it may increase as the tissue gets harden and the small vessels loose the compression of surrounding tissue. This is especially true when large cutting needle is used for myomectomy or suturing of uterine perforation that occurs during suction and evacuation. The side ports should be far enough from inferior epigastric vessels to avoid injury to them while insertion and removal of needle.

Suturing is one of the occasions to exhibit best of hand-eye co-ordination, sensory and motor orientation, imagination and anticipation. Though now technically simplified with the help of good needle holders, barbed sutures, auto sutures, clips and readymade loops, imagination of the endpoint/final picture at its best is the starting point for laparoscopic suturing. Suturing urinary bladder and intestines are very rare incidences in a gynecologist's practice. Tissues should not get pulled under tension and strangulated. The structure to be sutured should be stabilized with an appropriate a traumatic grasper. A short length of suture is more appropriate as it may cut through the tissue while pulling.

BIBLIOGRAPHY

1. Al Fallouji M. Surgical Laparoscopy and Endoscopy. 1993;3(6):477-81.
2. Clarke HC, Laparoscopy - new instruments for suturing and ligation. Fertil, Steril. 1972;73:274-7.
3. Reich H, Clarke HC, Sekel L. A simple method for ligation in Operative Laparoscopy with straight and curved needles. Obstet: Gynaecol. 1992:79:143-7.
4. Semm K. Operative pevliscopy. Br Med Bulletin 1986;42:284-95.

CHAPTER 14

Hysteroscopy—An Art to Achieve Excellence with Safety

S Krishnakumar

Chapter Outline

- Hysteroscopic Anatomy of the Uterus
- Distending Media for Hysteroscopy
- Distending Media Delivery
  - Instrumentation for Hysteroscopy
  - Office Hysteroscopy
  - Clinical Indications of Hysteroscopy
  - Contraindications of Hysteroscopy
- Technique of Panoramic Hysteroscopy
  - Operative Hysteroscopy
- Procedures (Technical nuances)
  - Targeted Hysteroscopic Biopsy
  - Removal of Intrauterine Foreign Bodies
  - Hysteroscopic Tubal Cannulation
- Metroplasty
  - Uterine Septum
- Lateral Metroplasty
- Lysis of Intrauterine Adhesions
  - Recommended Protocol Post-hysteroscopic Metroplasty and Adhesiolysis
- Leiomyomas and Endometrial Polyps
- Endometrial Resection (TCRE)
- Complications and Prevention
  - Mechanical
  - Electrosurgical and Gaseous Complications
  - Gas Embolism
  - Complications from Distention Media
  - Postoperative and Late Complications
- Do's and Dont's in Hysteroscopic Surgery

INTRODUCTION

Hysteroscopy is now considered a gold standard for evaluation of uterine cavity, detection of intrauterine disease and also offers surgical corrections which otherwise were very cumbersome and complicated, by the conventional method, and also has led to replacement of hysterectomy as a therapeutic procedure in specific cases of abnormal uterine bleeding.[1] However, not many gynecologists have integrated hysteroscopy into their operative spectrum.[2] Though the complication rates of hysteroscopy are low, varying from 0.012 percent for diagnostic hysteroscopy to 0.8 percent for operative procedures,[3-5] the art of hysteroscopy requires training and experience. Moreover, safety and outcome of surgical procedures are clearly linked to adequate training and adhering to safety recommendations. To achieve optimum surgical outcome, one has to understand not only the anatomy and physiology of uterus, but also has to have adequate knowledge of ideal instrumentation, the expected complications and their preventive steps. Before undertaking complex surgical procedures within the narrow uterine cavity, the surgeon should have complete mastery of the hysteroscopic anatomy of the uterine cavity.

HYSTEROSCOPIC ANATOMY OF THE UTERUS

The muscular anterior and posterior walls of the uterus are in close apposition and the uterine cavity is accurately described as potential cavity. The cavity of the uterus is flattened and has the shape of an inverted triangle **(Fig. 14.1)**, with the base formed by a line drawn between the tubal ostia and the apex at the isthmic opening. From top to bottom, this space measures 4 to 5 cm only.

The volume of fluid filling the cavity approximates 5 to 12 cc. The thick fundus lies above a line drawn between the tubal ostia. Frequently, the anatomic site is marked with a central ridge identifying the point where the Müllerian ducts have fused. This normal variant must not be confused with the more exaggerated subseptate uterus. The tubal ostia lie recessed in shallow depression at either extremity of the fundus (cornua) **(Fig. 14.2)**.

During hysteroscopy, there is some variation in the appearance of the ostia as well as in the depth and position of the cornual recesses. The cornual myometrium is thinner than the fundus or corpus muscle and measures 0.4 to 1 cm in thickness. During operative or diagnostic hysteroscopy, regardless of the location, the uterine cavity is stretched by the distending medium and thins by a factor of 50 percent to 60 percent. During hysteroscopic examination, the normal endometrium exhibits hue ranging from tan to pink and appears flattened when viewed during the proliferative phase. Regardless of the phase of the menstrual cycle, the endometrium is highly vascular[6] and bleeds with the slightest touch of endoscope **(Fig. 14.3)**.

Accurate determination of the position of the uterus is definitely essential to performing a successful hysteroscopic procedure. At the timing of vaginal examination, a severe anterior or posterior pointing of the cervix should alert the surgeon to suspect a displacement of uterus.

DISTENDING MEDIA FOR HYSTEROSCOPY

To convert the potential uterine cavity to a true cavity, one requires distension to view objects within the uterus when using the panoramic mode. Selecting the right media for hysteroscopy, diagnostic or operative goes a long way in ensuring safety in hysteroscopy. Amongst the distension media, liquid or gaseous, former

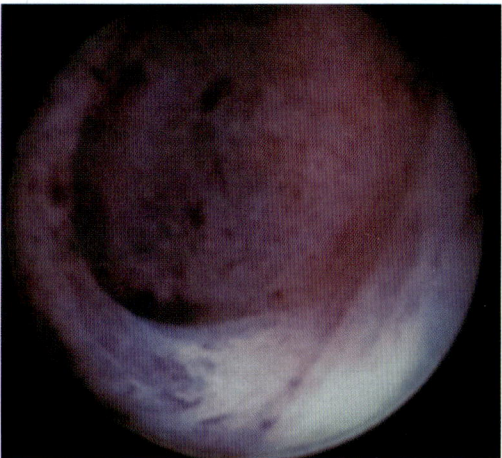

Fig. 14.2: Hysteroscopy-Uterine cornua

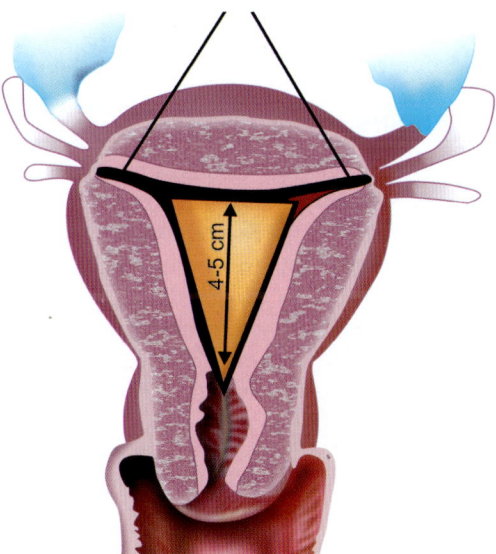

Fig. 14.1: Inverted triangle shape of uterine cavity

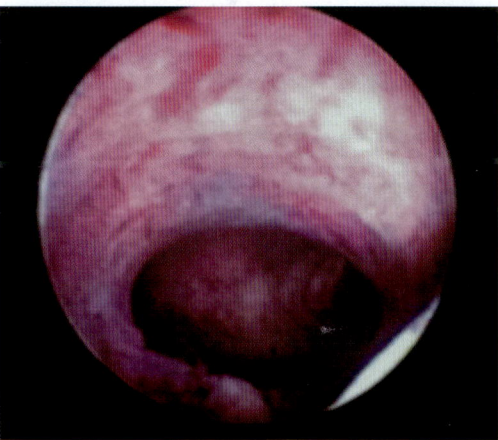

Fig. 14.3: Vascular pattern of the endometrial cavity

Table 14.1[7]: Advantages and use of the electrolyte and nonelectrolyte

Media	Operative	Office use	Misciblity (Blood)	Safety
Gaseous				
CO_2	+	+++	+	++
Liquid				
Nonelectrolytic (Monopolar)				
Glycine	+++	+++	++	+
Sorbitol	+++	+	++	+
Electrolytic (Bipolar)				
Normal Saline	+++	+	++	+++
Ringer Lactate	+++	+	++	+++

+: Unsatisfactory, ++: Average, +++: Highly advantageous

is most commonly used. The liquid distension media available for use in hysteroscopy is divided into electrolyte and non-electrolyte media **(Table 14.1)**.

Hykson, though not miscible with blood, is highly viscous, difficult to instill through narrow (5 mm) sheaths and with other disadvantages is rarely used today.

Amongst the low viscous fluid media, dextrose is rarely used, while glycine and sorbitol are more commonly used. Glycine is the most common distending media when using monopolar current as it is easily available. Whenever these agents are used, strict attention must be paid to the volume of medium used and the volume recovered, as these are hypoosmolar and can cause electrolyte imbalance, especially hyponatremia. Amongst the liquid media for hysteroscopy, only Ringer's lactate and normal saline match with osmolality of blood and are safer than the other media **(Table 14.2)**.

With these two media, hyponatremia does not occur even if there is fluid overload, but pulmonary edema can still occur. When using monopolar current for operative procedures, a non-electrolytic medium is to be used.

This permits sufficient current densities to exert a vaporization or coagulative action. Electrolytic fluids would result in the diffuse conduction of the electrons and dispersal of the electrical current (i.e., no thermal tissue action).

Table 14.2: Electrolyte content and osmolality of hysteroscopic distending solution

Solution	Na mEq/L	Cl mEq/L	mOsm/L
0.9% Sodium chloride	154	154	308
Lactated Ringers	130	110	275
0.45% Sodium Chloride	77	77	155
3% Sorbitol	–	–	178
1.5% Glycline	–	–	200
5% Mannitol	–	–	275
5% Dixtrose in water	–	–	250

DISTENDING MEDIA DELIVERY

The key to successful visualization of uterine cavity is to keep the visual field clear by continuously flushing the fluid through the uterine cavity. The safest way to administer distending media is by specially designed pumps for hysteroscopy **(Fig. 14.4)** which has correct adjustments for inflow pressure (120-150 mm Hg) and outflow pressure (50 mm Hg). For diagnostic and minor operative procedures, specialized simple devices like Medex bag can be used. But balance must be maintained to keep the necessary pressure gradient for separating the uterine walls (70 mm Hg).

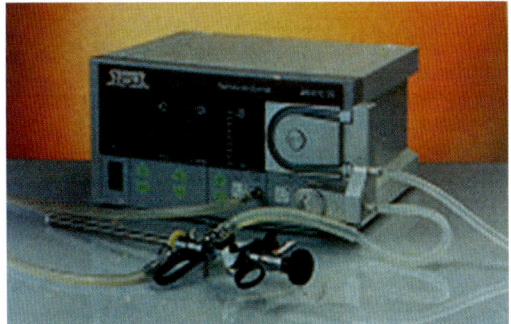

Fig. 14.4: Endomat

Instrumentation for Hysteroscopy

Selection of the proper and most appropriate instruments is one of the keystones for the performance of a successful hysteroscopic examination. Fine, skilled procedures should be performed with precision instrumentation. The two major elements of hysteroscopy are telescope and the sheath. One should have a 30 degree telescope for performing most of the procedures. Having a complete set of sheaths, should include continuous flow sheaths of:

1. The typical diagnostic sheath measures 5 mm OD (for a 4 mm hysteroscope) and will have only inflow channel **(Fig. 14.5)**. It is better to go for continuous flow sheaths (6-7 mm) for the clearance of blood tinged fluid inside the uterine cavity, for better and rapid vision.
2. Operative sheath come usually with diameter ranging between 7 and 9 mm OD and has an operating channel with a stopcock and a nipple to prevent loss of medium and distension when operating instruments are introduced **(Fig. 14.6)**.

The Resectoscope has a continuous flow system of two concentric sheaths, an outer sheath that provides the fluid outflow and an inner sheath that provides the inflow for continuous irrigation **(Fig. 14.7)**. Both concentric sheaths assembled permit the introduction of an optical system for viewing as well as the spring-loaded mechanism for manipulation of various electrodes.

The activation of the electrode is obtained by connection with a high frequency electro-

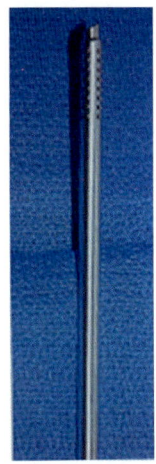

Fig. 14.5: Diagnostic sheath

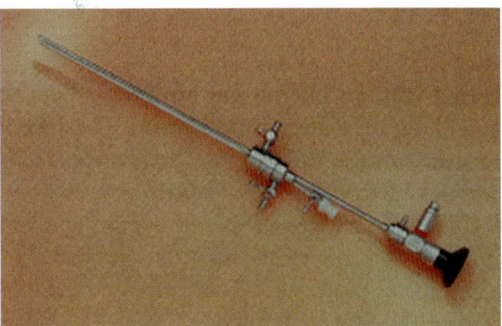

Fig. 14.6: Operative sheath

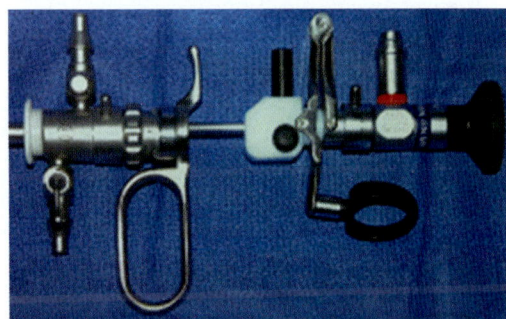

Fig. 14.7: Resectoscope

surgical unit; therefore, proper grounding of the patient is required when monopolar electrodes are being used.

Of late, bipolar resectoscope is also available, which requires the same two concentric sheaths of the monopolar resectoscope, but the active element is of different nature which permits the use of bipolar electrodes **(Fig. 14.8)**. With a bipolar resectoscope, the electrosurgical unit should have the facility of both bipolar cut and coagulation current **(Fig. 14.9)**.

Office Hysteroscopy

Telescopes are available with diameter of 1.9 mm versascope **(Fig. 14.10)**.

Bettochi with a diagnostic sheath of 2.9 mm OD, that permits visualization of the uterine cavity without cervical dilatation with minimum morbidity and inconvenience to the patient. Holding of the cervix is also not needed. A special bipolar generator (Versapoint-Gynecare) **(Fig. 14.11)**, if present, can be used for minor surgical procedures like, adhesiolysis, septal resection, removal of small fibroids and polyps can be carried out.

The disadvantages of these smaller devices are that, only 5Fr instruments can be passed, and the cost involved.

Clinical Indications of Hysteroscopy[8]

1. Evaluation of infertile patients with abnormal hysterograms and sonograms.
2. Abnormal premenopausal and postmenopausal uterine bleeding.
3. Diagnosis and surgical treatment of intrauterine adhesions.
4. Diagnosis and surgical treatment of symptomatic uterine septa.
5. Diagnosis and transcervical removal of submucous leiomyomas or endometrial polyps.
6. Location and retrieval of lost intrauterine devices and foreign bodies.
7. Transcervical resection of endometrium in patients with abnormal uterine bleeding unresponsive to hormonal therapy.
8. Tubal cannulation for cornual blocks of fallopian tube.
9. Evaluation of uterine cavity in patients with repeated pregnancy losses.
10. Tubal sterilization (Essure system).

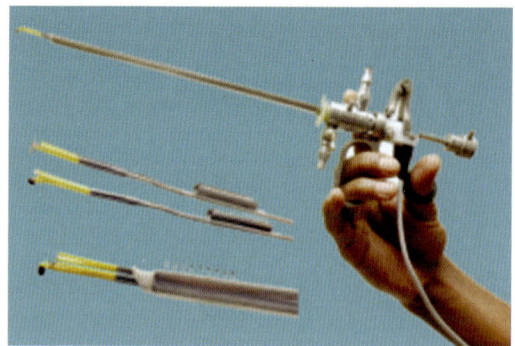

Fig. 14.8: Bipolar resectoscope

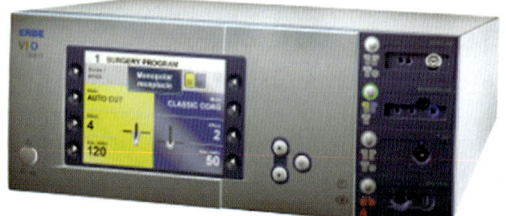

Fig. 14.9: Electrosurgical unit

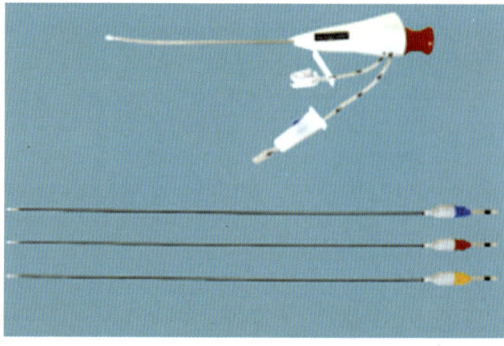

Fig. 14.10: Versascope and Versa point office hysteroscope

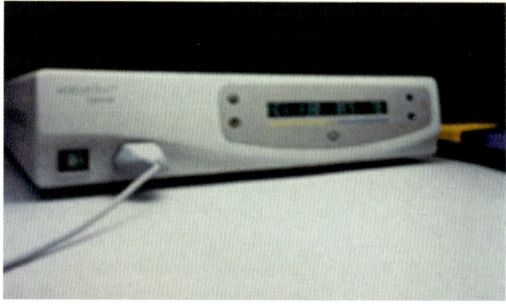

Fig. 14.11: Versapoint-Gynecare bipolar generator

Contraindications of Hysteroscopy

Absolute

a. Pregnancy.
b. Recent or existing uterine or cervical infection.
c. Profuse uterine bleeding.
d. Known cervical malignancy.

Relative

a. Marked cervical stenosis.
b. Operator's unfamiliarity with instrumentation, media and technique used.

TECHNIQUE OF PANORAMIC HYSTEROSCOPY

With appropriate selection of patients, hysteroscopy will offer a safe, simple, and efficient examination of the endocervical canal and uterine cavity. With the patient in dorsal lithotomy position and with all asepsis, per vaginal examination is carried out for correct position of uterus. For office hysteroscopy no cervical dilatation may be required, but for all other hysteroscopy cervical dilatation will be required. With the optics and the sheath appropriately attached to the camera system and light cable, the cervical canal is visualized in its totality, once the junction between the cervix and uterus is passed, the uterine cavity is observed first in its totality and systematically in each portion of the posterior wall, the left lateral wall with left tubal ostia, right lateral wall with right tubal ostia and last the anterior wall. These steps require manipulation of the light cable which is to be held in the opposite direction of the area being visualized. While the hysteroscope is slowly removed, it is used to examine again the uterine cavity and cervical canal.

Operative Hysteroscopy

Advantages

1. Rapid recovery and less pain.
2. Shorter operating time.
3. Risk of postoperative complications much less.
4. Avoids major incision on uterus for removal of intrauterine conditions like submucous fibroids, septae, etc.
5. Vaginal delivery possible after hysteroscopic metroplasty.

Diagnostic skills and mastery in learning to orient oneself within the intrauterine milieu must always precede intrauterine operative intervention. Every operative hysteroscopic procedure should be immediately preceded by a thorough diagnostic scan of the endometrial cavity.

General Aspects

A. **Preparation:** Every patient requires a complete preoperative evaluation starting with complete history and physical examination. All appropriate laboratory investigations should be carried out and a good transvaginal sonography should be carried out before complex surgical procedures. If indicated, hysterograms can be carried out and viewed by the surgeon.

B. **Concurrent Laparoscopy:** Simultaneous laparoscopy is indicated in:
   a. Infertility evaluation.
   b. Congenital anomalies of uterus.
   c. Tubal cannulation for blocked fallopian tube.

C. **Preparation of Endometrium:** Plan all surgeries within the uterine cavity in the early proliferative phase of the cycle. In patients with endometrial hyperplasia, waiting for TCRE, the endometrium can be prepared by gonadotropin-releasing hormone, Danazol or Oral Contractive pills.

D. **Cervical Softening:** Several studies have shown the beneficial actions of vaginal misoprostol and laminaria tents.

E. **Video Hysteroscopy:** Needless to say all operative procedures should be done with good camera system and complete recording of the procedure.

For prolonged procedures, it is advisable to dedicate an operation theater attendant to accurately record and read out the quantity of liquid medium used and the volume recovered. Additionally, it is important to inform the anesthesiologist about side effects of selected medium prior to surgery. It is always advisable to use isotonic electrolyte containing liquid media (Ringer's lactate, 0.9 percent saline) for distension. Bipolar current if available, should be the current of choice whenever electrosurgery is planned.

PROCEDURES (TECHNICAL NUANCES)

Targeted Hysteroscopic Biopsy

Direct hysteroscopic biopsies are carried out with biopsy forceps. The major disadvantage of this type of biopsy relates to the small volume of tissue obtained **(Fig. 14.12)**.

An alternative and acceptable technique uses the hysteroscope to identify the lesion to establish a presumptive diagnosis as well as to localize the site of the disease process. The endoscope is the withdrawn, a curette is directed to the known location of the lesion, and a plentiful sample could be removed.

Removal of Intrauterine Foreign Bodies

Not only can one see where the device is located, but also eliminates trauma of blind probing. With a 3 mm grasping forceps, the IUD string or the stem is grasped, and the hysteroscope is withdrawn, dragging the IUD with it through the cervix **(Fig. 14.13)**.

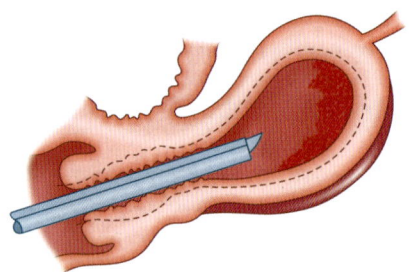

Fig. 14.12: Targeted hysteroscopic biopsy

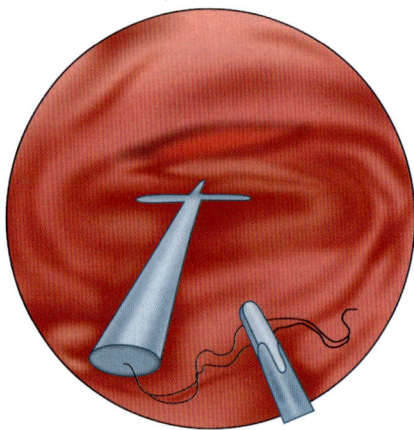

Fig. 14.13: Removal of IUD

Hysteroscopic Tubal Cannulation

The combined approach of hysteroscopy and laparoscopy for proximal tubal cannulation, allows the assessment of distal tubes and ovaries, and more accurate application of instruments into the tubal ostia. Laparoscope is to be done first to rule out distal and irreversible tubal damage, before attempting hysteroscopic tubal cannulation. A catheter device with terumo guide wire is passed through the operative channel of operative sheath, and under vision it is guided into the cornual cup and the end of the hysteroscope must be placed very close to the tubal ostium to provide extra stability for the guide wire **(Fig. 14.14)**.

The guide wire is then made to negotiate into the ostia and once it is guided into the tube without much pressure its position is documented by laparoscopy. The guide wire is then withdrawn and the patency is confirmed by the use of methylene blue. By this method at least one tube can be cannulated in 90 percent of cases and pregnancy rates reported is 45 to 50 percent.[9]

METROPLASTY

Uterine Septum

Septate uterus, most commonly seen in patients with recurrent pregnancy loss (13%), and seen with infertility evaluation, and various figures has been quoted about the relative risk of abortion or premature labor. Prior to the development of modern hysteroscopy, the accepted surgical techniques required laparotomy with

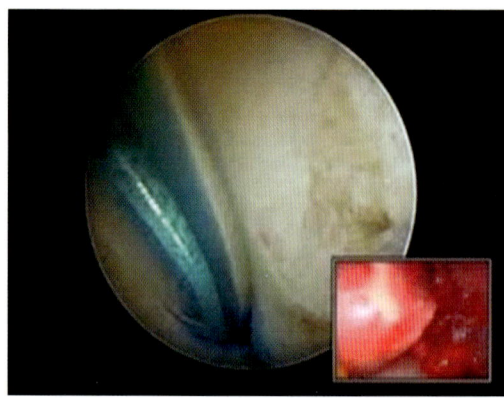

Fig. 14.14: Hysteroscopic tubal cannulation

incision into the substance of the uterus. Hysteroscopy offers great advantage as compared to the abdominal metroplasty **(Table 14.3)**.

The following methods are commonly employed to treat septum through the hysteroscope:

A. **Scissors:** A 3 mm scissors can be used through the operative channel of an operative sheath. Usually one should begin at the lower extremity on either the right or left side and progress upward towards the fundus with one arm of the scissor blade free (on the outer margin of the septum) and the other within the substance of the septum **(Fig. 14.15)**.

   Septae are usually fibrotic, hence very rarely bleed. From time to time it is wise to stop cutting in order to reorient the endoscope to the midline of the uterine axis and then continue the incising operation.

B. **Resectoscope:** The Collin's knife electrode is mounted on the resectoscope active handle with a power set at 60 to 100 W pure cutting current. One should always start at the tip of the septum and short bursts of current should be used, and the ostia should always be under vision, so that one does not drift too much posterior or anterior in to uterine wall. One should, from time to time reorient the resectoscope and both sides of the septum should be cut **(Fig. 14.16)**. It is always better to stop just below the line drawing the two tubal ostia.

   It is always better to slightly underperform the procedure particularly during the learning curve or when in doubt, reassess the residual septum by ultrasound and complete the procedure at a later date.

C. **Nd-Yag** laser can also be used to incise septa, but the cost involved is usually prohibitive, hence rarely used.

There are no prospective randomized studies to suggest which of the above methods is superior to the other. In general, scissors may be better if perforation occurs during the procedure, as thermal damage to the bowel can be avoided. If perforation occurs with resectoscope, it may be advisable to assess the abdominal cavity, to rule out damage to the bowel. Bipolar resectoscope offers better safety profile as compared to monopolar.

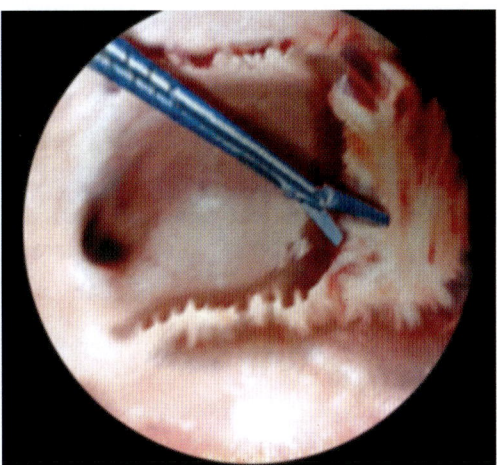

Fig. 14.15: Uterine septal resection with scissors

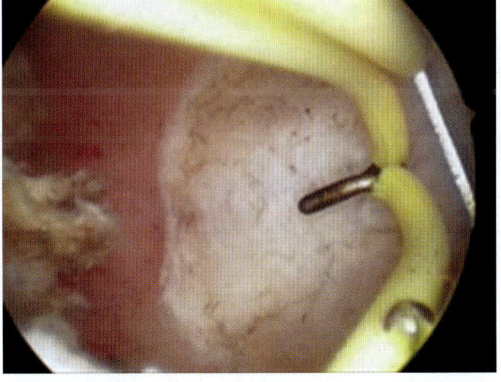

Fig. 14.16: Septal resection using Collin's knife

Table 14.3: Comparison of abdominal metroplasty and hysteroscopic incision of uterine septum

	Abdominal Metroplasty	Hysteroscopic Incision
Hospitalization	Yes	No
Surgery	Major	Minor
Avoid pregnancy	3 Months	1 Month
Delivery route	Cesarean section	Vaginal
Postop HSC or HSG	Yes	Yes

HSC hysteroscopy; HSG hysterosalpingography

LATERAL METROPLASTY

This was described by Naegel and Malo, to basically treat T shaped uterus. The procedure now consists of electrosurgical incision of the lateral walls of the uterine cavity with the help of a resectoscope using a Collin's knife, starting near the tubal ostia and extending proximally **(Fig. 14.17)**.

Care must be taken avoid incising the lateral wall in the region of the isthmus and internal os. The incision is done millimeter by millimeter till a normal uterine architecture is achieved and the underlying myometrium is seen. The end point is the visualization of both the cornual ends satisfactorily on panoramic hysteroscopy.

LYSIS OF INTRAUTERINE ADHESIONS

Intrauterine adhesiolysis is one of the most challenging procedures performed via the hysteroscopy route. Before treatment, it is important to classify the severity of the disease, for prognosis and comparison of results. The adhesions could be either central, marginal or both. Intrauterine adhesiolysis by hysteroscope becomes easier if either one or both tubal ostia are visible. Marginal adhesions are diagnosed when the uterine cavity viewed from the internal os is not symmetrical and one cornua is not visible **(Fig. 14.18)**. Complex adhesions with both central and marginal types may divide the uterine cavity into several chambers communicating by small orifices. In very severe cases, the uterine cavity is reduced to a small, narrow tunnel.

Normal endometrium has disappeared, and only fibrous tissue is visible.

Adhesions which break just by the tip of the hysteroscope are usually very thin, but most other adhesions will require either scissors, electrosurgery or laser beam. We, conventionally believe, a resectoscope is better suited for all cases of adhesiolysis and we prefer to use the operative sheath with scissors in very severe cases where gradual probing is done in to the cavity. Whichever method is employed identifying the tubal ostia, either one or both is always aimed at. In cases, where the tubal ostia cannot be identified, it may be worthwhile attempting to create an adequate cavity and in a subsequent re-look hysteroscopy, better anatomy may be seen.

Recommended Protocol Post Hysteroscopic Metroplasty and Adhesiolysis[10]

High dose estrogen therapy (5 mg of Conjugated estrogens) daily for 20 days followed by 10 mg Medroxyprogesterone daily for 5 days is commonly used.

IUDs have not shown to be of any benefit in preventing adhesions from reforming. A balloon or Pediatric Foley's catheter have been shown to be better and is usually kept for a period of 15 days.

LEIOMYOMAS AND ENDOMETRIAL POLYPS

Hysteroscopy is the procedure of choice for locating, and treating polyps as it can also locate the pedicle. Pedicles near the fundus may be

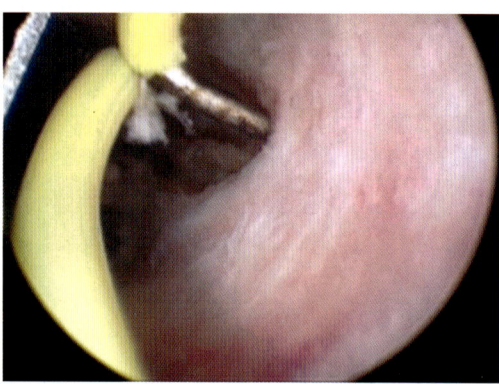

Fig. 14.17: Lateral metroplasty using Collin's knife

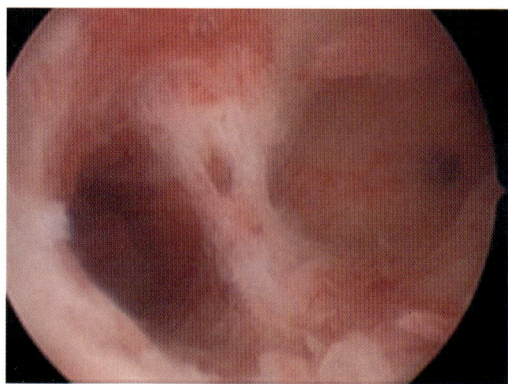

Fig. 14.18: Intrauterine adhesions

difficult to approach, and also pedicles of polyp on the posterior wall of the uterus may not be visible, and the operator may have to push the tip of the endoscope between the polyp and the posterior wall and lift it up. The resectoscope is now the most common tool used to remove uterine polyp.

The loop electrode is attached to the resectoscope and the movement of the loop should always be from fundus to the internal os. Intermittently, the resectoscope can be removed to clear the pieces of endometrial polyps with ovum forceps. Care should be taken to avoid damage to the adjacent endometrium during the use of resectoscope, and the current setting is of pure cutting current.

Before embarking upon the hysteroscopic management of submucous myomas, the exact size and exact projection into the cavity of the fibroid should be determined by either, saline infusion sonogram or MRI to plan the surgical approach and to estimate the likelihood of complete excision. Myomas, with > 50 percent extension into the cavity, are better managed hysteroscopically. Those myomas with a significant intramural component pose a challenge, and should not be attempted by hysteroscope. Removing tumors > 5 cm in diameter can be quite challenging and should not be attempted, as the time taken can be more, allowing large quantities of fluid to be absorbed into the body. Myomas that are present on opposing uterine walls deserve special consideration. Because the risk of adhesion formation is high if both surfaces are resected simultaneously, but one surface should be treated initially and the other one month later after the first operative site has healed.

Prior to beginning myoma resection, the vessels that course over the surface of the myoma are coagulated to reduce the amount of bleeding and the amount of fluid absorption. The loop electrode is passed to the tumor, the electrode is activated and then it is drawn towards the operator **(Figs 14.19 and 14.20)**. The electrode should be in view during the entire time of current flow. Often myometrial contractions cause more of the myoma to be extruded into the cavity as the surgery progresses. Intermittent release of intrauterine pressure will also help in more of myoma projecting into the uterine cavity. Open vessels are coagulated as the procedure progresses. If some portion remains, it may be extruded into the cavity over the ensuing months, and a second hysteroscopic procedure may be needed for complete resolution. The tumor fragments are intermittently removed for better vision. At the completion of the procedure, the cavity is inspected, and bleeder vessels if any, should be coagulated. Resection of submucous myoma is one of the most difficult hysteroscopic procedures and the following safety steps should be strictly followed:[11]

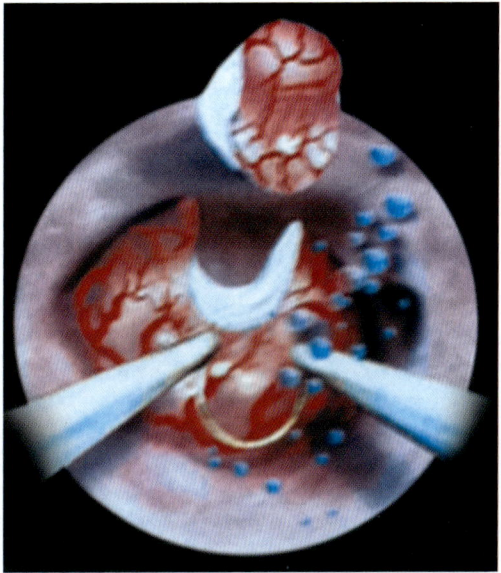

Fig. 14.19: Uterine polyp

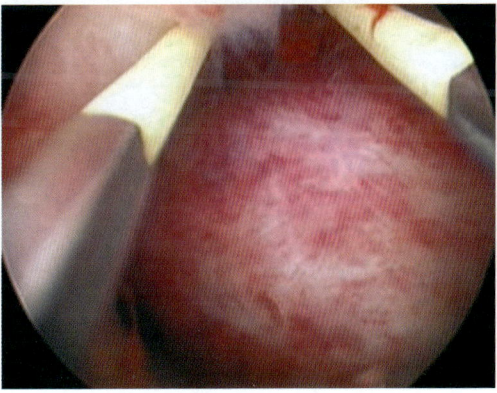

Fig. 14.20: Uterine fibroid

a. Operate in follicular phase.
b. Inspect cavity.
c. Avoid opposing wall myomas.
d. Coagulate surface vessels.
e. In large myomas, dilute vasopressin can be injected in the paracervical region.
f. Resect myoma.
g. Coagulate cut vessels.
h. Coagulate center of residual myoma.
i. Evacuate chips.
j. Re-inspect cavity.
k. Follow-up hysteroscopy if needed.

ENDOMETRIAL RESECTION (TCRE)

Hysteroscopic ablation of the endometrium is a relatively noninvasive method that can accomplish the treatment without removing the uterus. It should be reserved for patients who cannot be managed by medical treatment. Most of these patients have dysfunctional uterine bleeding and are therefore amenable to hormonal management. With the advent of lesser invasive methods for endometrial ablation, TCRE is rarely performed today, because of its potential complications. Total amenorrhea is observed in 60 percent of the women treated and scanty menstrual flow in 30 percent. The overall success rate reported is 90 percent.[12]

Proper selection and preparation of patients is mandatory for good results. Resectoscope with either bipolar or monopolar working element can be used **(Figs 14.21 and 14.22)**.

The cutting loop electrode resects 3 to 4 mm thick strips of endometrium and myometrium. Power settings of 60 to 100 W create rapid tissue vaporization and cutting. The straight cutting-loop is used to accomplish fundal resection. The cornual regions should be ablated first by roller ball to decrease the risk of perforation. The cutting loop is then introduced, with the resection of the anterior wall, beginning where the wall intersects with the fundus and working downward towards the internal os of the cervix. The reason for performing the ablation of the anterior wall first is based on the fact that debris and bubbles rise to the anterior wall. Next, the hysteroscope is rotated to the right and then to left to ablate the upper lateral walls of the uterus. Then, the fundus is resected with straight loop electrode. Finally, the posterior and posterolateral walls are resected. The resection is avoided in the cervical canal, as it would lead to sealing of the endometrial cavity. At the end of the procedure, a panoramic view of the cavity is obtained to ensure completion of the procedure. In skilled hands, TCRE is completed in 20 to 30 minutes.

COMPLICATIONS AND PREVENTION

Mechanical

a. Inability to insert the hysteroscope: This may be caused by acutely anteflexed or retroflexed uterus, stenosed or nulliparous cervix, or previous surgery on cervix.
Inserting a laminaria tent the evening before surgery or vaginal misoprostol 200 µg inserted vaginally, will help to ripen the cervix allowing easier dilatation.

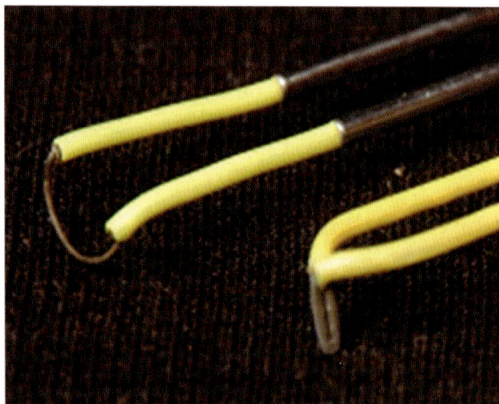

Fig. 14.21: Monopolar loops

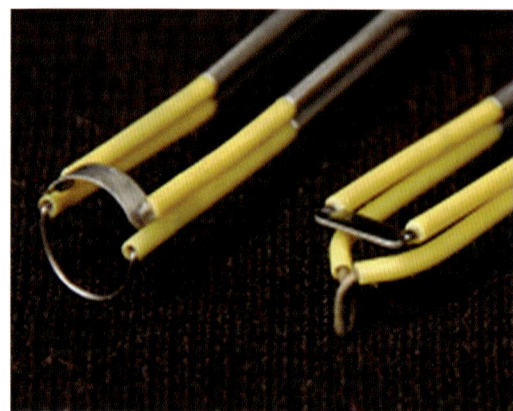

Fig. 14.22: Bipolar loops

b. A false passage can be created while entering the uterus. If muscle fibers are visible and the tubal ostia are not visible, assume the passage is false. Slowly remove the hysteroscope and identify the true cavity for confirmation. Discontinue the procedure if true cavity is not identifiable. Delay repeat hysteroscopy for 2 or 3 months. To avoid false passage, dilate the cervix with slow steady pressure and stop as soon as the internal os opens. If dilatation is not possible to the desired number, simply turn on the resectoscope's inflow with the outflow shut off, and let the fluid pressure dilate the cervix.
c. Perforation of the uterus: Most perforations, even those involving large dilators usually do not require treatment, but further assessment may be required to rule out bowel injury. When perforation occurs during the use of thermal energy, laparoscopy is necessary to assess the organs overlying the site.
d. Bleeding from lower uterus or cervical canal can obscure the view. Bleeding usually stops, coagulation with the electrode may be necessary when bleeding is heavy.
e. Intraoperative bleeding: Bleeding is more common when endometrial or fibroid resection is performed with loop electrode. Bleeding sufficient to require intervention occurs at a rate of 0.5 percent to 1.9 percent in several reported series. To achieve hemostasis, the vessel can be coagulated, if seen. If a bleeder is not identifiable, one can either pack the uterus with ribbon gauze soaked with diluted vasopressin or a Foley's catheter with balloon inflated with 15-20 ml of fluid for 2 hour. To reduce intra operative bleeding during operative hysteroscopy, Phillips et al[13] demonstrated a marked decrease in blood loss by injecting very dilute vasopressin (0.2 ml) in 60 ml of normal saline, directly into the cervix 2 cm deep, at the 4 and 8 o'clock positions. A vaporizing electrode may prevent significant blood loss during myoma resection (Versapoint). Preoperative Danazol or GnRH agonists decrease the thickness and vascularity of the endometrium and shrink fibroids.

Electrosurgical and Gaseous Complications

a. Perforation with an active electrode: This occurs when current is applied as the electrode is extended or the resectoscope is moved toward the fundus. It can be avoided if the electrode is activated only when moving it toward the operator.
b. Diversion of current: Electrode insufflation failure, which allows current to jump to the outer sheath of the resectoscope. To avoid this, inspect all the electrodes thoroughly before surgery.
c. To avoid return-pad injuries, keep the patient's thigh completely dry, ensure that the pad is flat against the skin at application.
A major step towards safety will be to switch to using bipolar resectoscope and a generator which generates bipolar cutting current.

Gas Embolism

Sources of gas embolism: room air, carbon dioxide, carbon monoxide, and other gaseous products of combustion. The anesthetist will be the first person to identify the following signs:
a. Sudden fall in oxygen saturation.
b. Sudden hypotension.
c. Hypercarbia.
d. Arrythmias, Tachypnea or a mill wheel murmur.

If gas embolism develops, stop the procedure immediately and ventilate the patient with 100 percent oxygen.

To reduce risk of gas embolism:
a. Avoid trendlenburg positioning.
b. Remove last dilator just before inserting the resectoscope.
c. Limit repeated removal-reinsertion of the resectoscope.
d. Vaporizing myomas eliminates the need to remove fibroids.
e. Intracervical injection of vasopressin may block gas from entering circulation.

Complications from Distension Media

Excess absorption of distension media is one of the most frequent complications in operative hysteroscopy. Especially when using monopolar electrosurgical instruments, electrolyte containing fluid is incompatible, and where 1.5 percent glycine is used, which can lead to dilutional hyponatremia and hypo-osmolality.[14] These conditions may have catastrophic consequences if they are not recognized promptly. The brain swells as it attempts to become iso-osmotic with the vascular system. If swelling exceeds 5 percent, the risk of severe neurological damage increases dramatically. This problem gets exaggerated in premenopausal women because of the inhibition of the sodium pump. Classic clinical features of hyponatremic hypovolemia include apprehension, confusion, fatigue, headache, mental agitation, nausea, visual disturbances, vomiting and weakness. These complications are more readily apparent when regional anesthesia is used rather than general anesthesia.

Guidelines for Distension Media

1. Use bipolar resectoscope, where isotonic electrolytic fluid, Ringer's lactate or 0.9 percent saline can be used.
2. Draw preoperative serum electrolytes for a baseline in all patients undergoing major monopolar resectoscopic surgery and evaluate electrolytes (Na$^+$) status of procedure and patients condition, if deficit is more than 1000 ml.
3. Continuously record inflow and outflow using the electronic monitor with deficit alarm set at 500 ml. If electronic device is not present in the operation theater, one attendant should be given the job of monitoring the amount of liquid infused and the amount that is drained in the suction bottle, he should alarm the surgeon of the deficit.
4. Discuss with the anesthetist (e.g. procedure, IV fluids, vital signs, pulse oximetry, patient's risks).
5. Consider epidural anesthesia in high-risks patients.
6. Keep the distension fluid at body temperature and monitor the patient's core temperature continuously.
7. If the fluid deficit reaches 750 ml, immediately give 20 to 40 mg of intravenous frusemide and draw serum sodium.
8. Interrupt the procedure for 5 to 10 minutes to allow the uterus to contact and to seal off small blood vessels.
9. Discontinue the procedure if the fluid deficit reaches 1,500 ml or if the serum sodium level is below 125 mEq/L.

The use of bipolar devices in normal saline prevents dilutional hyponatremia, but fluid deficits must still be monitored. Large fluid deficits can lead to pulmonary edema and death.

Postoperative and Late Complications

a. Infection rate, reported is 0.3 percent to 2 percent.
b. Hematometra.
c. Iatrogenic adenomyosis.
d. Post-ablation pregnancy.

DO'S AND DONT'S IN HYSTEROSCOPIC SURGERY

Do's

1. Always select the patients properly, paying attention to indications and contraindications.
2. Counsel the patient properly, regarding the procedure being attempted, their realistic results and the complications.
3. Get all the investigations necessary, like HSG, Transvaginal Sonography and have them evaluated just prior to the beginning of the surgery.
4. Keep all the equipment and instruments ready, before the surgery. The surgeon must know how to assemble and dismantle all the instruments himself and check their smooth functioning, just before the commencement of the surgery. Use good standard instruments and equipments.
5. Follow all the safety precautions recommended, like the inflow pressure, current settings, etc.
6. Try to use isotonic electrolyte containing solutions for all hysteroscopic surgeries.
7. Switch over to bipolar current as modality of choice in resectoscopic surgeries. If using monopolar current always use non-ionic electrolyte free solutions.

8. Have an attendant dedicated for monitoring the fluid deficit in all hysteroscopic surgeries.
9. Avoid Trendlenberg's position during hysteroscopic surgeries.
10. Use cervical softening agents like vaginal misoprostol for easy cervical dilatation.
11. Before embarking upon difficult surgeries like intrauterine adhesiolysis, submucous myoma resection, do sufficient diagnostic and simple hysteroscopic surgeries, to be well adjusted to all the steps.
12. At the beginning of surgery, always inspect the cavity of the uterus and identify the normal uterine anatomy.
13. In the event of fluid overload or any other complications abandon the procedure, identify the complication and immediately rectify them.
14. Always remember the surgery can be completed at a second sitting.
15. Keep proper record of all the procedure done and document all steps.
16. Inform the patient about the complications, if any and the need for subsequent follow up.

Dont's

1. Do not start surgery if instruments are malfunctioning.
2. Do not use unsafe pressure devices for delivering fluid.
3. Do not give deep head low positions.
4. Do not over dilate the cervix.
5. Do not begin or continue surgery if the anatomy is not clear.
6. Do not use electrolyte containing solutions for monopolar resectoscopic surgeries.
7. Don't exceed the recommended fluid the deficit during hysteroscopic surgeries.

REFERENCES

1. Dongen H, Kolkman W, Jansen FW. Hysteroscopy: Perspectives on skills training. J Am Assoc Gynecol Laparosc. 2007;4:121-5.
2. Lethaby A, Shepperd S, Cooke I, Farquhar C. Endometrial resection and ablation versus hysterectomy for heavy menstrual bleeding. Cochrane Database Syst Rev. 2000;CD000329
3. Sowter MC, Singla AA, Lethaby A. Pre-operative endometrial thinning agents before hysteroscopic surgery for heavy menstrual bleeding. Cochrane Database Syst Rev. 2000;CD001124.
4. Hill D, Maher P, Wood C, et al. Complications of Operative hysteroscopy. Gynaecolog Endosc. 1992;185-9.
5. Jansen FW, Vredevoogd CB, van Ulzen K, Hermans J, Trimboss JB. Complications of hysteroscopy: a prospective, multicenter study, Obstet Gynecol. 2000;96:266-70.
6. Aydeniz B, Gruber IV, Schauf B, Kurek R, Meyer A, A Multicenter survey of complications associated with 21,676 operative hysteroscopies. Eur J Obstet Gynecol Reprod Biol. 2002;104:160-4.
7. Baggish MS. Distending Media for Panoramic Hysteroscopy: 16,201-12.
8. Valle RF. Hysteroscopy, Visual perspectives of Uterine Anatomy, Physiology and Pathology, 3rd Edition:17: 213-25.
9. Letterie GS. Surgery, Assisted Reproductive Technology and Infertility.2nd Edition: 13:351-73.
10. March CM. Hysteroscopy for Infertility. Hysteroscopy, Visual perspectives of Uterine Anatomy, Physiology and Pathology, 3rd Edition:28: 417-50.
11. Debirashrafi H, Mohammed K, Moghhadami-Tabirzi N, et al. Is estrogen therapy necessary after hysteroscopic incision of uterine septum? J Am Assoc Gynecol Laparosc 1996;3 623-5.
12. Magos AL, et al. Experience with the first 250 endometrial resections for menorrhagia. Lancet. 1991;337:1074-8.
13. Philips DR, Nathanson HG, Milil SJ, et al. The effect of dilute vasopressin solution on intraoperative blood loss during operative hysteroscopy: a randomized control trial. Obstet Gynecol. 1996;88:761-6.
14. Istre O, Shajja K, et al. Changes in serum electrolytes after transcervical resection of endometrium and submucous fibroids with the use of 1.5 percent glycine for irrigation. Obstet Gynecol.1992;80:218-22.

CHAPTER 15

Safe Management of Female Urinary Incontinence

Prakash H Trivedi, Maya Prasad, Neha Rani

Chapter Outline

- Magnitude of the Problem
  - Essentials for Safe Management of Female Urinary Incontinence
- Safety Points for Laparoscopic Burch
- Trivedi's Adjustable Tape

MAGNITUDE OF THE PROBLEM

With advancing age; due to better health care of females we have a larger section of women with good longevity, of course, this comes at a price. Taking care at 40 plus becomes prevention and later due to advanced age it has to be cured or treated.

It is estimated that almost 16 million women in India have urinary incontinence of different types. Quite often, they are tossed up between general practitioner, gynecologist and urologist. Very often beyond antibiotic, vaginal cream and urine alkalinizers are prescribed, with no benefit. One may have lack of knowledge in the subject or has knowledge but feels it's trivial and small for focused attention.

The woman suffers in silence and it doesn't become a laughing matter as they leak urine on a hearty laugh. There may be more than 130 surgeries for treatment for stress urinary incontinence and unlike in the past, other incontinence—urge, bladder instability, frequency, etc. can be now dealt with newer medications quite effectively.

Essentials for Safe Management of Female Urinary Incontinence

1. Complete knowledge on the subject.
2. To carry out necessary investigations, urodynamic studies, etc. when needed.
3. Most important is accurate history taking. Without going into elaborate details sufficing it to say that whether she has burning while passing urine or pain or fever may suggest cystitis, if she had many deliveries or forceps delivery and on cough, laugh, change in movements leaks small quantity of urine then this is stress urinary incontinence (SUI). The same takes place around menopause. SUI may be withheld for short time on medications by selective serotonin norepinephrine reuptake inhibitor (SSNRI) which acts as a medical sphincter, till she plans surgery if GSUI or sphincter deficiency persists. Urgency, frequency and urge incontinence has enough queries but can be distinguished by proper history. Corrected by medical treatment with commonly used drugs tolteridine, rolefenacin, solifenacin, darifenacin, etc.
4. Clinical examination and investigation.

The patient should be told to keep bladder partially full. On clinical examination she is asked to cough and watch for any demonstrable leak, even of small quantity of urine, then it is stress urinary incontinence **(Fig. 15.1)**.

If not in supine position, ask her to stand with legs apart and occasionally with knees bend and legs apart. We can see demonstrable small quantity of urine leak then it is stress

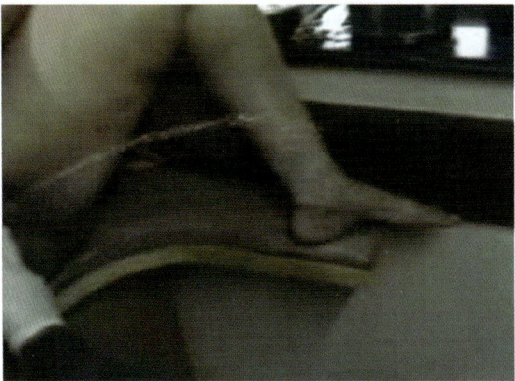

Fig. 15.1: Demonstrable stress urinary incontinence

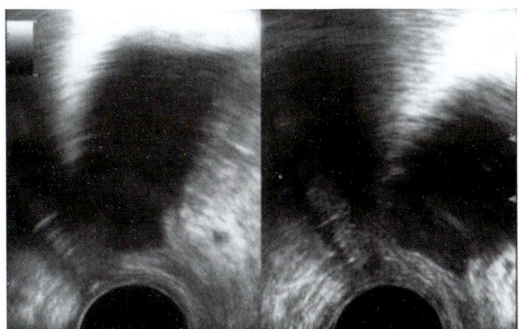

Fig. 15.2: Stress urinary incontinence

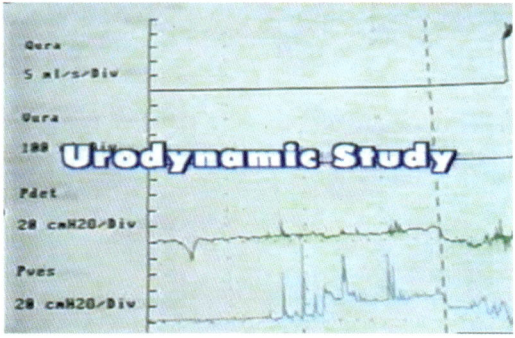

Fig. 15.3: Urodynamics study strip

incontinence. A large leak or less severe jet of urine on clinical examination can be picked up as genuine SUI or intrinsic sphincter deficiency on urodynamic study.

A simple clinical evaluation of raising the mid urethra with two fingers upward gently pressed towards symphysis or with opened sponge holder correcting leak of urine on cough or sneeze, suggest urethral hypermobility. Evaluate presence of cystocele, prolapse, etc. In a Q-tip test, a long bud or a stick just entering the bladder, if the tip goes upwards on cough or sneeze, it suggests urethral hypermobility. The same can be picked up by transvaginal sonography **(Fig. 15.2)**.

Urodynamic study **(Fig. 15.3)** is very useful but not compulsory in all cases, but in case of doubt of mixed incontinence, intrinsic sphincter deficiency, bladder instability or failed procedure.[1]

5. If surgery needed, choice of:
   a. Open burch/tape-sling procedure.
   b. Laparoscopic burch sutures/tape.
   c. Transabturator sling outside in. Monarch, Trivedi's obturator tape.
   d. TVT- O inside out.
   e. Miniarc, TVT secure.
   f. Bulking injections.

Anti-incontinence surgery can be done with or without any associated procedures like hysterectomy or anterior or posterior compartment defect corrected by open, laparoscopic or trans perineal new mesh, though currently the Trans obturator sling is preferred with different products.

SAFETY POINTS FOR LAPAROSCOPIC BURCH

Modified lithotomy position with possible adjustable leg rest, fill the bladder by 250 ml of fluid, identify the upper limit of the bladder **(Fig. 15.4A)**, make incision above it to enter Space of Retzius **(Fig. 15.4B)**.

Laparoscopic CO_2 insufflation creates planes by bubbles between bladder and space of retzius laterally. Harmonic scalpel is necessary and enhances by cavitational effect.

Once the para urethral space is dissected, the bladder with catheter is seen and free space created around midurethra **(Fig. 15.5)**.

The most important part now is to empty bladder, with the needle and goretex no. 2 sutures on curved needle are introduced through ports. Next, the operator puts his or her own fingers to elevate mid urethra while taking helical stitches 2 cm below and lateral to the bladder neck **(Fig. 15.6)**.

Then same suture on the Cooper's ligament from the needle holder on the same side **(Fig. 15.7)** to avoid injury to aberrant obturator vessel which may present.

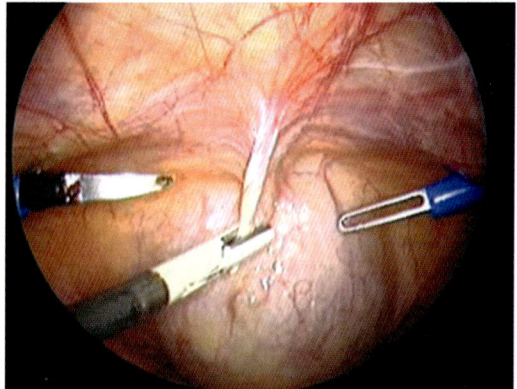

Fig. 15.4A: Upper limit of the distendes

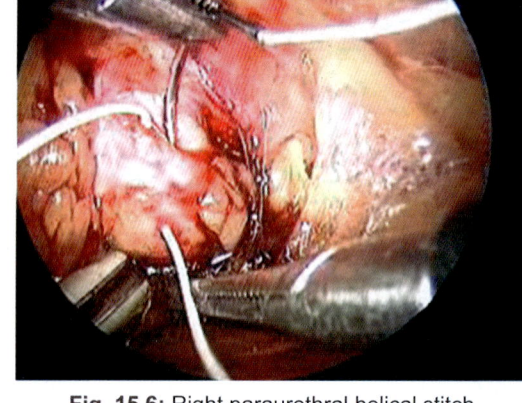

Fig. 15.6: Right paraurethral helical stitch

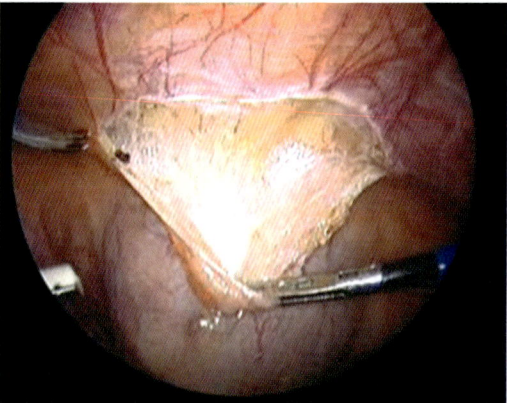

Fig. 15.4B: Entry into space of retzius bladder

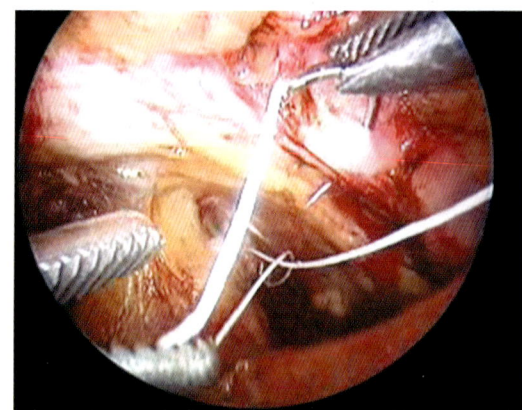

Fig. 15.7: Right Cooper's ligament stitch

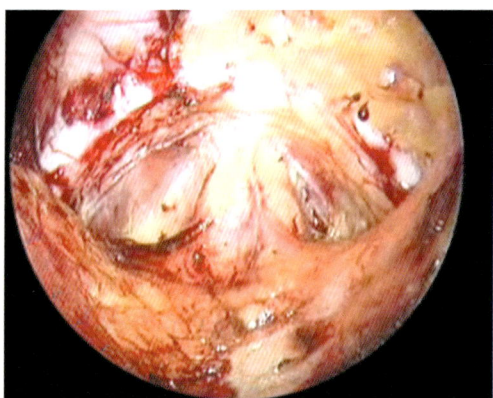

Fig. 15.5: Space of retzius dissected urethra, bladder neck and Cooper's ligament

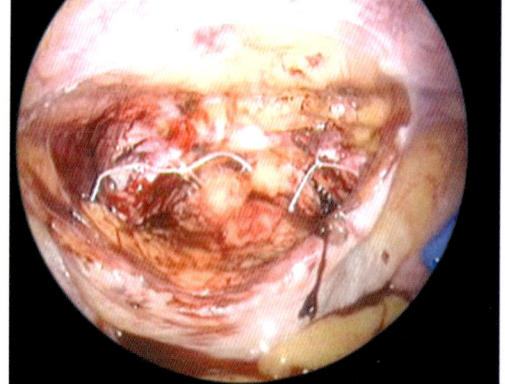

Fig. 15.8: Burch-bilateral colposuspension

The knots are tied with goretex suture as hammock on both sides **(Fig. 15.8)** not too tight.

A Mersilene tape is used by many and tuckers are used especially at Cooper's ligament and not ideally on vagina. The space of Retzius and peritoneum is closed to avoid bowel adhesion. Burch should not be done if there is intrinsic sphincters deficiency. The sling tape has replaced Burch for both GSUI and ISD.

Role of Sling—New Tapes—TVT, TSUIT, Monarc, TrOT, TVT-O, Miniarc, TVT Secure

As midurethra is to be supported on which the bladder rocks back on cough or sneeze. As the suburethral first group of sling were good but higher complication rate, were replaced by transobturator sling/tape.[2] We will give more points of safety for transobturator sling like Monarc or TrOT, outside-in technique **(Figs 15.9 to 15.11)**.

Placement of TrOT

Patient is under spinal, epidural, saddle block or short general anesthesia, patient in normal lithotomy position. There is no need for catheter or cystoscopy. The vaginal dissection is started by infiltration of a combination normal saline with 0.25-0.5 percent sensorcaine and 3-4 drops of adrenaline. Vaginal incision is 1.5 cm from the external urethral meatus a vertical incision of 1.5-2 cm is taken **(Fig. 15.12)**. Dissect the vagina and the finger enters the space below the sub pubic angle easily by blunt dissection.

Small saline adrenaline soaked gauze is kept in the dead space. Now the important landmark for the outside in technique, identify the adductor longus tendon and below that the obturator foramen's upper and medical most point close to the thigh crease, a 4 mm incision is made with 11 no. knife after infiltrating with 5 ml of 0.25-0.5 percent sensorcaine undiluted to reduce pain postoperative **(Fig. 15.13)**.

The Monarc or TrOT **(Fig. 15.11)** outside-in needle is first inserted perpendicularly to perforate obturator membrane **(Fig. 15.13A)**, then with index of the other hand in the vagina and the thumb of the same hand guiding the needle, the handle which is angulated by 45° **(Fig. 15.13B)** pushing the needle and gradually

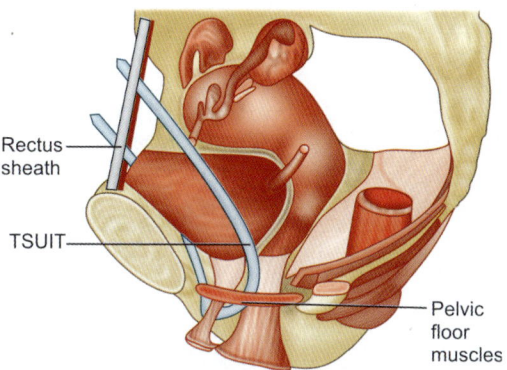

Fig. 15.9: Dynamic action of TVT/TSUIT/TrOT/Monarc on cough

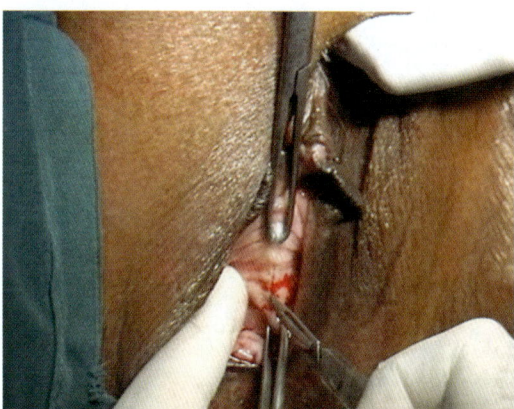

Fig. 15.11: Vaginal vertical incision of 1.5 cm

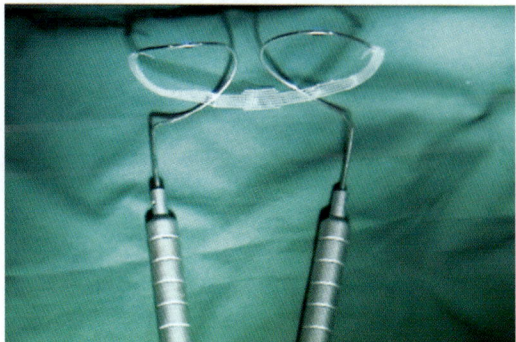

Fig. 15.10: Monarc, TrOT

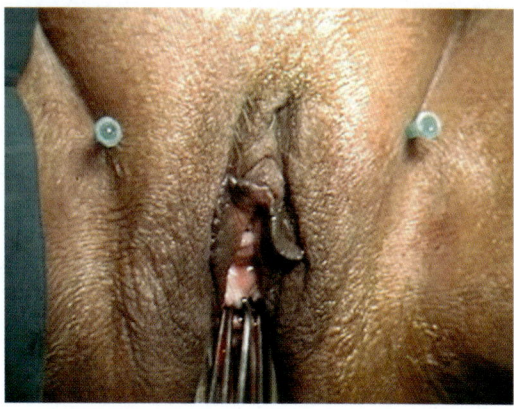

Fig. 15.12: Important landmarks for outside in technique

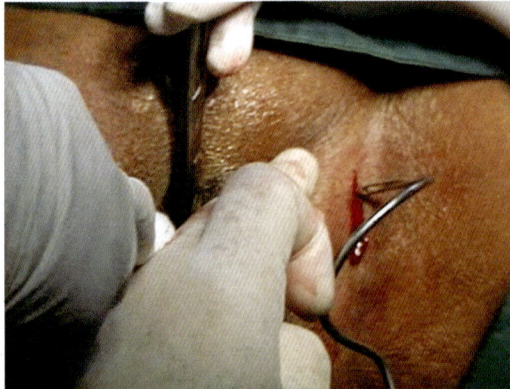

Fig. 15.13A: Perpendicular entry of Monarc or TrOT needle

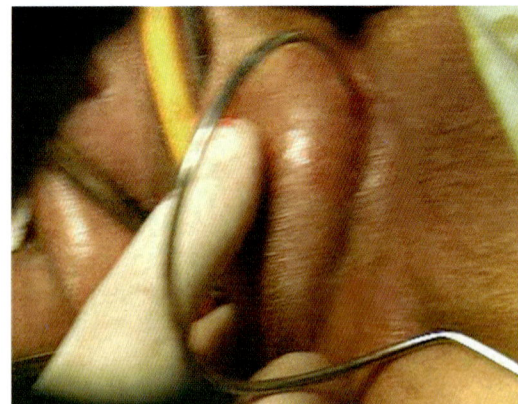

Fig. 15.13B: A 45 degree angulation of the shaft pushing the needle

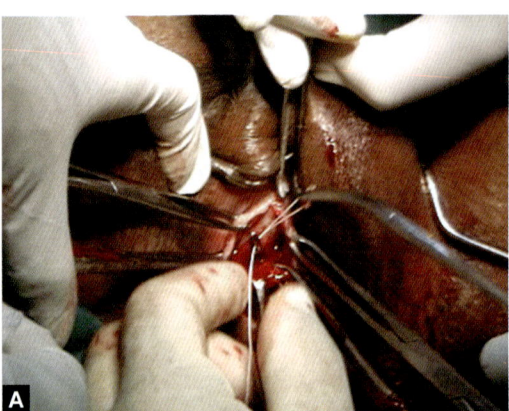
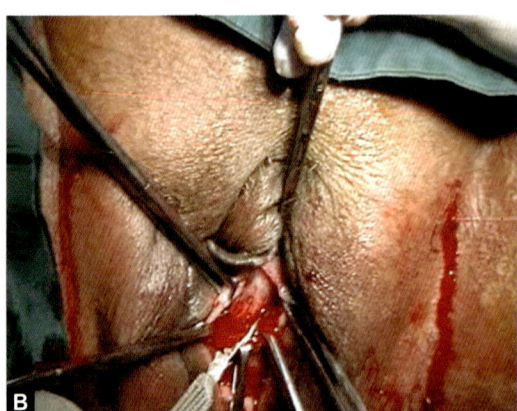

Figs 15.14A and B: TrOT tape tied in the eye of needle pulled out of obturator foramen

comes out in the vagina below the subpubic angle below the vagina dissected and out from the area with tip of the needle pointing the urethra.

The Monarc tape is anchored or TrOT is tied at the eye of the needle carrying back the tape or sling—Monarc/Trivedi's tape on one side and the same on opposite side **(Figs 15.14 and 14.15)**.

The tape/sling is kept tension free in the mid urethra. The vagina is closed and extra tape outside the obturator foramen is cut and skin pulled so the tape sinks in subcutaneous tissue **(Fig. 15.16)**. The results are on the spot and so are failures. In SUI the tape may not erode but can herniate through opening of vaginal suture with relief from SUI because fibrosis is already developed, in that case the tape can be cut and vagina closed fresh again.

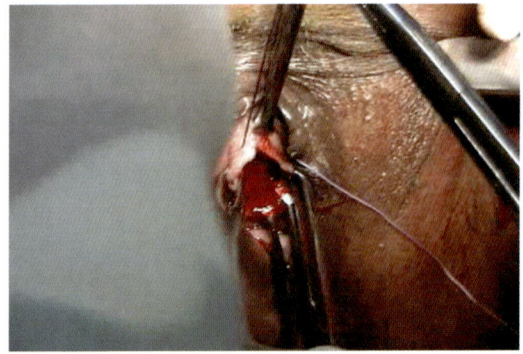

Fig. 15.15: Tension free TrOT

The chance of entering bladder is insignificant with TrOT or obturator route unless there is a cystocele; hence no cystoscopy or catheterization is needed.

Procedures like miniarc and TVT-secure are not elaborated as their long-term results are not good and still in research.

TRIVEDI'S ADJUSTABLE TAPE

This is like TrOT but has specially woven nonabsorbable threads which allow us to tighten or loosen the tape till 48-72 hours after surgery and these four nonabsorbable threads can then be pulled out easily. The procedure is shown in **Figures 15.17A to C**. Few more refinements would make this as the standard tape or sling for GSUI or ISD.

TVT or TSUIT the vaginal SUI Sling used less nowadays was a sling placed sub midurethra and coming out of the abdomen **(Fig. 15.18)**.

The original TVT and TSUIT needed a 20 French Foley's catheter to pass a metal guide to take the bladder on the opposite side where the

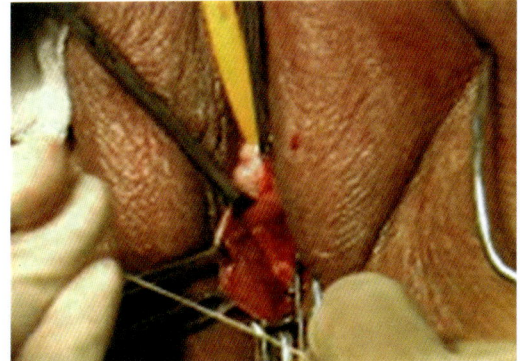

Fig. 15.17B: Needle seen coming out below the midurethra

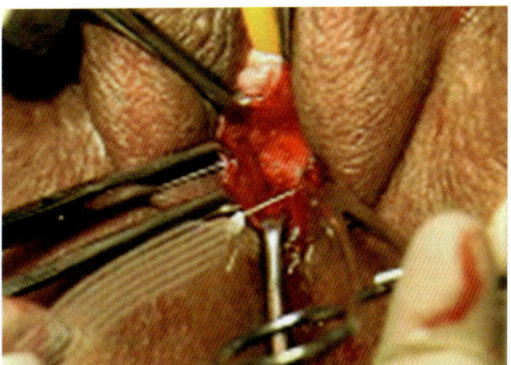

Fig. 15.17C: Loading of Tr-O tape on the TrOT needle's eye

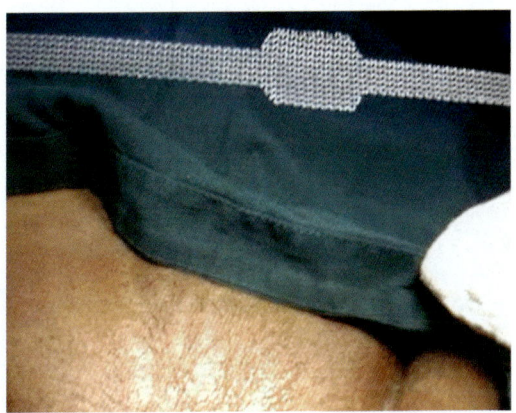

Fig. 15.16: Trivedi's adjustable tape

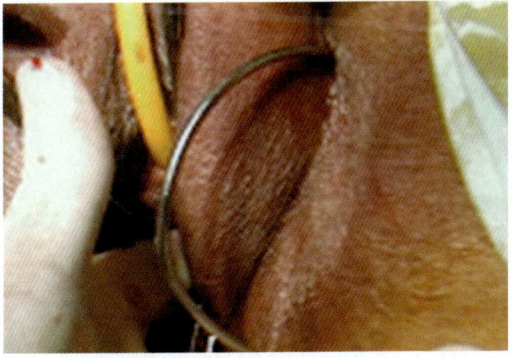

Fig. 15.17A: Left needle insertion at the upper and medial most area of obturator foramen

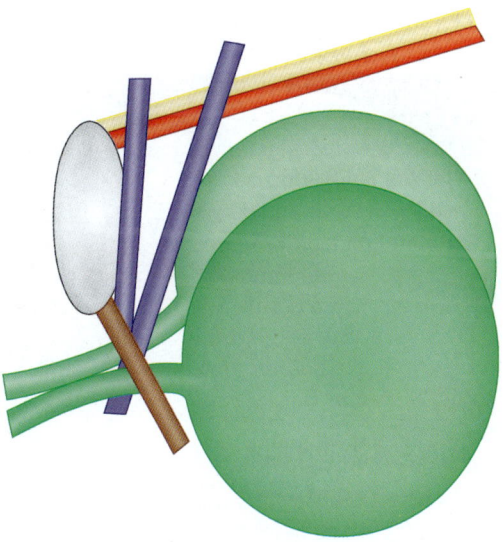

Fig. 15.18: Mechanism of action of midurethral application of TVT/TSUIT

needle were used usually from below upwards coming 3 cms lateral to the midline i.e. the posterior part of pubic tubercle.

Further on 70° cystoscope with a Fore oblique shape was necessary to identify the bladder injury or placement of the mesh in the musculature of bladder.

There were complications of retention. Also entry into the bladder **(Figs 15.19A to C)** and other structures around could be injured.[3-5]

Vaginal dissection is like TrOT but the needle goes from the vagina entering through space of Retzius, coming out 3 cms away from the midline in the abdomen as the metal guide takes the empty bladder away. Attached tape is also pulled up **(Figs 15.20A to C)**. The same

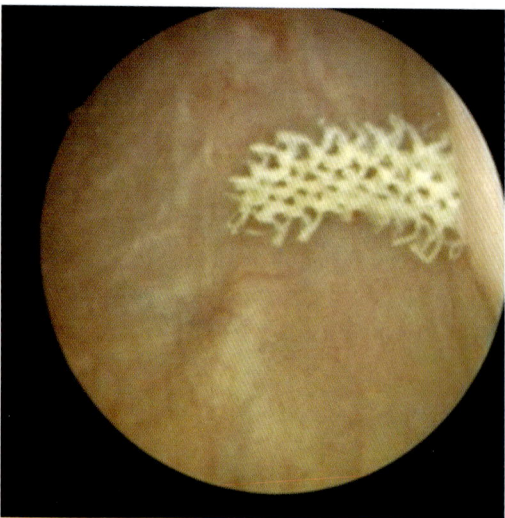

Fig. 15.19C: Last part of tape in bladder

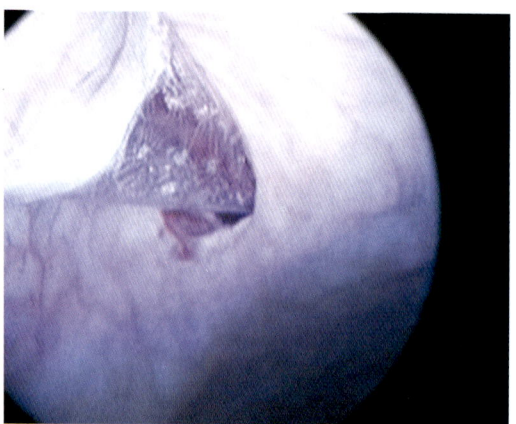

Fig. 15.19A: Bladder perforation of TVT/TSUIT

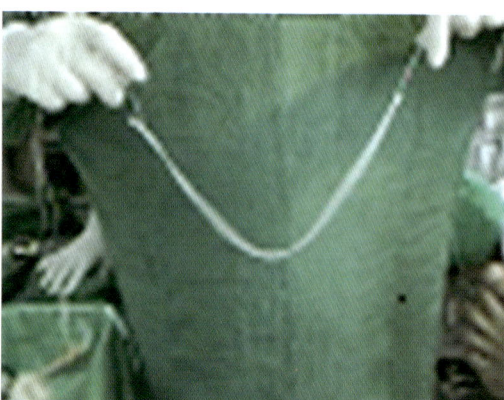

Fig. 15.20A: TSUIT tape

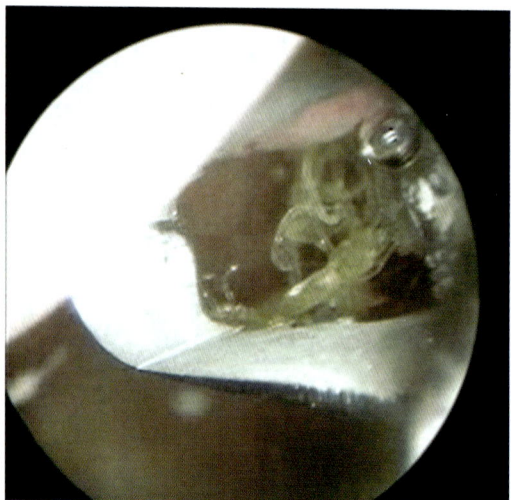

Fig. 15.19B: Calcified tape in bladder

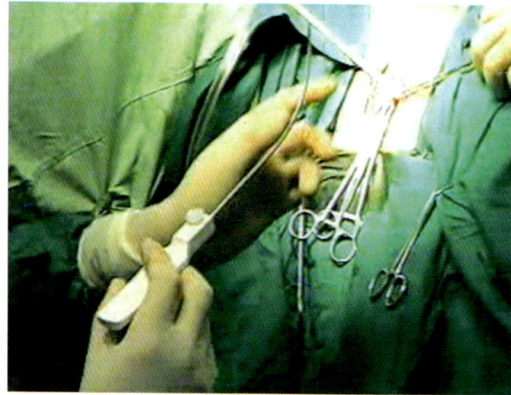

Fig. 15.20B: TSUIT tapes pulled out on both sides

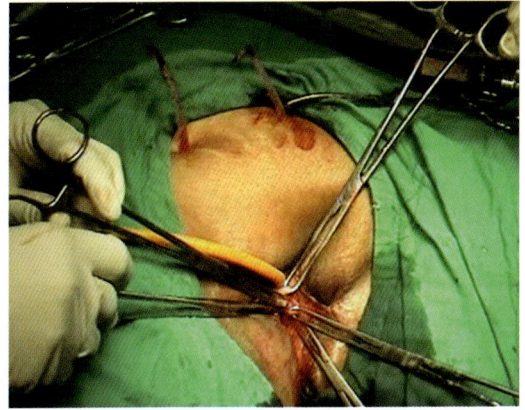

Fig. 15.20C: TSUIT needle

is repeated on the other side. Vagina is closed with continuous Vicryl 2-0 or Vicryl Rapide.

CONCLUSION

Urinary problems, especially frequency, urgency, urge incontinence, bladder instability–detrussor dysynnergia, genuine stress urinary incontinence, intrinsic sphincter deficiency affect millions of women who come more often to gynecologist and general practioners, less to urologist directly. First four conditions are corrected by medicines very effectively. GSUI and ISD needs surgery, now a trans obturator sling which is quick, easy and has excellent results and need for catheter, cystoscopy being absent, having minimal complications have replaced burch or Marshal Marcheti Krantz and other thread suspension procedures. The new Trivedi's adjustable tape can reduce post operative retentions or poor outcomes, holds promise for future. Female urinary incontinence is to be managed by urogynecologist, i.e. ether gynecologist or urologist having focused attention for the subject and experience.

REFERENCES

1. J Christian Winters, RA Appell, Practical Urodynamics, Nitti, Chapter 16,184-96, 1998.
2. Delorme E, Trans obturator urethral suspension: mini invasive procedure in the treatment of SUI in women. Prog Urol 2001; 11:1306-13.
3. Kuuva N, Nilsson CG. A nation wide analysis of complications associated with TVT procedure. Acta Obstet Gynecol Scand 2002;81:72-7.
4. Tsivian A, Mogutin B, et al. TVT procedure for the treatment of female SUI: Long term result. J. Urol 2004; 172:998-1000.
5. Canis Sanchez D, Bielsa Gali O, et al. Results and complications of TVT procedures in the surgical treatment of female SUI. Actas Urol Esp.2005;29:289-91.

CHAPTER 16

Performing Safe Multicompartment Mesh Replacement Surgery

Ajay Rane, Jay Iyer

Chapter Outline

- General Considerations for Mesh Surgery
  - Assessment
  - Investigations
  - Preoperative Stategies
  - Clinical Governance
  - Intraoperative Considerations
- Mesh Extrusions/Erosions/Sexual Sysfunction
- Specific Considerations for Mesh Surgery
  - Anterior Compartment
  - Apical Compartment
  - Posterior Compartment

INTRODUCTION

The life expectancy for women has almost doubled through the 20th century. With the significant increase in our postmenopausal female population, there is a growing demand for improved quality of life and management of pelvic floor dysfunction.[1] Surgery for pelvic organ prolapse has evolved over the past two hundred years and continues to be influenced by dynamically changing concepts involving not just newer approaches to the difficult problem of recurrent pelvic organ prolapse but also by a renewed understanding of pelvic floor anatomy.

It is important to remember that ones approach towards surgery for pelvic organ prolapse (POP) be dictated by patient symptoms. A significant prolapse, of any of the three compartments, is defined as one that reaches the hymenal ring, i.e. points Ba, C or Bp are at '0' by the POP-Q classification. Indeed operating on 'asymptomatic' patients is best avoided because the only thing she will get postoperatively are 'symptoms'![2-4]

Richard Te Linde famously commented "the patient should ask the gynecologist for relief; the gynecologist should not urge the patient to have corrective surgery if she does not feel sufficiently uncomfortable to request it" (Rock and Howard, 2008).

GENERAL CONSIDERATIONS FOR MESH SURGERY

Assessment

Assessment of prolapse needs to done mindful of the day-to-day situations that aggravate it; for example examining a woman after a bout of exercise. The dorsal or the lithotomy position may not reveal an enterocele, whereas a squatting or a semi-crouching position might be useful (Rock and Howard, 2008). One should never hesitate to perform a rectal or bidigital examination that is not only useful in distinguishing between enteroceles and rectoceles but also effectively evaluates damage to the perineal body. Involve the patient by using mirrors to help understand what is it that bothers the patient and also to explain what you plan to do and what she should expect from her operation.

Investigations

Investigation modalities like ultrasound, MRI and defecation proctography are underutilized albeit being extremely useful adjuncts in preoperative planning especially in recurrent genital prolapse and often reveal hitherto unrecognized defects in anatomy and function.[5-8]

Preoperative Stategies

Counseling and Education

Adequate preoperative patient education and postoperative support is essential to help reduce readmission rates when performing prolapse operations in ambulatory day surgery. It is important to appreciate that results of mesh repair, be they 'augmented' or 'replacement' grafts, are always good in the short term and only studies with longer than a years follow-up reveal the true picture (A Rane et al, 2008). So one should be wary of promising 'too much too soon'. It is appropriate to use preoperative vaginal oestrogen and advise pelvic floor physiotherapy that ideally should continue postoperatively as well.[9] It is desirable to employ strategies that reduce chronic pelvic floor stress like ensuring weight loss, treating constipation and chronic cough.[10]

Sexual Function

It is often forgotten that the vagina is not just a copulatory organ but also moves dynamically during defecation and voiding. The natural tissue planes that allow for this may become stiff and less compliant when mesh is used inappropriately. Always consider 'His' and 'Her' pareunia whilst planning surgery – male dyspareunia seems invariably associated with stiff graft material exposure whilst female dyspareunia seems to be more associated with excessive graft tensioning or with shortening and narrowing of the vaginal canal.[2,11,12]

Concomitant Incontinence

About 50 percent of women with vault prolapse will have occult stress urinary incontinence and thus there may well be a role for preoperative urodynamics.[13,14]

Underdiagnosis and Consenting Issues

Another issue that needs consideration is the under diagnosis of severity of POP that can occur in about a third of cases in outpatient assessments. Preoperative assessment under anesthesia is invaluable and when the true severity of prolapse is revealed, the pelvic surgeon should have numerous choices available to correct the prolapse without compromising the consent for surgery. When the use of mesh is contemplated it follows that there should be an inherently flexible plan in place to cover for dealing with unforeseen compartmental defects.

Appropriate Training

Every needle, every kit is different- helical needles, open curve needles, self retrieving needles, needles with inner and outer sheaths all require a detailed knowledge of anatomical safety–preferably demonstrated on cadavers first. Understanding the needle curvatures, the directional reversals of the needle tips with respect to the handles and last but perhaps most importantly their spatial relationships within the three dimensionality of female pelvic anatomy is foremost in preventing major visceral and vascular injuries.[15] It is vital that replacement mesh surgery be performed per protocol established by the manufacturer as any deviations from the accepted technique can cause untold damage to the woman besides being medicolegally indefensible. One needs to have knowledge of complications that could potentially result with pelvic reconstructive surgery and importantly be capable of managing these; especially the severe ones.

Clinical Governance

There has been an unprecedented 'explosion' in various kinds of mesh delivering kits with biotech companies aggressively marketing these. This relatively new technology has not had the benefit of many robust randomized controlled trials or case controlled studies done to address the pros and cons.[16,17] The proliferation of different types of synthetic and biologic meshes without comprehending their individual biodynamics could lead to delayed complications.[18] There is also a tendency among biotech companies to change meshes in their kits with little or no warning or information to end users.

Intraoperative Considerations

Positioning

Patient positioning should be supervised by surgeon–it is too awkward to change mid operation especially when the vaginal route is being employed. Anatomy also changes with changing patient position and major complications could result if this fact is not appreciated.

Graft Augmentation or Graft Replacement

There seems a clear difference appearing in the outcomes of these two separate methodologies – most reported studies are on graft augmented surgery – augmentation appears to be extrafascial whilst replacement surgery is necessarily intrafascial with graft placed close to the viscus.[15]

Hydrodissection

It is good practice to use hydrodissection with local anesthetic mixed with diluted epinephrine. Not only does it help in developing the natural relatively avascular tissue planes in the pelvic floor, it facilitates proper mesh placement, reduces the incidence of visceral or neurovascular damage and is of immense benefit in carrying the dissection through the full thickness of the vagina.[15] The tissue planes between the viscus and the lateral pelvic wall can usually be developed efficiently with a combination of blunt and sharp dissection **(Fig. 16.1)**.

Deeper Dissection

The latter ensures that the mesh lies directly abutting the prolapsing viscus. This markedly reduces the chance of mesh erosion besides meeting the core requirement of reducing the prolapse of the affected organ; not of its enveloping fascia[15] **(Fig. 16.2)**.

Skin Excision

In this crucial point one sees a departure from the conventional surgical belief that has led generations of surgeons to believe that skinning the vagina clear of its fascia is essential to a good repair. This, added to the fact that no or minimal vaginal skin is excised in mesh surgery, makes the whole concept counter-intuitive. The operated area often looks, as it should, visually unpleasing, as if the prolapse has not been reduced at all this is in fact an indirect indicator of appropriate mesh tensioning (Muffly and Barber, 2010).[15] **(Fig. 16.3)**.

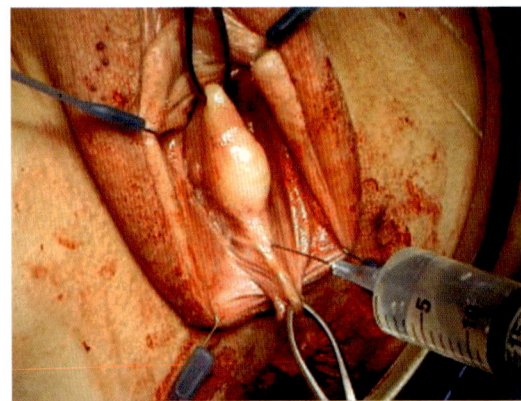

Fig. 16.1: Hydrodissection

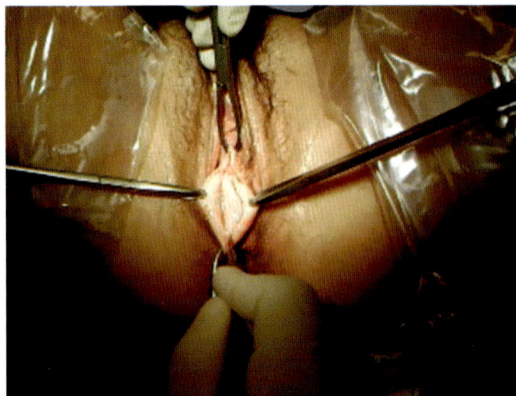

Fig. 16.2: Full thickness vaginal dissection

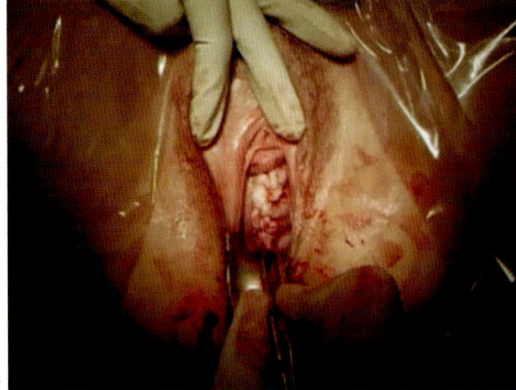

Fig. 16.3: End result of anterior elevate for cystocele: apparently prolapse still present

Vaginal Remodeling

Herein lies the beauty of mesh surgery it factors in the concept of vaginal remodeling that allows surrounding tissues to restructure in much the same way the vagina involutes to its pre-pregnancy state following vaginal birth.[19,20] In our unit we do not excise "excess" vaginal tissue even in cases of advanced procidentia because at the end of the day the prolapsing organ, namely the bladder, rectum or the vault as the case may be, has been reduced by the mesh. Any attempt to make the vagina appear "taut" is almost always as a result of excessive mesh tensioning or vaginal skin removal. In a recent study in our unit we have been able to demonstrate that there is no histopathological difference in vaginal quality in prolapsed and non-prolapsed tissue. This further confirms the fact that the vagina in fact does 'remodel' and the concept that prolapsed tissues are stretched or devitalized- therefore can be 'sacrificed', no longer holds any water!

Anchorage

Pivotal to the success of mesh replacement surgery is the key factor of 'Anchorage'. Robust anchorage carries the day where suture anchorage invariably tends to fall through. Currently the sacrospinous ligament lies at the heart of mesh surgery it is relatively avascular, has a fixed anatomic location with well-circumscribed boundaries, identifiable even in obese women and acts as a sturdy anchor. The anterior approach to the sacropinous ligament is an art that requires some degree of relearning and is quintessential to mesh surgery[21] **(Fig. 16.4)**.

Multicompartmental Prolapse

It is important to address prolapse of each compartment as a separate operation chiefly because they deal with different prolapsing organs that need individually tailored solutions. It is good practice to approach each compartment through separate colpotomy incisions, irrigate tissues during repair, lay the mesh as flat as possible on the abutting viscus carefully avoiding excessive tension in the mesh limbs and rolling of mesh edges.[22] The latter can be achieved using a couple of anchoring sutures to the underlying fascia.

Vaginal Closure

Additionally a two-layered vaginal closure makes mesh erosion less likely as much as it reduces dead space preventing hematomas (A Rane, personal communication).

Dose of Mesh

It is useful to think of mesh as a medication that needs to be used in the 'correct dose' - so trim the mesh to meet individual requirements.[23] **(Fig. 16.5)**.

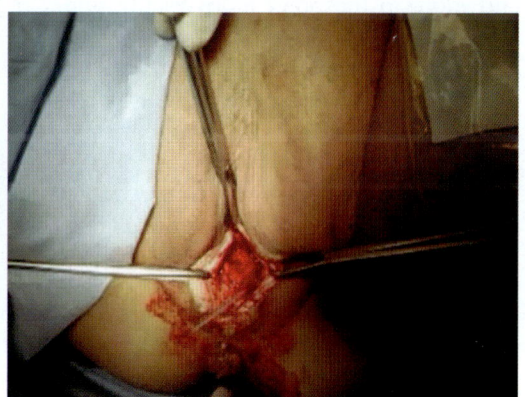

Fig. 16.4: Sacrospinous anchor in place

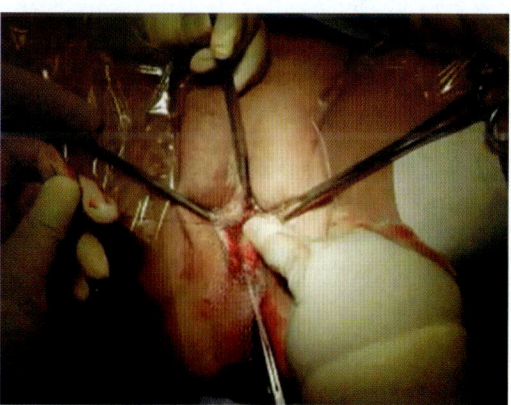

Fig. 16.5: Posterior mesh elevate to be trimmed to patient's requirement

MESH EXTRUSIONS/EROSIONS/SEXUAL DYSFUNCTION

The anterior compartment is most prone to mesh failures and mesh erosion, the latter usually an effect of an overtly tensioned graft.

A word about mesh erosion - it is important to remove as much of the visible mesh as possible before performing a layered closure.[24] Mesh-related complications after mid urethral slings and mesh sacrocolpopexies with monofilament polypropylene are uncommon. Even so up to a 26 percent mesh erosion rate and up to 38 percent dyspareunia rate with vaginally introduced mesh for pelvic-organ prolapse repair has been reported. Concurrent hysterectomy seems to increase mesh erosion rates.[25,26]

SPECIFIC CONSIDERATIONS FOR MESH SURGERY

Anterior Compartment

Mesh augmented surgery, i.e. placing a mesh on the cystocele and attaching it to fascia around it is doomed to fail as the lateral attachments to the arcus tendineus fascia pelvis is not addressed. Even the so-called vaginal para-vaginal repairs are unable to adequately address level 2 support mainly on account of poor anchorage. The sacrospinous ligament has been the pivotal structure in the pelvis around which all the recent needle driven mesh technology has evolved.

The Perigee™/Anterior Prolift™ system has two helical needles designed specifically to be driven through two entry points in access portal viz. the obturator foramen. The needles pass through the arcus tendineus providing level 2 support. These exit through the vagina when the mesh is attached to it and retrieved by reversing the needles through the same track. It is evident that this technique allows for arcus-to-arcus suspension of the bladder thereby treating the cystocele. The FDA notification and NICE statement alluded to have forced the biotech majors to change tack and devise a way to achieve the same objective without transgressing the obturator foramen thereby reducing complications that were associated with needle driven procedures.[27] Invented by Professor Rane – the 5 years data on 350 cases of Perigee™, which is the longest follow-up to date, shows a low rate of cytocele recurrence of 5.71 percent and mesh erosion rates of 11 percent falling to 2 percent especially in the later years of follow up. Sexual function was unimpaired or improved in almost 93 percent of the women and satisfaction rates were high.

The Anterior Elevate™ was developed to offset the perceived disadvantages of the transobturator perigee or prolift procedure. This new system utilises a single colpotomy incision to drive an anchor into the sacrospinous ligament that in turn will be used to fix and lock in the mesh. The mesh is also attached through an in-built anchor to the obturator internus muscle in close proximity to the arcus tendineus. Thus the Anterior Elevate™ system addresses two levels of support, apical or level one via the sacrospinous ligament and level two at the arcus tendineus. So it is also effective in the subset of cases that have a cervical/vault descent or enterocele co-existing with a large cystocele. Interestingly the mesh is not directly attached to the sacrospinous ligament, which provides surrogate anchorage, and thus there is no deviation of the vaginal axis unlike that seen with a classical sacrospinous colpopexy.

Apical Compartment

The apical compartment deserves special mention because it often co-exists with the more obvious anterior or posterior vaginal prolapse and more to the point is invariably under or inappropriately treated. Although it is usually addressed adequately with a McCall's culdoplasty or a sacrospinous hitch, it may necessitate a sacrocolpopexy (SCP)/hysteropexy especially in a woman with a short vagina all too often following overzealous vaginal trimming; the bane of older 'AP' repairs. The Anterior Elevate™ is an alternative worth considering in this situation.

Sacrocolpopexy

Bowel dysfunction is not uncommon following a SCP and this may suggest that is an operation that inherently involves "over correction". The laparoscopic approach to a SCP is preferred although it requires advanced skills that have a steep learning curve. It is preferable to use a light weight polypropylene mesh for SCP's and important to efficiently anchor the graft to both ends remembering these are the commonest sites for mesh 'fracture' leading to recurrences.

Posterior Compartment

Fascial repair of rectocele has stood the test of time and whether one does a standard colporrhaphy, a site specific repair; attach the rectovaginal fascia to the uterosacral or ileococcygeus fascia the results are consistently good at over 85-90 percent success.[25,26] So only in a small subset of patients with very large rectocele or when a concomitant enterocele is invariably present in this setting does the patient need mesh surgery. As in the anterior compartment mesh augmentation has absolutely no role, as the rates of recurrence and mesh erosion are unacceptably high. It is here that an APOGEE™ or a Posterior Prolift™ or more recently the Posterior ELEVATE™ can be considered. All of these mesh systems help in not only reducing the prolapsed rectal wall but also effectively suspend the apex.

In conclusion every pelvic surgeon should define his or her 'comfort zone' while considering a procedure for a patient.

A word from the wise - do it when you believe in it and more importantly are trained for it (B Schull, personal communication)! One should desist from succumbing to pressure from ones peers as much as from the compelling persuasive tactics employed by the industry.

REFERENCES

1. Cardozo, Linda; Staskin, David. Textbook of Female Urology and Urogynecology. Informa Healthcare, 2nd edition, 2006.
2. Altman D, Elmér C, Kiilholma P, Kinne I, Tegerstedt G, Falconer C. Sexual dysfunction after trocar-guided transvaginal mesh repair of pelvic organ prolapse. Obstetrics and Gynecology 2009;113(1):127-33.
3. Hampton BS. Pelvic organ prolapse. Medicine and Health Rhode Island. 2009;92(1):5-9.
4. Kiilholma P, Nieminen K. Gynaecological Prolapses.Duodecim 2009;125(2):199-206.
5. Barry C, Dietz HP. The use of Ultrasound in the evaluation of pelvic organ prolapse. Reviews in Gynaecological and Perinatal Medicine 2005;5(3):182-95.
6. Dietz HP, Lekskulchai O. Ultrasound assessment of pelvic organ prolapse: the relationship between prolapse severity and symptoms. Ultrasound in Obstetrics and Gynecology 2007;29:688-91.
7. Dietz HP, Haylen BT, Broome J. Ultrasound in the quantification of female pelvic organ prolapse. Ultrasound in Obstetrics and Gynecology 18(5):511-4.
8. FM Kelvin, DS Hale, DD Maglinte, BJ Patten, JT Benson. Female pelvic organ prolapse: diagnostic contribution of dynamic cystoproctography and comparison with physical examination. American Journal of Roentgenology 1999;173:31-7.
9. Felding C, Mikkelsen AL, Clausen HV, Loft A, Larsen LG. Preoperative treatment with oestradiol in women scheduled for vaginal operation for genital prolapse. A randomised, double-blind trial. Maturitas 1992;15(3):241-9.
10. Bela I. Kudish, Cheryl B. Iglesia, Robert J. Sokol, Barbara Cochrane, Holly E. Richter, Joseph Larson et al. Effect of weight change on natural history of pelvic organ prolapse. Obstetrics and Gynecology 2009;113(1):81-8.
11. Feiner B, Jelovsek JE, Maher C. Efficacy and safety of transvaginal mesh kits in the treatment of prolapse of the vaginal apex: a systematic review. British Journal of Obstetrics and Gynaecology 2009;116(1):15-24.
12. Feiner B, Maher C. Vaginal mesh contraction: definition, clinical presentation, and management. Obstetrics and Gynecology 2010;115(2):325-30.
13. Gallentine ML, Cespedes RD. Occult stress urinary incontinence and the effect of vaginal vault prolapse on abdominal leak point pressures. Urology 2001;57(1):40-4.
14. Martan A, Svabík K, Masata J, El-Haddad R, Pavlikova M. Correlation between stress urinary incontinence or urgency and anterior compartment defect before and after surgical treatment. Ceska Gynekologie 2010;75(2):118-25.
15. M Muffly, Tyler, Barber Matthew D. Insertion and removal of vaginal mesh for pelvic organ prolapse. Clinical Obstetrics and Gynecology 2010;53(1):99-114.
16. Davila GW, Drutz H, Deprest J. Clinical implications of the biology of grafts: conclusions of the 2005 IUGA grafts roundtable. International Journal of Urogynecology and Pelvic Floor Dysfunction 2006;17 Suppl 1:S51-5.

17. Galloway NT. Words of wisdom. Re: the perils of commercially driven surgical innovation. European Urology 2010;58(1):179.
18. National Institute for Health and Clinical Excellence IPG Number: IPG267 http://www.nice.org.uk/IPG267.
19. Alperin M, Moalli PA. Remodeling of vaginal connective tissue in patients with prolapse. Current Opinion in Obstetrics and Gynecology 2006;18(5):544-50.
20. Committee on Gynecologic Practice, American College of Obstetricians and Gynecologists. ACOG Committee Opinion No. 378: Vaginal "rejuvenation" and cosmetic vaginal procedures. Obstetrics and Gynecology 2007;110(3):737-8.
21. Cespedes RD. Anterior approach bilateral sacrospinous ligament fixation for vaginal vault prolapse. 2000;4;56(6 Suppl 1):70-5.
22. Drutz HP. The first century of urogynecology and reconstructive pelvic surgery: where do we go from here? International Urogynecol Journal 1996;7(6):348-53.
23. Brubaker L. Editorial: partner dyspareunia (hispareunia). International Urogynecology Journal 2006;17(4):311.
24. Jacquetin B, Cosson M. Complications of vaginal mesh: our experience. International Journal of Urogynecology and Pelvic Floor Dysfunction 2009;20:893-6.
25. Baessler K, Maher CF. Mesh augmentation during pelvic-floor reconstructive surgery: risks and benefits. Curr Opin Obstet Gynecol. 2006;18(5):560-6.
26. Maher C, Baessler K. Surgical management of posterior vaginal wall prolapse: an evidence-based literature review. Int Urogynecol J Pelvic Floor Dysfunct. 2006;17(1):84-8.
27. FDA public health notification. Serious Complications Associated with Transvaginal Placement of Surgical Mesh in Repair of Pelvic Organ Prolapse and Stress Urinary Incontinence. http://www.fda.gov/MedicalDevices/Safety/AlertsandNotices/PublicHealthNotifications/default.htm, 2008.

CHAPTER 17

Training and Credentialing in Endoscopic Surgery

Shyam V Desai

Chapter Outline

- Objectives of a Training Program
- Course Contents
  - Lectures
  - Video Demonstrations
- Seminars and Symposia
- Ward Rounds and Case Presentations
- Practical Training

Several practicing Gynecologists are now carrying out diagnostic hysteroscopy, laparoscopy and tubal ligation procedures across our country, however when it comes to operative procedures not many can perform advanced procedures efficiently.

As gynecological endoscopic surgery gains popularity amongst gynecologists all over the World it is no wonder that more and more emphasis be placed upon the proper training and certification of those who embark on this fascinating sub speciality gynecological endoscopy and minimal access surgery has advanced rapidly in last two decades and there is a growing need to have gynecologists comprehensive and extensive training in this field to have a complete knowledge of the subject.

Gynecologists should enhance their skills to a level to actually be able to perform simple to moderately advanced gynecological endoscopic surgery in a center, which is properly equipped with the infrastructure of instruments and equipments for safe endoscopic surgery.

Having attended a training program and watched several procedures being performed does not constitute adequate training the duration of any good course should be for a period of 6 months. The period is structured to give the candidate increased responsibility systematically.

OBJECTIVES OF A TRAINING PROGRAM

The candidate at the end of the training will acquire skill; full knowledge of advanced technology and shall be able to:

1. Perform basic to moderate level of gynecological endoscopy and minimal access surgery pertaining to his/her field of speciality.
2. Adapt various technologies of minimal invasive therapy that supplement each other and act together to decrease patient morbidity.
3. Perform safe laparoscopic, hysteroscopic and minimal access surgeries.
4. Appreciate the benefits, limitations and complications of the newer techniques.
5. Be aware of various instruments ~ equipments and their applications that are coming into vogue in the field of minimal invasive surgery.
6. Detect and manage complications that may occur with these types of surgeries.
7. Practice, ethical and evidence based medicine.
8. Develop communication skills to present papers, lectures, etc. at various platforms.
9. Physiological and kinetic changes associated with pneumoperitoneum for short or long duration needed for laparoscopic surgery and also the changes related to uterine distension media for hysteroscopic surgery.

Basic knowledge of the anesthesia and multiparameter monitoring related to basic to advanced laparoscopic and hysteroscopic surgery.
10. Role of diagnostic laparoscopy, microlaparoscopy, hysteroscopy, microhysteroscopy and contact hysteroscopy or gynecological pathologies and conditions which are correctable by laparoscopy along with intrauterine pregnancy like ovarian cyst, concurrent ectopic pregnancy, appendicectomy, etc. conserving uterine pregnancy and reducing chances of abortion.
11. A comprehensive details of pathologies correctable by endoscopic surgery like endometriosis, fibroids and adhesions, etc.
12. A complete knowledge of all instruments and equipments used for laparoscopic and hysteroscopic surgery along with proper sterilization, proper usage and proper maintenance of the same for effective and continuous functioning for safety.
13. A complete knowledge of electrocautery and electrosurgery, the new energy sources, vessel-sealing devices, harmonic scalpel, lasers along with surgical or technical risks, complications and management of the same.
14. A full working knowledge of alternative procedures for endometrial ablation, thermal balloon techniques, etc.
15. Two work station regularly available for laparoscopic inanimate exercises, hysterotrainer, endosuturing lab. Given at discretion of teacher. Adequate amount of hours of training and practice should be filled in a logbook signed and supervised by the teacher.
16. A thorough clinical evaluation with adequate sonographic and hormonal assay levels for clinical correlation to give proper treatment to the patient.
17. After 6–8 weeks of exposure to live surgery, adequate knowledge and reading the trainee will scrub with the teaching personnel as second and later first assisting surgeon to get hands on tissue feeling and confidence to operate independently later.
18. Maintenance of a logbook with proper record of full management of laparoscopic and hysteroscopic surgical cases, which includes 60 cases in total.
19. A complete knowledge with literature data and centers own data for fertility enhancing endoscopic surgery and also when not to do endoscopic surgery for a given patient.
20. One subject can be taken by the delegate as a research activity or a comparative data analysis related to laparoscopic or hysteroscopic surgery or MIS in SUI/prolapse.
21. A proper knowledge and live surgery observation of laparoscopic and alternative methods of treatment of stress urinary incontinence and prolapse and pelvic floor defect.
22. Experience and expertise in endoscopic, minimal access and open surgery for various gynecological pathology and conditions affecting women's health.
23. A proper knowledge with complete hands on experience of laparoscopic sterilization with fallope rings and also cases with bipolar coagulation with small tubal segment excision confirmed on histopathology and also video recorded.
24. Experience and knowledge of medico legal and ethical aspects of gynecological endoscopic and minimal access surgery.
25. Research, statistics and audit of success, morbidity and mortality if any.
26. Role and place of laparoscopic Microsurgery theoretical, practical and comparative knowledge with skill enhancement.
27. Optimum knowledge of crisis management in gynecological endoscopic and minimal access surgery.
28. Adequate knowledge to interact, discuss and learn from teachers, colleagues on all finer aspects of gynecological laparoscopic surgery.
29. Full details of postendoscopic surgical care, follow-up advice.
30. Knowledge of future technology like robotic surgery, NOTES, telemedicine.
31. The trainee on finishing a 6 months phased course in gynecological endoscopic and minimal access surgery after getting the certificate should continue to expand his skills further.

The end point for this course is that the person attending has a definite complete knowledge, skill to do the gynecological endoscopic and minimal access surgery in a properly equipped setup.

COURSE CONTENTS

The course should be structured so that the following aspects are covered:
1. The theory behind various kinds of laparoscopic surgeries.
2. Knowledge about specialized instrumentation and their maintenance.
3. Operative details about the various operative procedures.
4. Indications, limitations of procedures and contraindications based on evidence based medicine.
5. Use of computers and various software to maintain surgical audit, prepare presentations, maintain website browse the net, to perform digitization of videos and edit them and use of telemedicine and virtual reality.
6. Evaluation of data based on surgical audit.
7. Topics which includes ethical, legal and social responsibilities of surgeons.

The various topics that would be covered in detail include:

I. Basic laparoscopy
1. History of laparoscopic surgery.
2. Basic instrumentation.
3. Operating room layout and troubleshooting.
4. Anesthetic considerations..
5. Laparoscopic space access and physiological significance.
6. Gasless laparoscopy.
7. Sterilization and disinfections in laparoscopy.
8. Principles of laparoscopic hemostasis.
9. Laparoscopic tissue approximation.
10. Role of laparoscopic ultrasonography.
11. Retrieval system in minimal invasive surgery.
12. Complications of laparoscopic surgery.
13. Laparoscopy during pregnancy
14. Strategies for laparoscopic diagnosis of malignancy.
15. Laparoscopic surgery for various gynecological conditions.
16. Less invasive laparoscopy and alternative treatments.
17. Role of laparoscopy in abdominal pain syndromes.
18. Hysteroscopy and hysteroscopic surgeries.

II. Gyncological endoscopy and minimal access surgery
1. Diagnostic laparoscopy.
2. Laparoscopic sterilization.
3. Laparoscopic adhesiolysis.
4. Laparoscopic salpingostomy and fimbrioplasty.
5. Laparoscopic management of ectopic pregnancy.
6. Laparoscopic microsurgical tubal anastamosis.
7. Laparoscopic management of ovarian cysts.
8. Laparoscopic treatment of ovarian endometriomas.
9. Laparoscopic management of tubo-ovarian mass.
10. Polycystic ovaries, surgical management.
11. Laparoscopic uterine nerve ablation.
12. Laparoscopic surgery for pelvic pain
13. Laparoscopic myomectomy.
14. Laparoscopic hysterectomy.
15. Laparoscopic assisted vaginal hysterectomy.
16. Laparoscopic supracervical hysterectomy.
17. Laparoscopic colposuspension.
18. Laparoscopic repair of enteroceles and pelvic floor defects.
19. Laparoscopic treatment of advanced endometriosis.
20. Role of laparoscopy in gynecological malignancy.
21. Hysteroscopic surgery for intrauterine septum, adhesions, polyps, fibroids and tubal block.
22. Hysteroscopy endometrial ablation and resection.
23. Microlaparoscopy and microhysteroscopy.
24. Urinary incontinence and pelvic floor defects minimal access and new mesh surgery.

Skills

The candidate will be given an opportunity to observe (O), assist surgeries (A), perform with assistance (PA) and perform independently (PI) in various cases and the minimum participation of the candidate will be as per the table mentioned below:

Procedure	Category	Number
Diagnostic laparoscopy	O	10
Diagnostic laparoscopy	A	10
Diagnostic laparoscopy	PA	5
Diagnostic laparoscopy	PI	5
Laparoscopic sterilization	PA	5
Laparoscopic sterilization	PI	5
Ectopic pregnancy/salpingectomy	A	5
Ectopic pregnancy/salpingectomy	PA	5
Ovarian cystectomy	A	5
Ovarian cystectomy	PA	5
Endometriosis	A	5
Endometriosis	PA	5
LAVH	O	5
LAVH	A	5
LAVH	PA	5
TLH	O	10
TLH	PA	5
Ovarian drilling	PA	10
Ovarian drilling	PI	10
Hysteroscopic surgery	O	15
Hysteroscopic surgery	PA	20
Hysteroscopic surgery	PI	15
Advanced gynec surgery	O	50

Training methods: There will be regular training sessions for the candidates, as follows:
1. Lectures and pelvitrainer sessions.
2. Video demonstrations.
3. Seminars and symposia.
4. Panel discussions.
5. Ward rounds and case presentations.
6. Journal club.
7. Presentations of paper in conferences.
8. Publication in important journals.
9. Project work.
10. Practical training in inanimate trainers, computerized modules, virtual reality modules.
11. Assisting live surgeries.
12. Performing surgeries under supervision.

Lectures

Didactic Lectures

Selected common topics will be discussed during the first few months of the course and most of them will be introduced to the candidate to enable him increase his productivity during the course. These would include:
1. Biostatistics
2. Use of library
3. Research methods
4. Communication skills, etc.
5. Use of computers

Integrated Lectures

These are a combination of multidisciplinary talks given by experts in the respective fields the intention being that we need to react with our inter disciplinary colleagues and work with them.

These would include:
1. Emergency surgeries.
2. Management of multiple complications.
3. Management of multiple pathological conditions.

Video Demonstrations

There will be a series of lectures based on DVD's demonstrations of various laparoscopic surgeries. This will be from the vast compilation of DVD's (> 100's laparoscopic, hysteroscopic and minimal access surgeries performed by various gynecological endoscopic surgeons of international repute). Several points will be discussed during these sessions, which include:
1. The operative procedure details.
2. Problems that would be encountered during the surgeries.
3. Dealing with different situations and pathologies.
4. Various approaches to a given problem.
5. Different techniques of surgery that can be adapted.
6. Proper usage of various instruments and energy sources.

Seminars and Symposia

This will be held once in 3 month. The PG students are invited to attend and actively participate in discussion. The candidate will present on various topics at least twice in 6 months. There will be evaluation of the candidate based on his participation and contribution for the seminar.

Ward Rounds and Case Presentations

The candidate will be doing rounds of all inpatients in the department of gynecological endoscopic and minimal access surgery this will be teaching rounds with faculty in the department. Candidates will be entering relevant data in their logbooks every day. There will be case presentations by the candidate during the rounds.

Practical Training

a. **Pelvi-trainer sessions:** Practical training should be given on inanimate pelvitrainers. Various types of exercises are taught in these trainers, the actions of which mimic the various steps of surgical procedures. Even though the basic hand movements can be taught on a pelivitrainer it cannot replicate the actual surgery experience which can be obtained by performing the steps in a live situation.
b. Hysterotrainers and simulators for different pathologies.
c. Virtual reality training module optional.
d. **Assisting surgeries:** The candidate will be give opportunities to assist a number of surgeries. The assisting surgeries would include various surgical procedures, operating through the other ports other than what the surgeon is using and coordinating by holding the camera.
e. **Performing surgeries under supervision:** Based on the performance and the active involvement of the candidate he/she will be allowed to perform certain operations under supervision by senior faculty. The type of surgery and number of surgery will be decided upon based on the expertise that the candidate as acquired. The trainee should be first given simple surgical procedures to be carried out such as simple adhesiolysis, cannulation of tubes and septum incision after which more advanced surgeries such as ectopic pregnancy simple ovarian cysts and PCOD cauterization before moving on to myomectomies and hysterectomies.
f. A preceptor is one who observes and guides a candidate when he is performing the surgical procedure A preceptor is one who is adequately trained to teach the candidate and one who can assess the competence of the operator.

Evaluation

Credentialing means to evaluate the trainee in various aspects of endoscopic surgery and certify him. He may be granted temporary privileges and allowed to perform surgeries and evaluated upon the outcome of the procedures

The evaluation of learning outcome of trainees consists of:

Assessment plan during the course: There should be continuous monitoring and regular assessment of all academic activities of the candidate.

Formal evaluation is done by the staff of the department based on participation of students in various teaching/learning activities. The evaluation is structured on the basis of checklists that evaluate these various parameters.

The following aspects will be assessed:

i. Personal attitudes: It is pertinent to assess and guide the candidate in facing stressful conditions in the ward and operating room, to assess the candidate's ability to work as a team and to evaluate the leadership qualities, and coordinating abilities.

ii. Acquisition of knowledge: This will be done by evaluation of the candidate's performance during the journal club, seminars, symposia, interactive conferences and discussions during the ward rounds.

Checklist of Operative Skills

Parameters evaluated	Poor	Below Average	Average	Good	Very Good
	0	1	2	3	4
1. Preoperative preparation					
2. Setting up of equipment					
3. Creation of pneumoperitoneum					
4. Port placement					
5. Patient positioning					
6. Co-ordination with operating team					
7. Camera focusing					
8. Proper usage of instruments					
9. Overall dissection skills					
a. Dexterity of movements					
Dissection, Hemostasis					
b. Maintaining clear field of vision					
c. Usage of energy sources					
d. Suturing and knotting					
10. Safety measures during surgery					
Handling crisis					

iii. **Teaching skills:** A close watch and guidance will be provided regarding the skills in communicating and teaching during the presentations that the candidates would make.

Check-List for Evaluation of Teaching Skill

Parameters evaluated	Poor	Below average	Average	Good	Very good
	0	1	2	3	4

iv. **Clinical and operative skills:** This would include an evaluation of the candidate's sincerity, punctuality ability to diagnose correctly handling of the patient and relatives, the speed and effectiveness of the decisions taken in the outpatient department and the wards. The candidate's operative skills will be assessed based on performance in the operating room, and standard tests given in inanimate pelvi-trainer, hysterotrainer, minimal access models session and assisting during surgery.

Prime importance should be given to maintaining a proper record of events of teaching and experiences that the candidate has obtained in a logbook. Internal assessment will be based on the evaluation of the logbook. The record will include academic activities as well as the presentations and procedures carried out by the candidate.

Endoscopic surgery has a long learning curve and it is important that proper training be imparted so that operative mishaps are kept down to a bare minimum.

Any surgical procedure will have its complications and it is not realistic to say that no complications are expected. However by giving adequate and through training the morbidity and mortality following endoscopic surgery can be reduced.

CHAPTER

18

Conquering Complications of Laparoscopic and Urogynecologic Minimal Access Surgery to Make it Safe for Patients

Prakash H Trivedi, Shaily Jain, Anjali Gupta

Chapter Outline

- Complications of Veress Needle
- Complications of Trocar-Cannula
- Electrosurgical/Cautery Complications
- Bleeding and Poor Hemostasis
- Technical Complications with Instruments
- Conversion to Open Surgery
- Medical, Anesthesia or Non-Gynecological Reasons

"If you believe in surgery you will have complications, it's truly said that anatomical knowledge can come by cutting tissues apart but surgical wisdom comes by putting things together"

INTRODUCTION

Achieving safety with less complication is the corner stone for piling up thousands of cases with acceptable morbidity (<3%) and mortality (< 0.1%) in gynecological endoscopy and minimal access surgery.

Complications in laparoscopic surgeries can be as follows:

a. Improper patient selection.
b. Improper counselling of patients and relatives.
c. Anesthesia related.
d. Patient position related.
e. Inadequate operation theater set up.
f. Poorly qualified surgeon, assistant or nursing staff.
g. Accidental or overconfidence casual approach.
h. Veress needle or trocars, insufflation or distension related.
i. Technical problems with instruments.
j. Electrocautery or energy source related.
k. Related to the ports.
l. Hypothermia.

As many aspects are already covered elsewhere, we would focus on actual surgical complications, their prevention and management. Safety factors for operation theater set up, patients positioning and anesthesia-related complications are discussed in other chapters.

COMPLICATIONS OF VERESS NEEDLE[1]

Proper method of insertion is discussed in other chapter. Hence, only direct complications are dealt here.

The Veress needle can be either reusable or disposable. If it is introduced obliquely towards the pelvis or if without checking the position needle is moved in the abdomen, problems of surgical emphysema, pneumo omentum **(Fig. 18.1)**, rarely, entry into stomach or bowel and still rarely, vascular injury can occur.

If you are not sure of the position of Veress needle assessed by hanging drop of fluid on the hub, or by pressure shown on the electronic insufflators, it is better to remove and reintroduce. A fluctuating pressure of CO_2 suggests that you are in the wrong place like adhesions, lesser sac of omentum or bowel. After reinserting properly, observe any area of damage. Fall of pO_2 on the insufflators can be vasovagal due to stretching of peritoneum, usually corrected by deflation, giving atropine or glycopyrolate. A fall in E_TCO_2 suggests embolization, although rare with CO_2, as almost 300-400 ml of CO_2 can be absorbed per 100 ml of blood without any problem. If the anesthetist is watchful cardiac arrhythmia due to CO_2 insufflation or diaphragmatic irritation does not occur. A pressure cut of 15 mm of Hg and an adequate flow rate of CO_2 at about 12-15 liters/min does not cause any problem. Duration of surgery is important, but can be smoothened by good anesthesia, meticulous surgery and good postoperative analgesia. Many surgeons and gynecologist do a direct trocar entry or an open laparoscopy.

COMPLICATIONS OF TROCAR-CANNULA[2]

1. **Bowel injury:** Through rare, this can take place more with patients of previous abdominal surgery adhesions, or accidentally **(Fig. 18.2A)**.

In case of previous surgery, Veress needle can be inserted 4-5 cm above the umbilicus after passing a nasogastric tube to empty stomach. Palmer's point is also used by many at left upper quadrant to look for adhesions at the umbilicus, separate and then introduce the umbilical port. Injury to a small bowel should be identified and sutured into layers without constricting the lumen **(Fig. 18.2B)**.

A colonic injury with a prepared bowel preoperative can be sutured during laparoscopic surgery, keep the patient nil by mouth for few days till peristalsis establishes and the drainage is not significant. A sigmoid injury with electrocautery or picked up later needs a diverting colostomy and later closing after 2 months gives enough time for lower bowel to avoid peritonitis and grave fatal outcome.

Out of 25000 cases we had one injury of small bowel, one injury of transverse colon **(Figs 18.2A and B)** during trocar entry,[3] both closed laparoscopically and then finishing the surgery. One sigmoid injury, not due to trocar but scissor dissection needed diverting colostomy in an

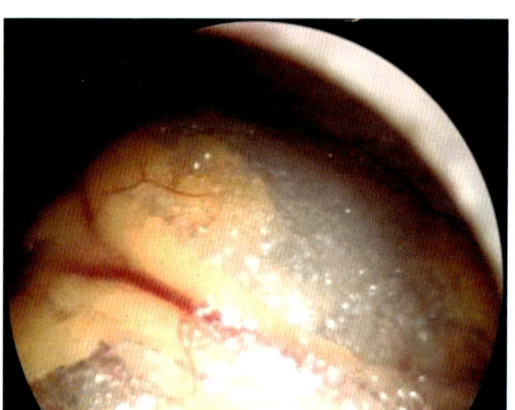

Fig. 18.1: Pneumo-omentum

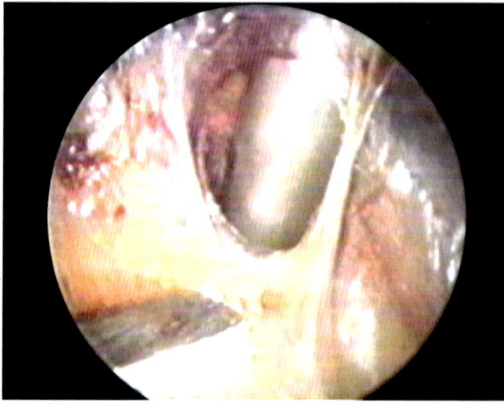

Fig. 18.2A: Umbilical trocar inside an adherent bowel

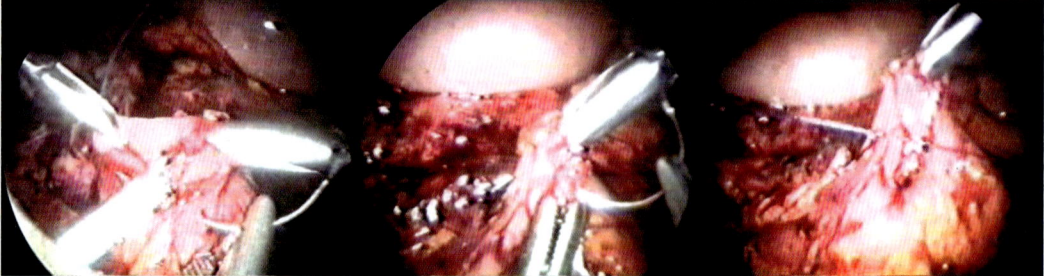

Fig. 18.2B: Bowel injured is sutured laparoscopically in two layers

extremely bad case of left sided endometriosis with bowel adhesions and an open surgery done for right side in an unmarried 20-year-old girl.

2. Vessel injury:

Ancillary trocars can injure small vessels, especially the epigastric vessel **(Fig. 18.4A)** (2-3/25000) treated by bipolar from the other port **(Fig. 18.4B)**, temporarily foley catheter **(Fig. 18.4C)** pressure (not needed) or through and through suturing **(Fig. 18.4D)** on a gauze sacrificing that port site.

The ancillary small 5/3 mm ports also can injure bowels and one has to be careful. After confirming port placement, sharp instruments like scissors needles, energy sources or electrocautery should be always kept under vision.

A blunt tip Termanium cannula is useful after pneumoperitoneum to enter under vision without any sharp trocar. A safety shield disposable trocar doesn't exist nor can the optiview prevent bowel injury.

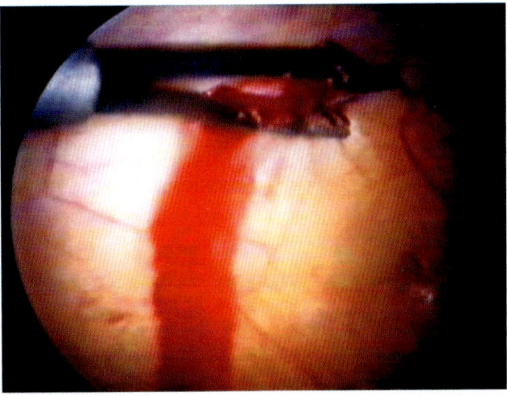

Fig. 18.4B: Bipolar coagulation-secondary trocar vessel injury (inferior epigastric artery)

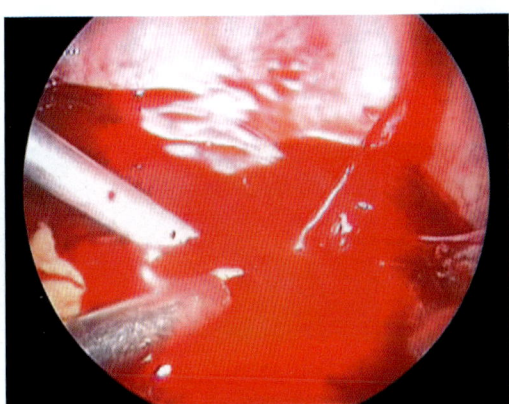

Fig. 18.3: Uterine artery bleeding

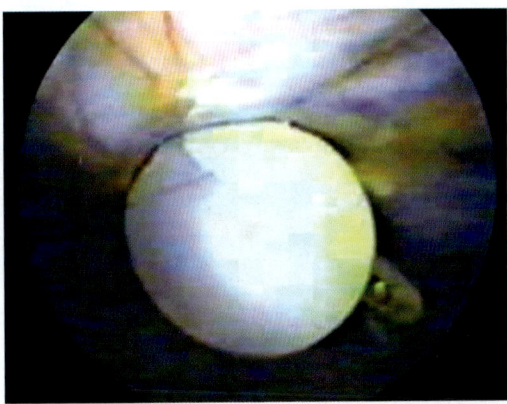

Fig. 18.4C: Foley's catheter tamponade-secondary trocar vessel injury (inferior epigastric artery)

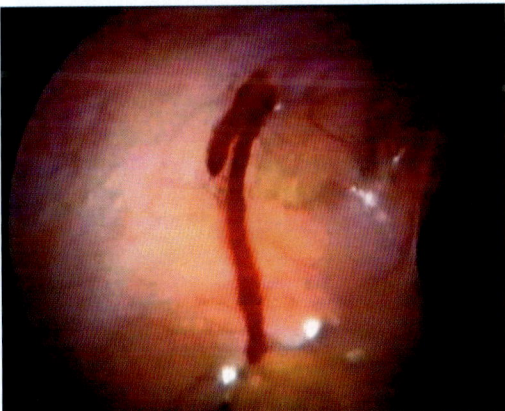

Fig. 18.4A: Secondary trocar vessel injury (inferior epigastric artery)

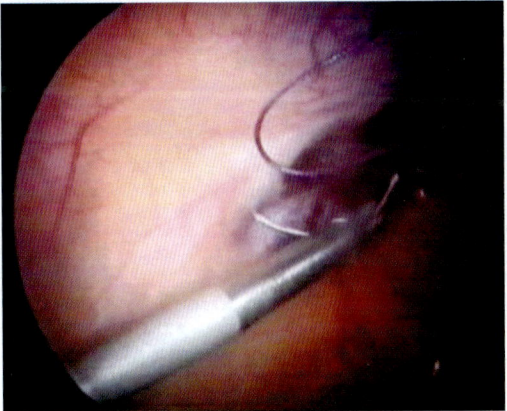

Fig. 18.4D: Intracorporeal ligation of inferior epigastric vessel

ELECTROSURGICAL/CAUTERY COMPLICATIONS[5]

If the earthing is not proper then there can be cautery burns at the reducing monopolar plate. If non-metal ancillary trocars are used capacitance burns takes place from an insulation leak to bowel or other structures.

Accidental stepping of a wrong foot switch can lead to injury and occasionally touching a hot cautery instrument tip to bowel or bladder after use can be dangerous. The point electrodes and hooks, etc. should always be retracted under the vision.

The availability of 5 to 6 vessel sealing devices or harmonic scalpel can cause injury due to lateral spread on to the ureter, bladder, etc. especially right ureter if you are not careful to push the bladder down, ureter away and lateral. We had all ureteric injuries (5/25000) on right side with new energy sources or in a case of double ureter **(Fig. 18.5A)**. The first injury occurred fourteen years after doing thousands of laparoscopic surgeries. Out of five, four were due to vessel sealing device and one with scissor all on right ureter. Ureteric DJ stenting was done under laparoscopic control **(Figs 18.5B to D)**.

Bladder injuries do take place during dissection or cutting of peritoneum, with energy source or scissors **(Figs 18.6A and B)**.

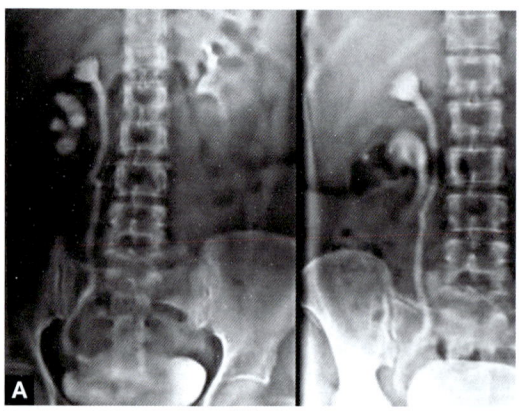

Fig. 18.5A: IVP showing double ureter on right side

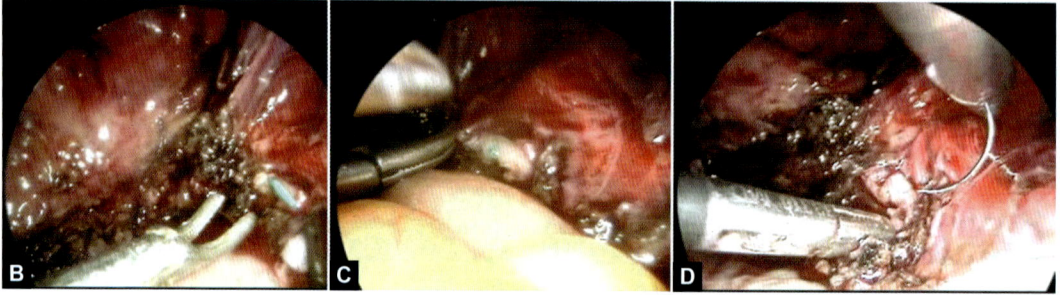

Figs 18.5B to D: Laparoscopy-ureteric DJ stenting; (B) Cystoscopic right ureteric stenting, (C) Two ends of ureter brought closer over stent, (D) Laparoscopic uretero-ureteric suturing

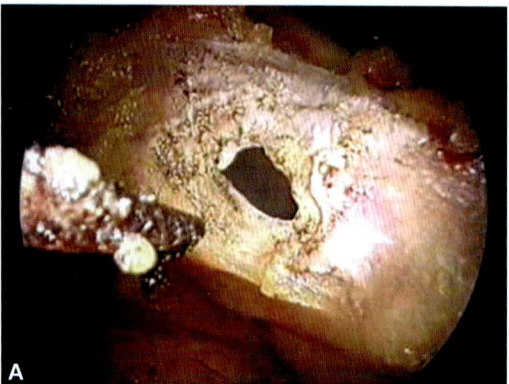 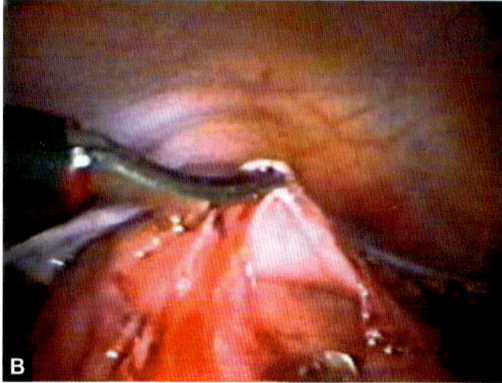

Figs 18.6A and B: Bladder injury during laparoscopic surgery

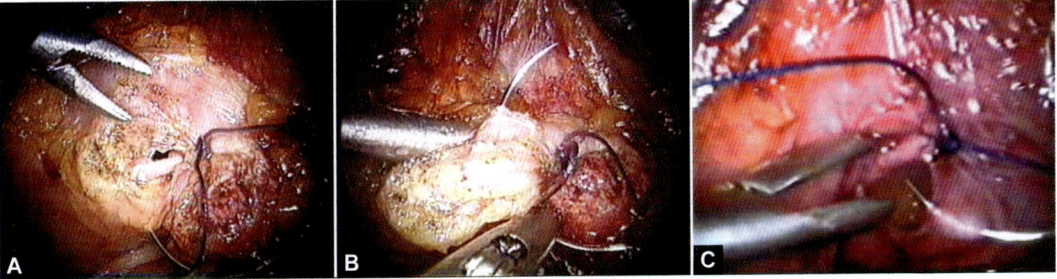

Figs 18.7A to C: Bladder suturing in two layers laparoscopically

The number of bladder injuries has decreased in the hands of expert but TLH can increase such injuries in the hands of an amateur surgeon.

The bladder injury, if identified is closed in two layers and catheter is kept for 8-10 days **(Figs 18.7A to C)**.

We had 7-8 bladder injuries, more in cases with previous cesarean section with the use of monopolar spatula or scissors which is reduced by the harmonic scalpel due to cavitational effects. Good planning, good assistants and proper manipulation of uterus can reduce bladder injuries. If the urinary bladder is accidentally injured, recognition of the injury should always be immediate intraoperatively.[4]

Injury to bladder takes place while dissecting urinary bladder away for safe colpotomy, when bladder is adherent to uterus extensively.

Bladder is closed in two layers by 3-0 Vicryl suture **(Figs 18.7A to C)**.

BLEEDING AND POOR HEMOSTASIS

Minimal blood loss and control of bleeding is of prime importance in laparoscopic surgery especially ectopic pregnancy, myomectomy, hysterectomy, etc.

In case of ectopic pregnancy and myomectomy, diluted vasopressin 2 ml in 100 ml of saline is injected, with a thin needle taking care of blood vessels into the ectopic-mesosalpinx and also at the point of incision for salpingotomy. If the ectopic is large or ruptured and with high hemoperitoneum it may be wiser to do a salpingectomy with bipolar or vessel sealing device or harmonic ace set at 2. Excision should

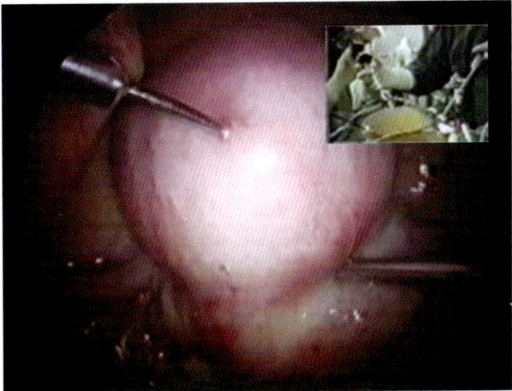

Fig. 18.8: Injection of dilute vasopressin in fibroid

be close to the tube and away from ovarian vessels, keeping less than 1 cm of the cornual end. The end is coagulated to avoid fistulas permitting sperms to go and lead to ectopic abdominal pregnancy. Though, generally its a belief that fastest way to reach bleeding ectopic pregnancy is open surgery but we disagree since by operative laparoscopy you can quickly reach the ectopic, suck out blood and achieve hemostasis. We haven't done any open ectopic pregnancy surgery since 1992 even if there is a large hemoperitoneum, rudimentary horn ectopic, etc.

In case of myomectomy, dilute vasopressin is injected to achieve temporary hemostasis **(Fig. 18.8)**, fibroid is separated and as the effect is wearing off, we suture the uterine defect till the dead space with Vicryl or barbed knotless sutures. When there are multiple fibroids, it is advisable to separate 3-4 fibroids, suture their dead space and then separating the others. This allows good effect of vasopressin, for next fibroids without having much blood loss. Remaining in the plane is important and detecting adenomyosis by preoperative sonography is good for planning the management.

Many gynecologists advocate suturing of the uterine vessel prior to myomectomy to reduce bloodloss, we don't prefer this as in simple cases its pointless and in very large difficult case you cannot reach uterus easily, further uterine vessel is not the only blood supply to the fibroids. Further, in patients desirous of future fertility, there is no need to suture uterine vessels. Occasionally, even injury to ureter in a clean benign case is not acceptable.

Bleeding during laparoscopic hysterectomy can take place at cornu, infundibulopelvic ligament, ascending or descending uterine artery or vein and the bladder plexus **(Fig. 18.3)**.

A good titrated bipolar 25-30 watts or a vessel sealing is good for cornu or infundibulopelvic but one should not be to close to the uterus to avoid back flow bleeding. Further also too close to infundibulopelvic pelvic ligament to dissect the bladder peritoneum down and laterally so ureter go away and uterine artery skeletonization is compulsory. After this, one can coagulate with bipolar or vessel sealing device or suturing the entire uterine knuckle, both ascending and descending. The uterines are then separated from the uterine wall to avoid avulsion bleeding on removing uterus. The bladder place is crucial to avoid bleeding from plexus and paravaginally treated with bipolar **(Fig. 18.9)**.

If the uterine artery or a major vessel slips during surgery then use suction irrigation and get the bladder coagulate with bipolar or rarely suture it.

If it is detected post hysterectomy on the table a meticulous lavage, identifying bleeders and coagulating them is necessary. For nonspecific generalized mild ooze surgicel is kept to form a clot. Nezhat et al[6] reported control of hemorrhage from the iliac artery following an injury by Verres needle by bipolar coagulation.

In case of small injury to a major vessel like iliac, use pulsed bipolar at low, 25 Watts as other methods may increase bleeding. Obviously, if it's a big bleeder not identified due to rapid hemoperitoneum, a laparotomy can be life saving.

Preventing bleeding is better than treating. A 16 French Ryle's tube drain in the positional cavity in fibroids or extensive tissue dissection surgery is useful to reduce postoperative pyrexia and not missing important bleeding. This is rarely needed in surgery for endometriosis, etc. which is a fibrotic disease.

Omental bleeders should be identified and coagulated. Injury to large major vessels or retroperitoneal if not increasing, it's fine but if worsening a quick laparotomy with surgeon or vascular surgeon is safe.

TECHNICAL COMPLICATIONS WITH INSTRUMENTS

There can be plenty of malfunctioning, as breakage of one of the blades or myoma screw **(Fig. 18.10A)**, which was removed laparoscopically **(Figs 18.10B and C)**.

A click line insert holding instrument can separate from the hand piece **(Figs 18.11 A to E)**.

Improper use and maintenance are both responsible for such problems. A good OT staff and technicians maintaining all instruments can help avoiding them.

A major concern can be with suction, electrocautery or needle holder not functioning properly. Insulations of all instruments should be meticulously looked upon and discard improper instruments.

Use of morcellator without experts' assistance and guidance can lead to injuries as it comes out of the fibroid strip dissected. Many morcellator have an auto safety withdrawal of

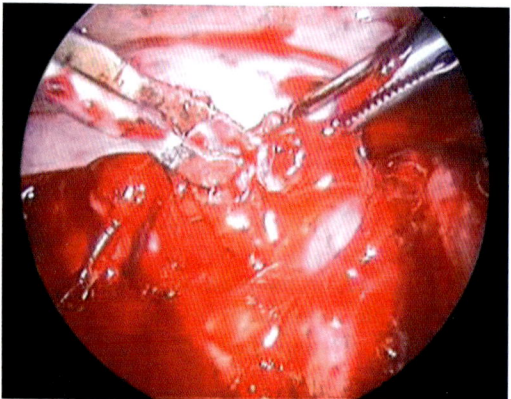

Fig. 18.9: Post hysterectomy bleeding controlled by bipolar

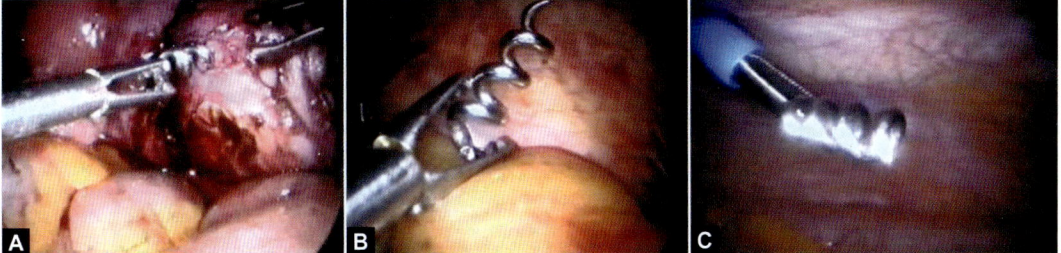

Figs 18.10A to C: (A) Broken myoma screw in the fibroid; (B and C) Laparoscopic removal of broken myoma screw

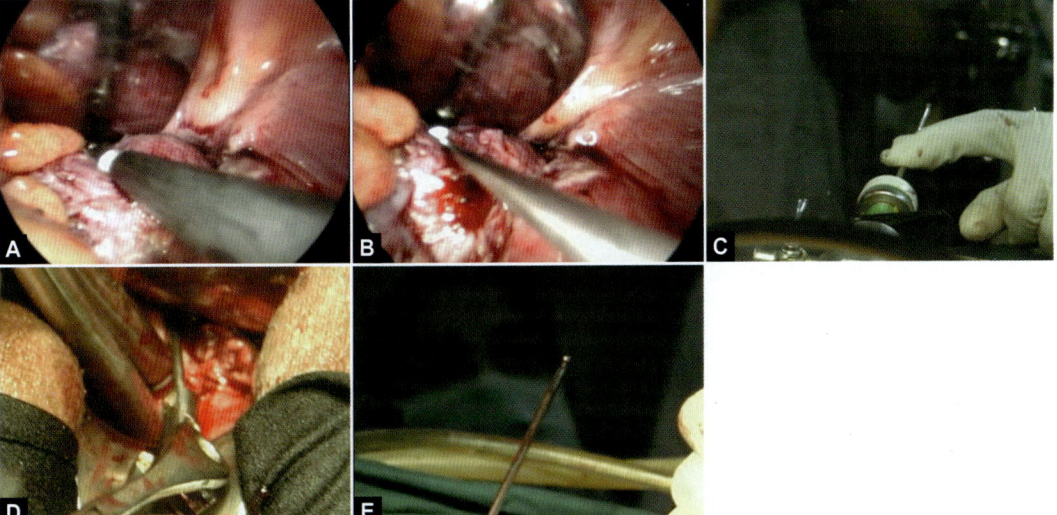

Figs 18.11A to E: (A) A click line insert holding instrument, (B) Instrument separate from the hand piece, (C) External view of detached insert of instrument, (D) Insert removed per vaginally with uterus, (E) Instrument seen after removal

the sharp blade once free of resistance of dissecting fibroid or uterus.

Having good practical attention and handling it carefully by removing the instrument under vision or in line with the trocar and removing enmass, documentation is important. Similarly, the curved needles, specimens, lap sac and the number of fibroids also should be systematically removed.

In unusual situations, like a morcellator not functioning well, a posterior colpotomy can be done in a parous patient. But, use of non-well functioning equipments is an act of negligence on the part of the surgeon and can cost a lot.

CONVERSION TO OPEN SURGERY

This is not a complication but quiet often is thought to be inability of the surgeon to do competently. This is totally incorrect as in all cases of laparoscopic surgery; consent for open surgery is always taken. When there is need to open, call the relative in the OT to inform why you need conversion and counsel him/her to avoid medico legal problem.

Conversion is not a defeat or complication but it is a prudent judgment in favor of safety of patient, which helps your wisdom to control your extreme desire or fantasizing to do laparoscopically.

We had 22 cases of conversion out of 25000 surgeries. The common reason was bad case selection, conversion in the first 2-3 minutes and not after hours of struggle. Occasional conversion is for bleeding and patient's worsening, rarely extensive bowel injury needing attention. Quiet often, previous surgery leading to lot of bowel adhesions can be a reason. Rarely, if you are not operating in your set up and are not comfortable with the instruments, equipments, assistants, or anesthetist for safe surgery, conversion is necessary.

MEDICAL, ANESTHESIA OR NON-GYNECOLOGICAL REASONS

In spite of doing all investigations and preoperative safety profile, more common in men than women, there can be factors which are either medical or anesthesia related for e.g. consistent drop in PO_2, fall in BP, cardiac arrhythmias, pulmonary vessel embolization, bronchospasm and unexplained cardiac arrest. You may convert to open or abandon the surgery.

Most of the gynecological endoscopic surgeries are done by entrepreneurs who don't have a surgical medical ICCU, which in few cases are mandatory. But they should have all the multiparameter monitors, good anesthesia machines, Cardiologist or Physician standby but still there can be unexpected reasons to convert a surgery.

"Safety is of prime importance and a true surgical genius is not borne in crisis but he or she exhibits in crisis."

REFERENCES

1. Kaloo P, Cooper M, Molloy D. A survey of entry techniques and complications of members of the Australian Gynaecological Endoscopy Society. Aust N Z J Obstetrical Gynaecol 2002 Aug; 42 (3): 264-6.
2. Cravello L, Banet J, Agostini A, Brettlee F, et al. Open laparoscopy: analysis of complications due to first trocar insertion; Gynecol Obstet Fertil 2002 Apr; 30(4):286-90.
3. Granata M, Tsimpanakos I, Moeity F, Magos A. Are we underutilizing Palmer's point entry in gynecologic laparoscopy? Fertil Steril. 2010 Dec;94(7):2716-9.
4. Classi R, Sloan PA. Intraoperative detection of laparoscopic bladder injury. Can J Anesth 1995 May; 42(5Pt 1): 415-6.
5. Vancaillie TG. Electrosurgery at laporoscopy guidelines to avoid complications. Gynecological Endoscopy 1994;3:143-50.
6. Nezhat F, Brill A, Nezhat C, et al. Traumatic hypogastric bleeding controlled by bipolar dessication during operative laparoscopy. J American Association of Gynecological Laparoscopist 1995;2:171-3.

CHAPTER 19

Resist Temptation or to Try New Techniques for Experience Before Evidence

B Ramesh, BV Bharathi

Chapter Outline

- Is Sils Future of Minimally Invasive Surgery
- Vessel Sealing Devices
  - Conventional Endosuturing/Endostitch/Barbed Suture (Myomectomy)
- Barbed Sutures
- Morcellators: Gynecare vs Rotocut G1
- Stress Urinary Incontinence
  - Advantages of the Single Incision Mini-Sling
- Company Pressure/Temptation

Never resist temptation: prove all things: hold fast that which is good-George Bernard Shaw

INTRODUCTION

The Portuguese navigator Vasco da Gama led an expedition at the end of the 15th century that opened the sea route to India by way of the Cape of Good Hope at the southern tip of Africa, assumed to be an impossible feat as it was believed that the Indian Ocean was not connected to any other seas.

Minimally invasive surgery has become a standard of care for the treatment of many benign and malignant gynecological conditions resulting in shorter hospital stays, improved quality of life and improved surgical outcomes when compared with open abdominal surgery.[1-3] With the goal of improving morbidity and cosmesis, continued efforts towards refinement of laparoscopic techniques is constantly stirring the minds of gynecological endoscopists.

During the last 25 years, the role of gynecologic laparoscopy has evolved from a limited surgical procedure used only for diagnosis and tubal ligation, to a major surgical tool used to treat a multitude of gynecologic indications.

IS SILS FUTURE OF MINIMALLY INVASIVE SURGERY

Ever since the first laparoscopic hysterectomy (LH) was performed in January 1988 by Harry Reich in Pennsylvania, USA, there was a growing interest to reform this conventional multiport LH to minimize the size and number of ports required for these procedures.[4] This led to the evolution of single incision laparoscopic surgery (SILS) **(Fig. 19.1)**. Laparoendoscopic

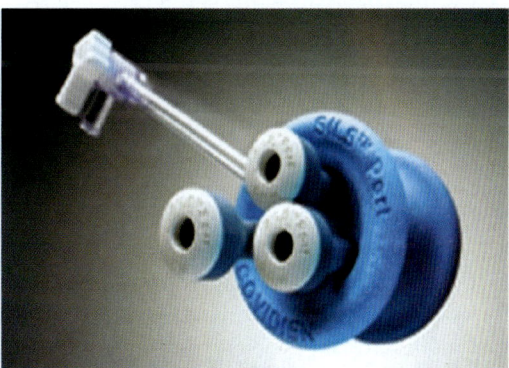

Fig. 19.1: SILS Port (Covidien, Mansfield, MA)

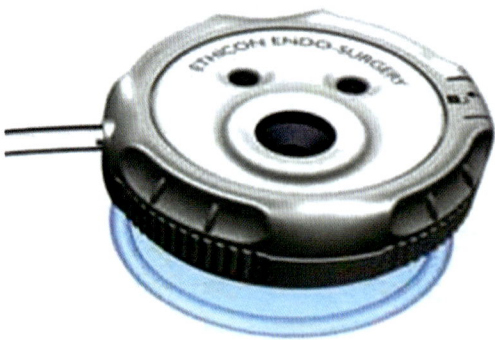

Fig. 19.2: Single site laparoscopy access system (ethicon endosurgery)

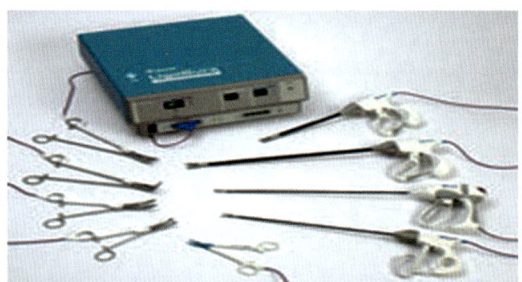

Fig. 19.3: Vessel sealing device ligasure

single site surgery (LESS) **(Fig. 19.2)** is a recently proposed surgical term used to describe various techniques that aim at performing laparoscopic surgery through a single, small-skin incision concealed within the umbilicus.[5] In the last 5 years, there has been a surge in the development of surgical technology and techniques for LESS surgery. LESS is a promising surgical innovation that results not only in improved cosmesis, but also, in many cases, a shorter convalescence period and decreased postoperative analgesia requirements when compared with patients treated with conventional laparoscopic approaches. Two of the biggest caveats that limit use of the LESS technique are instrument crowding and lack of triangulation. The recent surge in the number and variety of LESS cases has been facilitated by the introduction of new instrumentation and access devices. Improvements in access devices, optics and instrumentation have driven the dissemination of this new format of laparoscopic surgery.

Application of the LESS technique to hysterectomy has been described for both total laparoscopic hysterectomy (TLH) and laparoscopic-assisted vaginal hysterectomy (LAVH). LESS is also advocated in adnexal surgery for benign pathologies, including unilateral or bilateral salpingo-oopherectomy, adhesiolysis, excision of endometriosis and ovarian cystectomy. There is an agreement that these techniques provide improved cosmesis; however, standardized measures have not yet been employed to scientifically verify these findings. The routine application of LESS in gynecology not only requires evaluation of safety but also of cost-effectiveness, and these studies must all be performed in larger, prospective studies to definitively answer questions regarding the clinical and economic impact of this novel surgical approach.

The fishermen know that the sea is dangerous and the storm terrible, but they have never found these dangers sufficient reasons for remaining ashore—Vincent Van Gogh.

VESSEL SEALING DEVICES

Vessel sealing using bipolar electrosurgery is a development pioneered by the Ligasure system **(Fig. 19.3)**. Vessel sealing system seals vessels using both controlled energy and mechanical pressure, unlike other energy sources (monopolar, bipolar and ultrasonic dissectors) which relies only on the energy and produces a proximal thrombus for hemostasis. More recently other manufacturers have developed devices capable of achieving a similar surgical outcome. Three systems (Martin, Bowa arc, Enseal) use general purpose electro surgical unit (ESU) with specific modes designed for specialist vessel sealing instruments. The others require specialist bipolar ESUs.

The introduction of vessel sealing based on bipolar electrosurgery undoubtedly has led to a higher efficiency of open and laparoscopic surgical procedures. The newest generation of high-frequency bipolar systems uses active feedback to optimize output power and uses specific thermal engineering techniques to minimize collateral tissue damage. The bipolar LigaSure vessel-sealing device (Covidien-Valleylab, Boulder, CO) has demonstrated efficacy in a variety of procedures. A drawback of this device is that its instruments are disposable and therefore expensive. Recently, a new bipolar vessel-sealing device (MarSeal; KLS Martin, Tuttlingen, Germany) has been developed, which is a reusable instrument and thus may be less expensive. Every device now on the market claims to "seal" vessels. The ideal vessel sealing device produces minimal thermal spread, is effective on vessels upto[7] mm in diameter, works quickly, produces consistent results, and can be used multiple times.

The consensus? The best device depends on the case at hand, the skill of the surgeon, economic concerns, and other variables. Ideal instrument for vessel sealing also varies, depending on the surgical situation. All of the devices are roughly equivalent. Fortunately, almost all of the commercially available, energy sources that utilize bipolar radiofrequency or ultrasonic energy will perform the desired function if the surgeon understands the technology and utilizes the instruments properly. These devices perform best when tissue tension is reduced to maximize vessel sealing. Despite the fact that these devices provide audible feedback to signal the electrosurgical endpoint, the surgeon must also gauge tissue color, retraction, and the emission of steam before advancing the cutting blade.[6]

Only the ligasure advance provides both coaptive coagulation and spark cutting via an electrode on the tip of one blade; therefore, an adjunctive mechanical or energy based device must be employed to perform culdotomy during TLH when enseal or the plasma kinetic (PK) cutting forceps is used. The ability to efficiently and hemostatically cut through tissue of variable mass with minimal plume, predictable thermal margins, and the retention of tissue color make the harmonic scalpel first choice for laparoscopic resection of endometriosis, extensive adhesiolysis, myomectomy, cervical amputation during supracervical hysterectomy, and culdotomy during total hysterectomy.

Unlike other vessel sealing devices available, enseal tissue sealing device **(Fig. 19.4)** offers controlled temperature technology. The advanced jaw design restricts lateral energy flow, thus resulting in minimal thermal spread. And it achieves reliable vessel seal strength up to 7 times systolic pressure for vessels ≤ 7 mm.

Use of any energy-based device does not preclude the need for skill. Before adding any of these devices to your surgical armamentarium, appropriate training should be acquired in a skills lab using living tissue or with a laparoscopic trainer using a tissue surrogate. The ease of use, multiple functions for a single instrument, tissue safety, and minimal residual traumatized tissue are the reasons many prefer the mechanical energy of the harmonic ACE as primary laparoscopic energy source.

The bottom line is *"it's not the wand, it's the magician."*

Conventional Endosuturing/Endostitch/Barbed Suture (Myomectomy)

During lap myomectomy, repair of the uterine defect is a relatively difficult task and is considered the most important part. Obviously, a skillful laparoscopic suturing technique is indispensable for the close reapproximation of the uterine defect.

Well-reapproximated uterine wound during laparoscopic myomectomy is crucial for satisfactory postoperative recovery. It is still a thorny issue for laparoscopists regarding laparoscopic repair of the uterine defect because of the fact that this procedure required highly skillful suturing technique of the surgeon.

BARBED SUTURES

Bidirectional barbed suture **(Fig. 19.5)** (Quill self-retaining system; angiotech pharmaceuticals, inc., vancouver, british columbia) is a

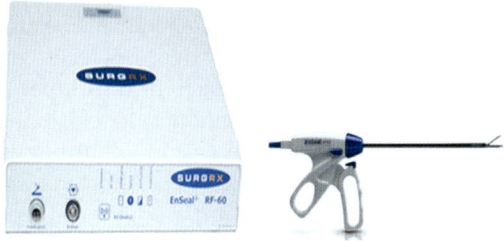

Fig. 19.4: Enseal PTC VSD

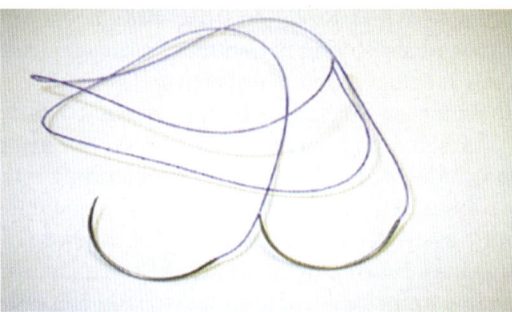 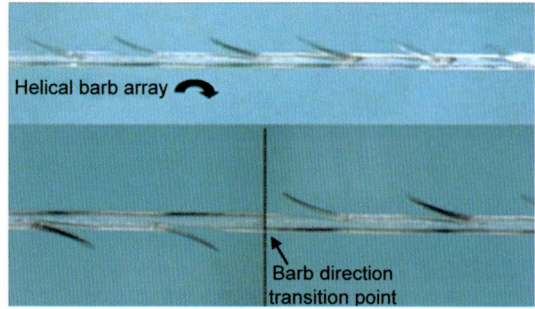

Fig. 19.5 : Bidirectional barbed suture

new design that incorporates tiny barbs spaced evenly along the length of the suture cut like a helical array set facing in opposite directions from the midpoint with a needle on each end. It greatly facilitates myometrial closure because there is no need to tie knots and there is no back-sliding of the suture, which enables continuous wound closure with even distribution of tensile strength throughout the repair. These benefits of barbed suture are especially valuable in single-incision surgery because intracorporeal knot tying can be more challenging than with the multiport approach. Also it is immensely helpful for budding laparoscopic surgeons who are not proficient with intracorporeal knotting, it will encourage them and will boost their morale.[7]

Limitations: Though it appears very promising, it still needs to be evaluated in huge myomas with deep myometrial defects, and postoperative follow up with respect to incidence of hematomas, and scar integrity has to be assessed.

Endostitch: Endo stitch laparoscopic suturing device **(Fig. 19.6)** (Auto Suture Company, division of US Surgical Corp, Norwalk, CT) combined with a running, locked suture technique enables the surgeon to achieve a secure multiple-layer closure of deep defects via laparoscopy. The endo stitch 10 mm laparoscopic suturing device enables to close the uterus with interrupted and continuous locked sutures. This instrument shortens the operative time when compared to conventional endosuturing.

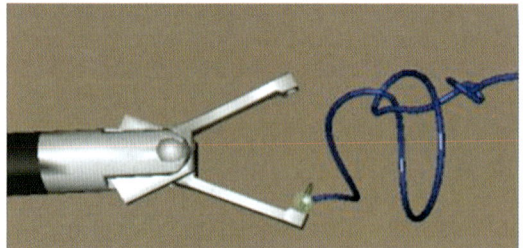

Fig. 19.6: Endo stitch

Conventional endoscopic suturing of the uterus often fails to provide a smooth serosal surface, thus creating additional focal points for the formation of adhesions. The endo stitch allows the surgeon to apply continually firm tension to the suture while the next stitch is placed. If a running suture is attempted with traditional methods, the uterine defect may be closed incompletely, since it is often impossible to maintain the proper tension on a large defect when suturing thick uterine tissue. The mechanical efficiency of the endo stitch 10 mm laparoscopic suturing device allow easy and secure multiple-layer closure of deep defects and endometrial cavity. In addition to the endometrial cavity, posterior and lateral defects were easily and securely sutured with the endo stitch.[8] Compared with traditional extracorporeal and intracorporeal suturing and knot tying,[9] endo stitch techniques are technically easier and less time consuming. The knot appears as secure as those we produced with traditional techniques and the uterine suture line appears more secure.[9]

Endo stitch loaded with barbed suture material will be excellent for endosuturing in LESS (TLH/Myomectomy) surgeries.

MORCELLATORS: GYNECARE VS ROTOCUT G1

Tissue retrieval plays an important role in laparoscopic myomectomy. Here comes the role of morcellators, surgeon is handicapped if he doesn't have a morcellator while performing laparoscopic myomectomy, as one of the limiting factors for laparoscopy is the volume of tissue that must be removed. Next comes the type of Morcellator to be selected.[10]

Currently, the Rotocut G1 morcellator (Karl Storz GmbH and Co. KG, Tuttlingen, Germany) and Gynecare Morcellex (Ethicon, Inc., Somerville, NJ) are probably the most frequently used instruments for morcellation. The Rotocut G1 is reusable and has a foot-pedal control, whereas the Gynecare Morcellex is disposable and is activated using a hand-trigger. The hand-trigger activation could be responsible for the rapid learning curve because of the absence of the foot-pedal control, which requires hand-foot coordination. The Gynecare Morcellex has an ergonomic handle that could simplify tissue morcellation for female surgeons. In terms of cost-effectiveness, in centers in which laparoscopy is performed routinely, the Rotocut G1 is preferred. It can be used indefinitely with periodic replacement of the cutting blade. However, where laparoscopy is not performed routinely, use of highly expensive instruments such as a reusable tissue morcellator is not justified, and the Gynecare Morcellex may be considered an effective, safe, and less expensive option. The Gynecare Morcellex **(Fig. 19.7)** device costs about € 500, the cost of a reusable instrument the Rotocut G1 **(Fig. 19.8)** is about € 15 000. Given its easier handling and lower costs, Gynecare Morcellex could be chosen in centers with a low rate of laparoscopic interventions followed by tissue extraction.[11]

Ideal requirements for a new morcellator include proper handling and ergonometrics, improvement of the safety aspects with the rotating knife visible during morcellation, maintenance of pneumoperitoneum, the possibility of removing tissue masses weighing several hundred grams in a short time, and decreased operator effort. Variety of morcellators being available in market, the ideal morcellator for the case at hand or for your set up has to be selected, in order to be cost effective.[12]

STRESS URINARY INCONTINENCE

There are only two procedures that are proven to have effective long-term cure rates for the treatment of stress urinary incontinence (SUI). These procedures are the abdominal burch colposuspension or (MMK) and the vaginal sling procedures. However, in the past, the sling procedure was far from standardized. There have been multiple different descriptions using different materials for the sling, different anchoring points, and different methods to adjust the tension of the sling.

Procedures were done under general anesthesia, patients required prolonged hospitalization, required a suprapubic catheter and many patients suffered high rates of voiding dysfunction following these slings.

However the introduction of the tension-free vaginal tape procedures in the late 90's

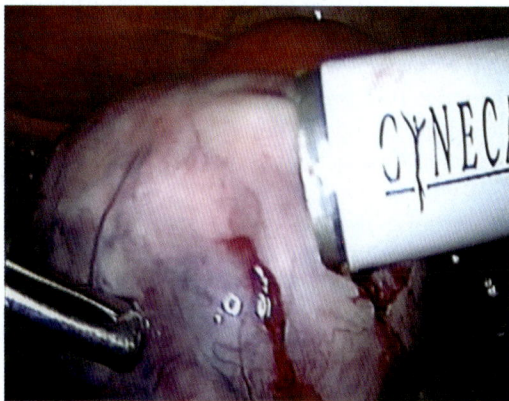

Fig. 19.7: Gynecare

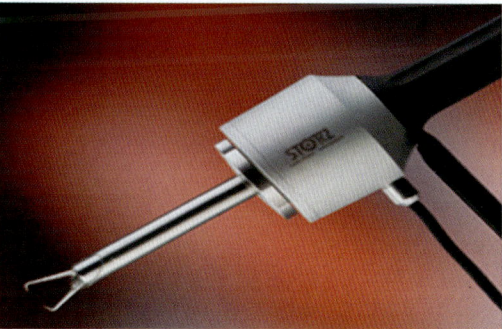

Fig. 19.8: Rotocut G1

revolutionized the treatment of SUI. It introduced a standardized sling procedure that could be completed safely in 20 minutes under local anesthesia, utilizing 3 very small incisions with minimal dissection, a cough test for tension adjustment and produced excellent cure rates.

Despite its relative safety, the original tension free vaginal tape procedures require the blind passage of needles through 2 small incisions in the abdomen just above the pubic bone. The retropubic space that the needle has to pass through to get to these abdominal incisions is also a very vascular space with venous plexuses and the potential for injury to large blood vessels in the pelvis. Secondary to this and the areas that the needle has to pass to place the mesh tape, there is potential for complications such as injury to the bladder, intestines, or nerves in the pelvis and/or abdomen.[13]

The transobturator sling was developed to help reduce the risks of retro pubic needle passage. Dr Moore and Miklos were two of the first surgeon's to utilize this newer, safer approach to the tension free tape sling procedure instead of passing needles blindly through the abdomen, the TOT procedure involves passing needles through the groin to place the sling, which is a safer approach, with much lower risks than TVT with similar cure rates.

Despite its improved safety profile and excellent cure rates, the procedure still involves passing needles through the groin, which in certain patients can result in groin pain. Although the risk is very low, especially with the outside-in approach like the Monarc TOT sling, the risk still exists.[14] Secondary to this, a new procedure involving only one incision vaginal, and NO incisions in the abdomen or groins and NO needle passages through the abdomen or groins has been developed. Single Incision Mini Sling represents next step in minimally invasive treatment of stress urinary incontinence.[15]

Advantages of the Single Incision Mini-Sling

No retropubic or groin needle passage, minimal risk of bowel or bladder injuries, safer, faster, less morbidity, very efficient, less bleeding, retains same anatomic position as tape.

This position has been shown to have the same cure rates of the TVT sling, however it is a less acute angle that mimics the natural position of the pubo-urethral ligament and therefore there is less risk of urinary obstruction (which requires long-term catheter use).[15]

However, it would be premature to conclude, that Mini-sling **(Figs 19.9 and 19.10)** is better than (or as good as other tension free slings), without long term studies.

The reasonable man adapts himself to the world; the unreasonable one persists in trying to adapt the world to himself. Therefore, all progress depends on the unreasonable man—George Bernard Shaw.

COMPANY PRESSURE/TEMPTATION

Technology and innovation are changing the ways in which companies build and sustain their brand. Customers expect their experience to be pleasant, fast, and free. If a company fails to meet their expectations (or exceeds them) the customers will blog, tweet, post comments, create facebook groups, and invent new ways to express their feedback using social media.

It is increasingly important for companies to pay full attention to that process and influence it positively by investing in proper customer service and in contributing to their own online communities. Today's angry customers are very loud, and happy customers are a company's best brand ambassadors.

Your customers are your ad agency-Jeff Jarvis

In the same way, medical representatives try to lure or influence medical professionals to

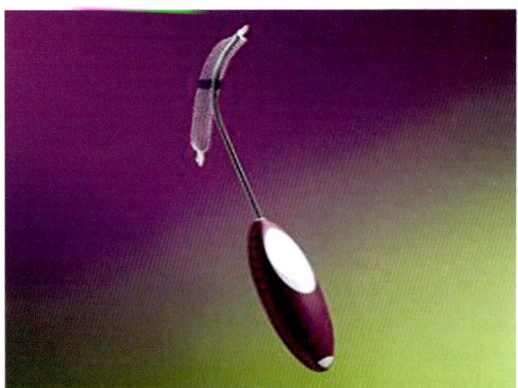

Fig. 19.9: Mini-sling

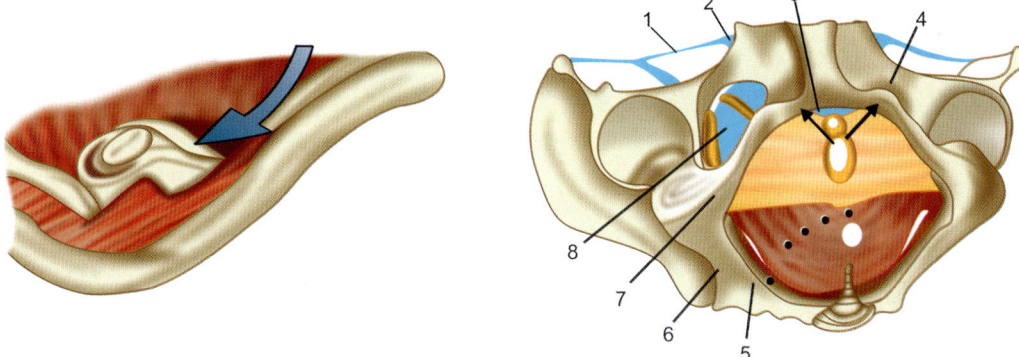

Fig. 19.10: Position of mini-sling duplicates position of pubourethral ligaments. This is a natural angle of the ligament and when the sling is placed in same position it is felt to reduce post op voiding dysfunction

buy their equipments. Do not succumb to pressure tactics and buy their products.

If you think something is not really useful, do not promote it. It is very difficult to resist temptation. Indeed, advertisements encourage us to buy. The buying impulses are generated by commercials, marketing campaigns or even our own entourage that make us envious and create a sense of need. Indeed, nowadays, advertising has crept into each nook and corner of our lives and around us: television, radio, computer, advertising signs, home, outside, everywhere. We are inundated by advertisements that encourage us to spend money. Moreover, advertising campaigns extolling the virtues of consuming products and make us believe in their usefulness, so they aim to create a need and a desire among consumers.

Personally, to resist temptation I try to stand back and wonder if the purchase is really necessary. I often think of everything I have. Moreover, when I have a sudden urge to buy then I ponder again the question of its necessity. It helps to clear the mind of temptation and unconsciously I say I can come back later and there is no reason to torment with decision. In conclusion, I think that it is not so difficult to resist temptation, we just must keep self-discipline.

Medical science is rapidly changing with emergence of new gadgets and techniques almost every day. Nothing is constant and evolution will continue in medical field too. Constant refinement of techniques ultimately adds to progress of our skill. So even if a new technique does not sustain, you can learn many lessons and it will show path for newer innovations.

Try new gadgets, as it is our duty to critically evaluate if these newer devices are genuinely good or bad.

Try newer techniques not to shoot into limelight or because of the indirect pressure from the rapidly expanding instrument manufacturing market, but in the best interest of the patient, in order to improvise technique, in terms of cure rates, shortened or time, minimal complications and cost-effectiveness.

To date all recent advances that have occurred in modern laparoscopy are due to the passion of enthusiastic surgeons to venture newer techniques, which has led us to this 21st century.

Never be afraid to try something new. Remember, amateurs built the ark. Professionals built the Titanic.

REFERENCES

1. Cho YH, Kim DY, Kim JH, Kim YM, Kim YT, Nam JH. Laparoscopic management of early uterine cancer: 10-year experience in Asan Medical Center. Gynecol Oncol. 2007;106:585-90.
2. Kalogiannidis I, Lambrechts S, Amant F, Neven P, Van Gorp T, Vergote I. Laparoscopy-assisted vaginal hysterectomy compared with abdominal hysterectomy in clinical stage I endometrial cancer: Safety, recurrence, and long-term outcome. Am J Obstet Gynecol. 2007;196:248.
3. Walker JL, Piedmonte MR, Spirtos NM, Eisenkop SM, Schlaerth JB, et al. Laparoscopy compared with laparotomy for comprehensive surgical staging of uterine cancer: Gynecologic Oncology Group Study LAP2. J Clin Oncol. 2009;27:5331-6.
4. Reich H, De Caprio J, McGlynn F. Laparoscopic hysterectomy. J Gynecol Surg. 1989;5:213-6.
5. Gill IS, Advincula AP, Aron M, Caddedu J, Canes D, Curcillo PG, 2nd, et al. Consensus statement of the consortium for laparoendoscopic single-site surgery. Surg Endosc. 2010;24:762-22.
6. Vessel sealing devices,Update technology Vol. 21 No. 9 | September | OBG Management.
7. Greenberg JA, Einarsson JI. The use of bidirectional barbed suture in laparoscopic myomectomy and total laparoscopic hysterectomy. J Minimn Invasive Gynecol. 2008;15:621-3.
8. Stringer NH: Laparoscopic myomectomy with the Endo Stitch 10 mm laparoscopic suturing device. J Am Assoc Gynecol Laparosc 1996;3:299-303.
9. Stringer NH, McMillen MA, Jones RL, et al: Uterine closure with the Endo Stitch 10-mm laparoscopic suturing device—A review of 50 laparoscopic myomectomies. Int J Fertil 1997;42(5):288-96.
10. Miller CE. Methods of tissue extraction in advanced laparoscopy. Curr Opin Obstet Gynecol. 2001;13:399-405.
11. Fulvio Zullo, Angela Falbo, Assunta Iuliano, Stefano Palomba, et al. Randomized Controlled Study Comparing the Gynecare Morcellex and Rotocut G1 Tissue Morcellators. J Minimn Invasive Gynecology 2010;17:192-9.
12. Brucker S, Solomayer E, Zubke W, et al. Anewly developed morcellator creates a new dimension in minimally invasive surgery. J Minim Invasive Gynecol. 2007;14:233-9.
13. Ward K, Hilton P, Minimally invasive synthetic suburethral slings: emerging complications, Obstet Gynaecol, 2005;7:223-32.
14. Moore RD, Miklos JR, Cervigni M, et al., Monarc Transtobturator sling: Combined analysis of one-year followup in nine countries with 266 patients, Int Urogynecol J Pelvic Floor Dysfunct, 2006;17:S203.
15. Moore RD, Mitchell GK and Miklos JR: Singlecenter retrospective study of the technique, safety, and 12-month efficacy of the MiniArc™ single-incision sling: a new minimally invasive procedure for treatment of female SUI. Surg Technol Int 2009;18:175.

CHAPTER 20

How to Make Ambulatory Endoscopist's Surgery Safe?

Prakash H Trivedi, Neha Rani, Anjali Gupta

Chapter Outline

- Consent, Expectation and Counseling
  - Set-up, Instrumentation, Wear, Tear and Sterilization
  - Need of your Assistants and Nursing Staff
- Complications
  - Postoperative Care
- Deficiency
  - By Ambulatory Surgeon
  - By Set-up
  - By Anesthetist
  - By Consent and Postoperative
  - Postoperative Care
- Medicolegal Aspects- Mortality, etc.

INTRODUCTION

As minimally invasive gynecological endoscopic surgery is popular in every corner; a desire is always there in patients, even in small towns, villages or cities, where adequate facilities or the required skill and expertise are not available, hence the birth of 'ambulatory endoscopic surgeon'. Often, these surgeons are established and popular thus synchronizing such activity is not difficult. The organizer wants to organize the surgery at their own center because generating patient is easy and for patients, it is service at door step - Welcome.

Though, many variables are the trouble shooting areas for such multiparty management practice, a center may call a less experienced person or surgeon having ample time so as to reduce the surgical charges. Even surgeons may, at times, ignore the need of good infrastructure, thus compromising the safety of the patient. Many non gynecological centers offer such endoscopic surgeries, further increasing the risk elements.

CONSENT, EXPECTATION AND COUNSELING

Inspite of the fact that the patient is getting operated in a center by a person coming only for a day or two and returning back, the organizing person promises miraculous outcome at an affordable price to the patient. This lacuna should be filled by proper counseling by ambulatory surgeon during preoperative evaluation. Explaining the realistic expectations, limitations, possible complications, also possibility of abandoning surgery, if found difficult and taking appropriate consent in a language patient understands and sign is necessary.

Set-up, Instrumentation, Wear, Tear and Sterilization

An ambulatory endoscopic surgeon visits different set-ups which vary from ill-equipped to the best. How is it then possible to do the same level of surgery?

The main requirement is well-maintained operation theater equipments, anesthesia machine, multiparameter monitors and a continuous flow of electricity. Back-up invertors or generators facility avoids damage to main equipments.

Amongst the compulsory requirements of any set up for an ambulatory endoscopist are the followings:
1. Full set of operative laparoscopy and hysteroscopy instruments(refer the chapters dedicated to this aspect). A 15 percent deficiency is manageable but not major deficiency.
2. A good endoscopy camera, preferably two TV monitors, electronic insufflators, xenon light source, good electrocautery, harmonic and vessel sealing device are optimal but a dedicated bipolar unit is mandatory, a good morcellator, proper supply of CO_2 cylinder and uterine distension media, an endomat or acceptable alternative for irrigation and suction.
3. Simple conventional instruments—A full set up of open surgery abdominal/vaginal instruments, more important are 1/2 mm Indian dilators, cervix holding slim forceps, simple ovum forceps, proper Tubal patency Rubin's/Spackman's or Rumi's cannula. It is surprising that many centers may not have proper vaginal speculum or retractors like Devers.
4. Disposable instruments and their brain units—If you are used to Harmonic ace, enseal vessel sealing device, Gyrus PICR, roles- Grasper, Ligasure or atlas make provisions. If using a sling or mesh for urinary incontinence or prolapse, confirm or make arrangements of all needed, apart from mesh/sling.
5. The anesthesia machine should be of a proper level with or without respirator but essentially with multiparameter monitor and a defibrillator, though, needed very rarely. You have to understand the level of each anesthetists which fortunately we have excellent in India. Group them into four types:
   A. Excellent, keen and, knows what endoscopy surgery needs.
   B. Excellent but deficiency in equipments.
   C. Excellent conventional anesthetist not convinced of endoscopic surgery or in hurry.
   D. Good but not used to endoscopic surgery.

You should be firm after 1 to 2 operating sessions that you want A and B only, C and D for vaginal minimal access procedure. Please remember a major morbidity or mortality due to anybody is written as your problem in the medical circle and also legally. Learn to say no to certain surgery, certain centers and certain anesthetist.

Need of your Assistants and Nursing Staff

Without any exaggeration, maximum amount of quality ambulatory endoscopic surgery in India is done by an endoscopist who insists and carries along with him/her best assistants and nursing staff of his/her center with the necessary and standby instruments.

We have been to centers, who claim to have excellent assistants for laparoscopic cholecystectomy hence good for gynecological endoscopic surgery, imaginary but totally involved. A good gynecologist with moderate endoscopic surgery knowledge is better than a surgeon or even a nonmedical assistant great for cholecystectomy.

Definitely it costs the ambulatory endoscopist but establishes the endoscopic surgeon in the new zone with the only disadvantage of addiction to this pattern of working, which is actually an advantage for the patient.

We also have to remember that the gap between surgeries being short, all instruments need to be sterilized and kept ready. Any damage or deficiencies should be quickly picked up, informed and rectified.

Sterilization of instruments is done by keeping it in cidex for 40 minutes or cidex OPA for 15 minutes, certain instruments can be kept in formalin chamber like morcellator but refer to chapter on this subject. Flash gas sterilization for long instruments is also suggested.

The wear and tear of instruments is the price an ambulatory surgeon pays in their interest in giving service to the patients and also popularizes endoscopic surgery in the country.
Many of the live workshops also falls under the preview of this same section and should be covered by respective organization.

COMPLICATIONS

If you are an ambulatory endoscopist working in different set-up with different teams, you are exposed to complications beyond your control. Hence, its imperative in the consent that the vicarious liability is with the chief of the set up wherein we do this surgery but the act of commission by the ambulatory surgeon remain his/her liability. Fortunately the complications in the hands of an expert are occasional.

"A true surgical genius is not born in crisis but exhibits in crisis." In case, a complication arise ambulatory endoscopist, knowing very well the advantages and limitations of the center, should remain cool and agile, swift and not disturbed and keep team under control. Proper communication with patient's relatives saves everything.

If we go on to the 'blame game' then we are inviting trouble for all of us. Hence, case selection, set-up, anesthetist, team, counseling and consent are equally important. Please note law experts you to deliver the best in any situation but does not accept acts of commission, omission and negligence. Be kind and responsible for any patient.

Postoperative Care

Postoperative instruction has to be dictated by the ambulatory endoscopist and written by the person in charge of the center. It is worthwhile to talk to the relatives after surgery, giving them a brief of how the surgery went, what precautions they should take and what results they expect out of the surgery. A separate person in charge of postoperative care should be allotted.

Removal of catheter, pack, drain, dressing, avoiding sexual relationship, bath, diet, etc. should be instructed clearly before patient discharge.

DEFICIENCY

The deficiencies in endoscopic surgery done by ambulatory surgeon are:
a. By ambulatory surgeon.
b. By set-up.
c. By anesthetist.
d. By consent.
e. By postoperative care.

By Ambulatory Surgeon

The deficiency can be failing to examine or informing the patient before surgery, compromise with operative procedure which is inadequate compared to what they would have done in their own set-up. Not informing the chief of the set-up of a possible problem or complication which can take place in a case which may be 1 out of 25.

By Set-up

Inadequacy for instruments, equipments, safety back up which can jeopardize our outcome. Complications can occur during the change-over of patients and immediate postoperative.

By Anesthetist

Informing the ambulatory surgeon very late, of an inadequacy in anesthesia set up or any anesthesia related problems, during surgery or when the patient is deteriorating. Taking surgery beyond the capacity of his/her capability. Shifting patient after surgery before necessary care.

By Consent and Postoperative

The Consent should not be exhaustive and should be in a language patient understands. The consent has to explain to the patient about the advantages, limitations, complications, need of open surgery and also clearly stating that operating team is going to stay for a day or two. Only pure surgical problem by the ambulatory endoscopist is his/her problem. A care has to be taken not to over promise success and results and also miraculous results with the complications. Preferably the signature should be of the inviting chief of the set-up, ambulatory surgeon, anesthetist, patient's and patient's relative. Filling up details of pre, post-and-intraoperative notes are mandatory with follow-up advice.

Postoperative Care

After doing 20 to 25 surgery, it is imperative that each patient be attended by a qualified person. In case of doubt, seniors or chief of the set-up, or ambulatory endoscopist is informed. Prompt action should be taken—law expects care not necessarily cure. Act of omission or commission should be in mind and always inform the relatives.

MEDICOLEGAL ASPECTS—MORTALITY, ETC.

Ideally, there should be a national registration of the ambulatory endoscopist or temporary state registration to avoid any lapses. Medicolegal safety comes from the consent clarifying major issues explaining patients and relatives. A detail review is given in the chapter of medicolegal aspects of endoscopic surgery.

But ambulatory endoscopist surgery and even live workshops by different organization needs special permission consent to safe guard all in medical fraternity.

Mortality in last 20 years though rare, can still be a setback and a medicolegal problem for both the organizer and ambulatory surgeon and anesthetist.

The safe method is to avoid blame game, work as a team, have convincing answers that you, your center and the endoscopist has taken sufficient precaution for the surgery. Also adequate care is taken in moment of crisis which can happen in any surgery but proper prompt care, information to patients relative, calling necessary experts keeping patients best health interest in mind is done and written on paper.

In today's time some patients may be violent, unhappy or instigated but you have to inform the chief of the center to be ready for such issues. Official formalities as per law of the land should be followed and always have an expert medicolegal lawyer in consultation and also see that the documentation and paper work is complete.

CHAPTER 21

Maintenance and Sterilization of Endoscopic and Minimal Access Surgery Instruments and Equipment

Anthony Lewis

Chapter Outline
- Maintenance and Sterilization
- Carrying Steam Sterilized Instruments Outside the Hospital

"A skilled craftsman always takes care of his or her tools. What a block of good marble is to an architect instruments are same to a surgeon."

Instruments and equipments are the heart and soul to any endoscopic and minimal access surgery operation theatre and surgeon. Equally or more important is the maintenance and sterilization of these instruments, which is very often looked after by an OT expert. We found that a person who is an expert who does this job even twice in a month, the remaining staff also picks up many aspects. The change it brings in your operation theatre and your work is not comparable in words or cost involved. This chapter is written by an expert and to the point without any jargons.

MAINTENANCE AND STERILIZATION

Odorless technique for disinfecting OT or IVF centers and nursing homes

Today maintaining a presentable, clean and aseptic condition in small and congested places is the need of the hour. Before the first surgical or diagnostic procedure of the day, cleaning of the OT, IVF and other important departments is essential.

Take 2 percent betadine scrub of 7.5 percent strength and 2 percent hydrogen peroxide 6 percent strength per liter of water and prepare 5 to 7 liters of solution **(Fig. 21.1)**. Take required quantity of solution in separate container to disinfect the OT light, table, trolleys and floor and discard the used solution. The above technique should be used to clean the department/section after every procedure. To maintain shine on the machines and equipments, one should use clean and well-squeezed duster. This solution not only disinfects, it also removes sticky and oily materials from the surface, corners of instruments and equipments.

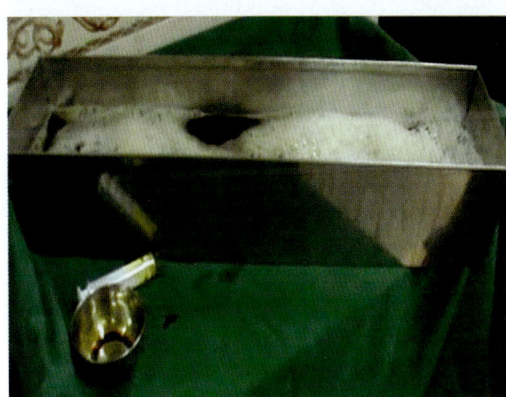

Fig. 21.1: Betadine scrub and hydrogen peroxide solution

Disinfecting or sterilizing with liquid chemical (CIDEX)

Although CIDEX has 14 days of shelf life the same should not be used liberally, especially by a busy institutions and departments. The new CIDEX or disinfecting solution must be prepared on a busy day to disinfect/sterilize instruments more effectively and quickly.

A busy institute or department which may have 3 to 4 procedures daily, must replace the solution after 7 days of use or before 7 days. Similarly, formalin tablets from instruments chamber must be replaced in 7 days (Maximum 14 days only).

The used instruments must be immersed in betadine scrub and hydrogen solution for a minimum of 5 minutes **(Figs 21.2A and B)**. Then the instruments should be brushed **(Fig. 21.2C)**, washed and kept on clean cloth **(Fig. 21.2D)**, shaken or held vertically to remove the water before immersing them in CIDEX **(Fig. 21.2E)**.

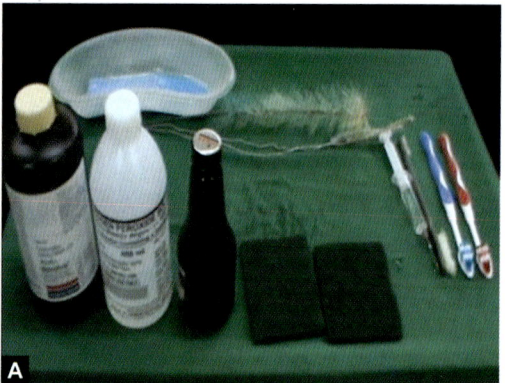
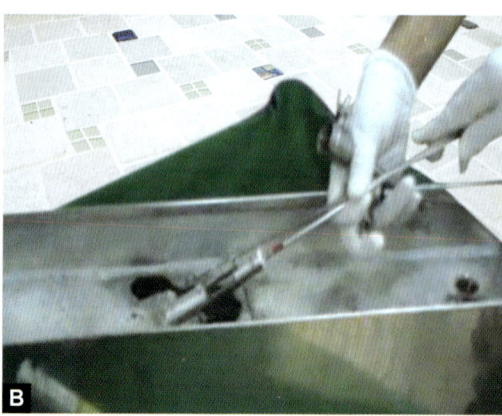
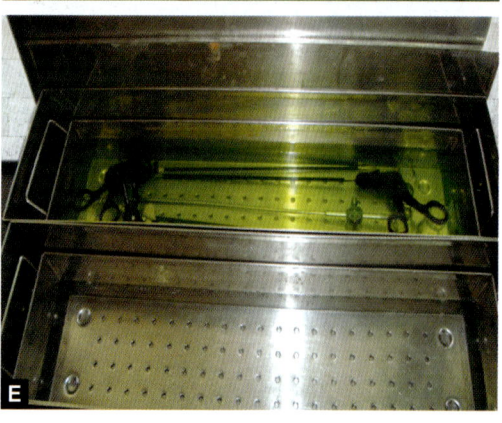
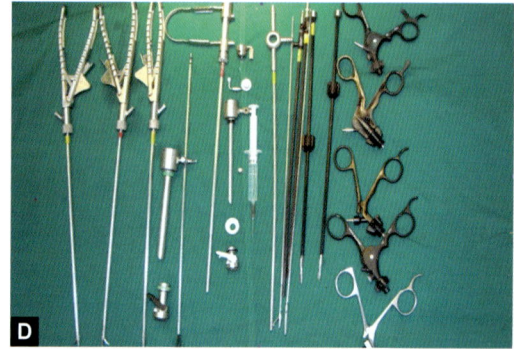
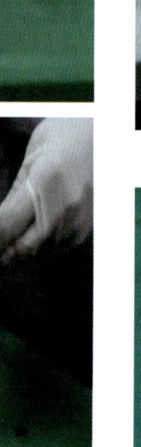

Figs 21.2A to E: Disinfecting/sterilizing through liquid chemical (CIDEX); (A) Disinfecting/sterilizing with liquid chemical (CIDEX), (B) Instruments cleaned in betadine scrub and H_2O_2, (C) Cleaning with brush and pad, (D) Instruments washed and kept on clean cloth (E) Immersing in CIDEX

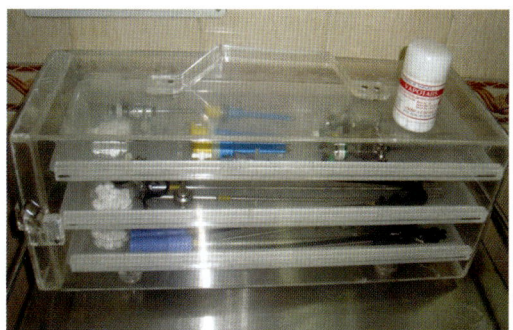

Fig. 21.3: Endo instruments carrying formalin chamber

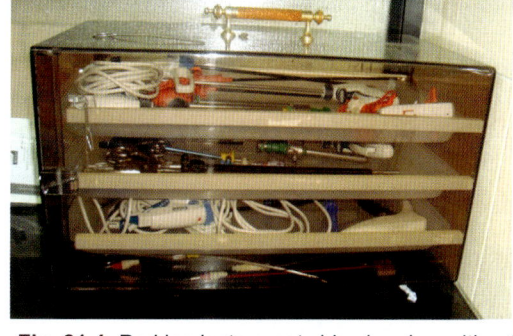

Fig. 21.4: Parking instruments big chamber without formalin

The instruments must be immersed in CIDEX for another 20 minutes. Thereafter, immerse these instruments in sterile water before using them for next procedure.

Disinfecting technique with formalin tablets for small nursing homes and clinics which do not have large autoclave to sterilize the laparoscopic instruments.

For a three tray acrylic laparoscopic instruments container use 90 to 100 tablets approximately 30 tablets in each tray. Open spread two gauze pieces, put 30 tablets in it, tie them together tightly and keep in each tray. Laboratory tests do show instruments cleaned in above solution and kept in the formalin chamber for 3 to 4 hours thoroughly get disinfected and are safe for direct use after thorough washing or rinsing in sterile water **(Fig. 21.3)**.

CARRYING STEAM STERILIZED INSTRUMENTS OUTSIDE THE HOSPITAL

Number of times, carrying special and personal instruments are essential. But they should be sterilized or disinfected in the same hospital in which it will be used. Carrying sterilized instruments, implants and devices in unsterile vehicles and carry bags is an open invitation for infection; particularly the cloth draped; which are not sealed airtight as such they are bound to get contaminated because they are transported in open environment. Therefore, if needed, it must be carried in special disinfected-air tight container with formalin tablets placed in four corners of the container (5 tablets in each corners). If required, use adhesive tapes to seal the container. The formalin tablets will help to maintain sterility of instruments to be used in another hospital. These small steps will help to prevent infection of instruments, implants and devices used in surgical procedure.

Clean instruments are kept in a big chamber without formalin tablets for easy removal **(Fig. 21.4)**.

Maintenance of rigid and flexible endoscopic or laparoscopic instruments in user friendly conditions.

Before actual use of endoscopic or laparoscopic instruments, take sufficiently long sterile empty tray, put one vial of 5 ml heparin 25000 IU in it, then pour 3 to 5 liters of sterile water, soak all instruments in it for 3 to 5 minutes, dry, wipe and use. Use of heparin prevents blood clotting inside the instrument rods and jaws. Retain this water and pour 2 percent of betadine scrub and hydrogen peroxide per liter in this water. Mix it properly and then soak the used instruments in this solution for 5 to 10 minutes before washing. Use any brush like nail brush, tooth brush etc. for cleaning the instruments.

Use of sterile camera cover on unsterile camera head to maintain sterility during surgical procedures.

This technique is unscientific or unsafe and does not give desirable protection from infection. This plastic camera cover cannot be sealed air tight on telescope. Therefore, infecting bacteria if any are allowed to travel from camera control unit, camera cord and head into the open cavity through telescope. Therefore, the camera head, light cord and CO_2 tube cautery cords kept in formalin chamber do disinfect entire imaging and connecting system. Namely from the camera, light, CO_2 and cautery control units to proximal and distal end of telescope and to connecting sockets of instruments **(Fig. 21.5)**. These items should be connected directly to the respective machines or units without wiping with sterile water, to retain the formalin effect and to detain the infecting bacteria at source. This technique maintains the sterility even when one requires changing or cleaning the telescope between the procedures.

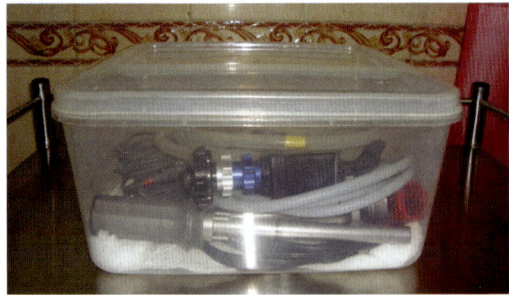

Fig. 21.5: Endocamera and morcellator kept in formalin chamber

In order to disinfect the above items for immediate next procedure, clean and remove the blood stains, if any. Use sterile water mixed with betadine scrub and hydrogen peroxide that is kept ready to clean the instruments. Wipe them dry. Thereafter, wipe and dry them with Sterillium or ordinary spirit and keep them in formalin chamber before initiating cleaning of instruments and floor. Allow them in formalin chamber till the second patient is anesthetized and draped. Since these are solid and jointless items and the CO_2 gas pipe remain untouched from inside 20 to 30 minute duration in formalin chamber is sufficient to disinfect these items, for use in next procedure.

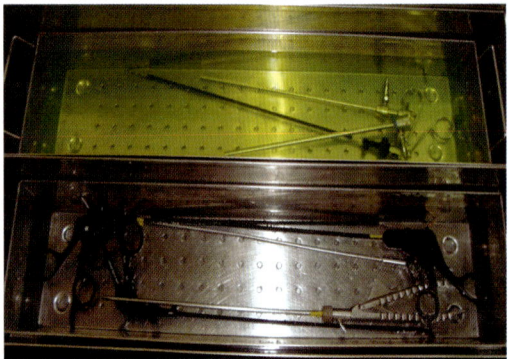

Fig. 21.6: Instruments washed in saline after sterilization in CIDEX

Note: Plastic camera cover is an obstacle for free adjustments and focusing of camera. But if still used then the plastic camera cover rolled on a camera head, light cord and CO_2 tube kept in formalin chamber may have added sterility and protection. Because all four, the camera, light cable, CO_2 tube and plastic camera cover remained sterile in respective sealed cover or chamber. Therefore, sterility is maintained even if one disconnects the camera head to clean or change the telescope during surgical procedure. The single tray container of these items must have 40 formalin tablets 20 each at both end or 10 each in four corners of container to disinfect them quickly and effectively.

Week end cleaning of instruments and imaging system of operating and IVF room.

Take a large tray and pour boiling water put betadine scrub and hydrogen peroxide at the rate of 2 percent per liter of water, dismantle or disconnect all possible instruments and use branded coconut oil or WD-40 spray to free the joints of instruments and keep them in this hot solution for 20 to 30 minutes and thereafter brush clean and wash under running water. Keep in a round straight container to drain and dry under the fan. Thereafter, if required dry them using oxygen or air jet and keep back in formalin chamber. The camera head, (if immersable) light cord, CO_2 tube, cautery cord etc. must be soaked for 10 to 20 minutes (with mild hot water) cleaned and dried identically.

Thorough weekend cleaning: The OT and IVF room cleaning must be carried out using above disinfecting solution. Even though this technique does give excellent result, fumigation of OT rooms is a must to disinfect the ceiling or roof and unreachable corners.

Very Important Information

Immersing the instruments in sterile water for 3 to 5 minutes before use, is very essential as CIDEX causes burning of hands and the fumes of CIDEX and formalin also irritate eyes **(Fig. 21.6)**. If this chemical content is allowed to enter in the open wound or cavity it will harm the internal organs and patient will experience increased postoperative pain, inflammation, irritation etc. The said pain does not mean the common surgical or interventional pain. This may prolong hospital stay; added discomfort and avoidable medication. Therefore, for the well being of patient, one must immerse the instruments in sterile water for 3 to 5 minutes, to remove chemical residuals from instruments before actual use.

Trouble shooting in rigid or flexible endoscopic procedures:

For blurred and unsatisfactary image

Keep dry gauze piece ready. Clean the camera head lens with wet gauze then immediately dry with clean dry gauze till the lens is crystal clear to the naked eye. Similarly, clean both end of telescope and ensure no visible filmy layer is seen. Alternatively, Sterillium can be used similarly. The CIDEX and soapy solutions if allowed to dry and not cleaned immediately and properly do produce a thin layer on telescope and camera lens.

CHAPTER 22

Medical Law—What is What and What is Not Medical Negligence

Gopinath N Shenoy

Chapter Outline
- Negligence and Rashness
- Standard or Degree of Skill and Care
- Criminal Negligence
- Accidents; Misadventures; Mishaps
- Error of Judgment
- Inherent Risks of Treatment
- Choice of Treatment—Discretion
- Guarantee and Warranty
- Vicarious Liability
- Deficiencies in Statutory Requirements

Law expects medical practitioners to render services which are free from "deficiencies".

The word "deficiencies" in services is defined by the Consumer Protection Act 1986 as:

"Deficiency" means any fault, imperfection, short coming or inadequacy in the quality, nature and manner of performance which is required to be maintained by or under any law for the time being in force or has been undertaken to be performed by a person in pursuance of a contract or otherwise in relation to any service. Presence of negligence in the services is actionable.

NEGLIGENCE AND RASHNESS

Negligence is opposite of diligence. Negligence and rashness usually go hand in hand. Eminent jurists and leading judgments have assigned various meanings to negligence. The concept as has been acceptable to Indian jurisprudential thought is well-stated in the Law of Torts, Ratanlal and Dhirajlal (Twenty-fourth Edition 2002, edited by Justice GP Singh). It is defined as:

"Negligence is the breach of a duty caused by the omission to do something which a reasonable man, guided by those considerations which ordinarily regulate the conduct of human affairs would do, or doing something which a prudent and reasonable man would not do."

In short, it can be an act of commission or an act of omission. An act committed which no reasonable prudent doctor (placed under the situation) would commit or an act omitted to be performed which a reasonable doctor would have undertaken.

According to Charlesworth and Percy on Negligence (Tenth Edition, 2001), the essential components of negligence are three: "duty", "breach" and "resulting damage", that is to say:
1. The existence of a duty to take care, which is owed by the defendant to the complainant.
2. The failure to attain that standard of care, prescribed by the law, thereby committing a breach of such duty.
3. Damage, which is both causally connected with such breach and recognized by the law, has been suffered by the complainant.

In Poonam Verma v. Ashwin Patel and Ors. (1996) 4 SCC 332 the Supreme Court has held that negligence has many manifestations—it may be active negligence, collateral negligence, comparative negligence, concurrent negligence, continued negligence, criminal negligence, gross negligence, hazardous negligence, active and passive negligence, willful or reckless negligence or negligence *per se*. Negligence *per se* is an act or an omission which is declared as negligence because it is in violation of a statute or valid ordinance, or because it is so palpably opposed to the dictates of common prudence.

In Indian Medical Association v. VP Shantha 1995 (6) SCC 651 it has been held that the following acts are clearly due to negligence:
i. Removal of the wrong limb.
ii. Performance of an operation on the wrong patient.
iii. Giving injection of a drug to which the patient is allergic without looking into the out-patient card containing the warning.
iv. Use of wrong gas during the course of an anesthetic, etc.
v. For negligence a medical practitioner can be taken to the Civil Courts, the Criminal Courts, Medical Councils or the Human Rights Commissions.

STANDARD OR DEGREE OF SKILL AND CARE

The degree of skill and care required by a medical practitioner is stated in Halsbury's Laws of England as under:

"The practitioner must bring to his task a reasonable degree of skill and knowledge, and must exercise a reasonable degree of care. Neither the very highest nor a very low degree of care and competence, judged in the light of the particular circumstances of each case, is what the law requires, and a person is not liable in negligence because someone else of greater skill and knowledge would have prescribed different treatment or operated in a different way; nor is he guilty of negligence if he has acted in accordance with a practice accepted as proper by a responsible body of medical men skilled in that particular art, even though a body of adverse opinion also existed among medical men. Deviation from normal practice is not necessarily evidence of negligence. To establish liability on that basis it must be shown: (1) that there is a usual and normal practice; (2) that the defendant has not adopted it; and (3) that the course in fact adopted is one no professional man of ordinary skill would have taken had he been acting with ordinary care."

MacNair, J in Bolam v. Friern Hospital Management Committee (1957) 2 All ER 118 (QBD held:

"Where you get a situation which involves the use of some special skill or competence, then the test as to whether there has been negligence or not is not the test of the man on the top of a clapham omnibus, because he has not got this special skill. The test is the standard of the ordinary skilled man exercising and professing to have that special skill. A man need not possess the highest expert skill ... It is well-established law that it is sufficient if he exercises the ordinary skill of an ordinary competent man exercising that particular art."

In Hucks v. Cole (1968) 118 New LJ 469, Lord Denning stated that a medical practitioner would be liable only where his conduct fell below that of the standards of a reasonably competent practitioner in his field.

Finally, Lord President Clyde in Hunter v. Hanley 1955 SLT 213 observed that the true test for establishing negligence in diagnosis or treatment on the part of a doctor is whether he has been proved to be guilty of such failure as no doctor of ordinary skill would be guilty of, if acting with ordinary care.

CRIMINAL NEGLIGENCE

For fixing criminal liability on a doctor or surgeon, the standard of negligence required to be proved should be so high as can be described as "gross negligence" or "recklessness". It is not merely lack of necessary care, attention and skill. The decision of the House of Lords in R. v. Adomako [(1993) 4 All ER 935; 15 BMLR 13; CA affirmed by (1994) 3 All ER 79 HL] relied upon on behalf of the doctor elucidates the said legal position and contains following observations:

"Thus a doctor cannot be held criminally responsible for patient's death unless his negligence or incompetence showed such disregard for life and safety of his patient as to amount to a crime against the State."

In Dr Suresh Gupta Petitioner v. Govt. of NCT of Delhi and Anr. Respondent [SC] 2004 AIR 4091, the Hon'ble Supreme Court has held:

Thus, when a patient agrees to go for medical treatment or surgical operation, every careless act of the medical man cannot be termed as 'criminal'. It can be termed 'criminal' only when the medical man exhibits a gross lack of competence or inaction and wanton indifference to his patient's safety and which is found to have arisen from gross ignorance or gross negligence. Where a patient's death results merely from error of judgment or an accident, no criminal liability should be attached to it. Mere inadvertence or some degree of want of adequate care and caution might create civil liability but would not suffice to hold him criminally liable.

This approach of the courts in the matter of fixing criminal liability on the doctors, in the course of medical treatment given by them to their patients, is necessary so that the hazards of medical men in medical profession being exposed to civil liability, may not unreasonably extend to criminal liability and expose them to risk of landing themselves in prison for alleged criminal negligence.

In Jacob Mathew v. State of Punjab and Anr. 2005(3) CPR 70 (SC), the Hon'ble Supreme Court has held:

In order to hold the existence of criminal rashness or criminal negligence it shall have to be found out that the rashness was of such a degree as to amount to taking a hazard knowing that the hazard was of such a degree that injury was most likely imminent. The element of criminality is introduced by the accused having run the risk of doing such an act with recklessness and indifference to the consequences.

ACCIDENTS; MISADVENTURES; MISHAPS

Courts have held that it would be wrong, and indeed bad law, to say that simply because a misadventure or mishap occurred, the hospital and the healthcare providers are thereby liable. It would be disastrous to the community if it were so (Hatcher v. Black (1954) Times, 2nd July).

A health-care provider is not an insurer; he does not warrant that his treatment will succeed or that he will perform a cure (Hunter v. Hanley (1955) SLT 213). Naturally he will not be liable if, a treatment which in ordinary circumstances would be sound, has unforeseen results. The standard of care which the law requires is not insurance against accident slips. It is not every slip or mistake that imports negligence. Law recognizes the dangers, which are inherent in surgical operations. Mistakes will occur on occasions despite the exercise of reasonable skill and care (Nathan, P C and Barrowclough, A R: Medical Negligence (1957).

ERROR OF JUDGMENT

An error of judgment does not of itself amount to negligence [Whitehouse v. Jordan (1981) 1 WLR 246]. Law allows errors of judgment which do not by themselves amount to negligence. The House of Lords in England held that some errors of judgment may be negligent and some may not. The error of judgment committed by a health-care provider may or may not be indicative of negligence, but the proper test to be applied is whether he abided by the standards laid down by his peers (Bolam's Test).

The courts have held "No human being is infallible and in the present state of science even the most eminent specialist may be at fault in detecting the true nature of the diseased condition. A practitioner can only be liable in this respect if his diagnosis is so palpably wrong as to prove negligence, that is to say, if his mistake is of such a nature as to imply absence of reasonable skill and care on his part, regard being had to the ordinary level of skill in the practitioner (Mitchel v. Dicksen 1954 APPD 519)."

With regard to junior health-care provider inexperience is no defense. He must meet the standard of care expected of his rank and status (Anesthesiology and the Law of Medical Negligence Dr Gopinath Shenoy and Dr Gayatri G Shenoy Ritanjan Publications 2002).

INHERENT RISKS OF TREATMENT

Every procedure has its own risk factors. Just because one of these factors becomes manifest does not mean that the health-care provider is negligent and his services defective. He can be held negligent only when the standard of care exhibited by him falls below the standards expected of a reasonable prudent health-care provider practicing under the circumstances he is placed in [Hatcher v. Black (1954) Times, 2nd July].

CHOICE OF TREATMENT—DISCRETION

Many medical problems can be managed or treated in more than one ways. Health-care providers have the discretion to choose the line of treatment they wish to adopt and can be faulted for the same only if their choice is palpably wrong and or dangerous to the patient. When there are two genuinely responsible schools of thought about the management of a clinical situation, the courts could do no greater disservice to the community or the advancement of medical science than to place the hall-mark of legality upon one form of treatment (Moore v. Lewisham Group Hospital Management Committee (1959) Times 5, February). A health-care provider is not liable for taking one choice out of two or for favouring one school rather than another (Hucks v. Cole and Anr. (1968) 118 NLJ 469). He is only liable when he falls below the standard of a reasonably competent practitioner in his field. In the realm of diagnosis and treatment there is ample scope of genuine difference of opinion and a health-care provider clearly is not negligent merely because his conclusion differs from that of other professional men, nor because he has displayed less skill or knowledge than others would have shown. If a health-care provider has followed a course of treatment or procedures accepted by and followed by a responsible section of the profession, he would not be guilty of negligence even if another section of the profession does not subscribe to that practice and follow a different course (AS Mittal v. State of UP. AIR 1989 SC 1570). A health-care provider has discretion in choosing the treatment which he proposes to give to the patient and such discretion is wider in cases of emergency, but he must bring to his task a reasonable degree of skill and knowledge and must exercise a reasonable degree of care according to the circumstances of each case (Laxman B. Joshi v. Trimbak Bapu Godbole and Anr. 1969 (1) SCR 2060.

GUARANTEE AND WARRANTY

Law does not expect health-care providers to guarantee the results of their services.

The Hon'ble Supreme Court in Jacob Mathew Petitioner v. State of Punjab and Anr. Respondent 2005(3) CPR 70 (SC) holds:

"He does not assure his client of the result. A lawyer does not tell his client that the client shall win the case in all circumstances. A physician would not assure the patient of full recovery in every case. A surgeon cannot and does not guarantee that the result of surgery would invariably be beneficial, much less to the extent of 100 percent for the person operated on. The only assurance which such a professional can give or can be understood to have given by implication is that he is possessed of the requisite skill in that branch of profession which he is practicing and while undertaking the performance of the task entrusted to him he would be exercising his skill with reasonable competence. This is all what the person approaching the professional can expect."

VICARIOUS LIABILITY

Liability which is incurred for, or instead of, another can be defined as vicarious liability. Every person is responsible for his own acts or omissions but there are circumstances where for the acts committed by a person, the liability comes to lie, not on that person, but on someone else. A master is liable for the acts or omissions of his servant and the principal is accountable for the acts of his agent. The hospital authorities are responsible for the whole of their staff, not only for the nurses and the doctors but also for the anesthetist and the surgeons. It does not matter whether they are permanent or temporary, resident or visiting, whole-time or part-time. The hospital authority is responsible for all of them. The reason is because even if they are not servants, they are the agents of the hospital to give the treatment. The only exception is the case of consultants and anesthetists selected and employed by the patient himself (Roe v. Minister of Health and Anr. Court of Appeal. (1954) 2 QB 66).

DEFICIENCIES IN STATUTORY REQUIREMENTS

To practice medicine without proper registration with the State Medical Council or the Medical Council of India would violate the provisions of law [Indian Medical Council (Professional conduct, Etiquette and Ethics) Regulations, 2002]. So also employing staff that is unqualified will violate the provisions of the Indian Medical Council (Professional conduct, Etiquette and Ethics) Regulations, 2002 as formulated by the Medical Council of India. Institutions where medical termination of pregnancy is undertaken must also be registered with the Appropriate Authority under the Medical Termination of Pregnancy Act 1971. Ratios of judge-made laws or precedents are also applicable and binding on the health-care providers and violation of the same also constitutes and offence that is actionable. Cross-pathy practice, that is, an allopathic practitioner prescribing ayurvedic drugs is bad in law (Poonam Verma v. Ashwin Patel and Ors. Supreme Court Civil Appeal No. 8856 of 1994. Decided on 10th May, 1996). Cross-speciality practice, that is, a surgeon undertaking a hysterectomy is also considered improper. Undertaking a tube ligation without the consent of the spouse is similarly actionable [Prasanth S. Dhananka v. Nizam's Institute of Medical Sciences and Ors. 1986-99 CONSUMER 3299 (NS)].

Lord Justice Denning explained the law on the subject of negligence against health-care providers and hospitals in the following words: "Before I consider the individual facts, I ought to explain to you the law on this matter of negligence against doctors and hospitals. Mr. Marvan Evertt sought to liken the case against a hospital to a motor car accident or to an accident in a factory. That is the wrong approach. In the case of accident on the road, there ought not to be any accident if everyone used proper care; and the same applies in a factory; but in a hospital when a person who is ill goes in for treatment, there is always some risk, no matter what care is used. Every surgical operation involves risks. It would be wrong, and indeed bad law, to say that simply because a misadventure or mishap occurred, the hospital and the doctors are thereby liable. It would be disastrous to the community if it were so. It would mean that a doctor examining a patient or a surgeon operating at a table instead of getting on with his work, would be forever looking over shoulder to see if someone was coming up with a dagger; for an action for negligence against a doctor is for him like unto a dagger. His professional reputation is as dear to him as his body, perhaps more so, and an action for negligence can wound his reputation as severely as a dagger can his body. You must not, therefore, find him negligent simply because something happens to go wrong; if, for instance, one of the risk inherent in an operation actually takes place or some complication ensues which lessens or takes away the benefits that were hoped for, or if in a matter of opinion he makes an error of judgment. You should only find him guilty of negligence when he falls short of the standard of a reasonably skilful medical man" (Hatcher v. Black (1954) Times, 2nd July).

ACKOWLEDGMENTS

Dr Gopinath N Shenoy is an Obstetrician/Gynecologist and a medicolegal consultant and specializes in the defense of doctors in the Consumer Forums/Commissions. He was a Member of the Consumer Court, Mumbai, Govt. of Maharashtra. He is an Honorary Assistant Professor of Obstetrics and Gynecology at the KJ Somaiya Medical College, Mumbai. He was also a Visiting Professor of Law at law colleges in Mumbai. Currently, he is a postgraduate examiner in law (LLM and PhD), Bombay University.

INDEX

Page numbers followed by *f* refer to figure

A

Abdominal
  ectopic pregnancy 67
  scars 25
  wall
    thickness 25
    vessels 25
Adenoma
  mapping 99*f*
  on hysteroscopy 97
  on laparoscopy 97
  with anterior adhesions 99*f*
  with fibroid 98*f*
  with posterior adhesions 99*f*
Adenomyoma 97*f*
  resection by elliptical
    incision 100*f*
Adhesiolysis 26
Advanced gynec surgery 144
Advantages
  and use of electrolyte and
    nonelectrolyte 114
  of single incision mini-sling
    160
AIDA video capturing system 8*f*
Allen stirrups 71*f*
Alligator forceps 16
Anesthesia
  for gynecological laparoscopic
    surgery 36
  for hysteroscopy 35
  pendent 5*f*
Anterior compartment 90*f*
Appearance of ovaries after
  reconstruction 76*f*
Appropriate training 135
Asherman's syndrome 26
Aspiration needle 17
Assisted reproductive
  technologies 59

B

Babcock/oval grasper 16
Barbed sutures 109, 157
Beginning of surgery 44

Betadine scrub and hydrogen
  peroxide solution 167*f*
Bettochi operative hysteroscopic
  sheath 23
Bidirectional barbed suture 158*f*
Bilateral proximal tubal
  occlusion 27*f*
Bipolar
  coagulation-secondary trocar
    vessel injury 149*f*
  forceps 19
  loops 122*f*
  resectoscope 116*f*
Bladder injury 88
  during laparoscopic surgery
    150*f*
Blood pressure 37
Bowel injury 88, 148
Broken myoma screw in
  fibroid 153*f*
Bulking injections 127
Bulky uterus with
  endometriosis 86

C

Calcified tape in bladder 132*f*
Cardiac arrhythmias 37
Case of previous cesarean
  section 85
Ceiling mounted instrument
  carts 6*f*
Cervical
  ectopic pregnancy 66
  softening 117
  stump being sutured 87*f*
Cervicoisthmic mesh fixation 92*f*
Circumferential incision around
  cervix 82*f*
Classification of adenomyosis 96*f*
Claw forceps 15, 15*f*
Clip applicator 20
Closure of uterine flap 54
CO_2 insufflator 11, 11*f*
Collin's knife 119*f*, 120*f*
Combination of regional
  anesthesia 41

Company pressure/temptation 160
Complications of
  laparoscopic surgery 143
  trocar-cannula 148
  Veress needle 147
Concomitant incontinence 135
Concurrent laparoscopy 117
Conservative medical therapy of
  ectopic pregnancy 60
Contraceptive devices 58
Contraindication
  for laparoscopic
    hysterectomy 79
  of hysteroscopy 117
Contralateral suturing 108
Cooper's ligament 128
Cornual
  resection 69*f*
    and salpingectomy
      technique 64
  suturing 69*f*
Correction of retroflexion of
  uterus 72
    with spill of chocolate
      material 72*f*
Creation of pneumoperitoneum 39
Criminal negligence 173
Culdocentesis 59
Cystectomy 74
Cystoscopic right ureteric
  stenting 150*f*

D

Debulking of uterus 83
Dedicated bipolar unit 13*f*
Deeper dissection 136
Degree angulation of shaft
  pushing needle 130*f*
Demonstrable stress urinary
  incontinence 127*f*
Dissecting forceps 16
Dissection of tissue around
  vessels with coagulation 81*f*
Distending media
  delivery 114
  for hysteroscopy 113

Double channel diagnostic
    hysteroscopic sheath 21f
Dysmenorrhea 100

E

Ectopic pregnancy 26, 58, 59, 69, 144
Electronic CO_2 insufflator 46f
Electrosurgical unit 116f
Endo stitch 158f
Endocamera and morcellator kept in formalin chamber 170f
Endomat 12
    inflow pressure 46f
Endometrial
    carcinoma 32f
    polypectomy 32f
    resection 122
Endometriomas 86f
Endometriosis 32, 86f, 144
Endoscope cleaning and storing 5f
Endoscopic surgery 26
Endosuturing 84
Endovision camera 10
Enterocele 93, 93f
Enucleation of cyst 74f, 75f
Equipment organization 8
Ergonomics in laparoscopy 7
Essentials for safe management of female urinary incontinence 126
Ethicon endosurgery 156f
Etiology of ectopic pregnancy 58
Excision of
    ectopic mass 67f
    horn 66f
Extraction of myoma 55, 55f
Extraperitoneal laparoscopic surgery 41

F

Fibroids 31
Fixed column gas outlet 4f
Foley's catheter 82
    tamponade-secondary trocar vessel injury 149f
Full thickness vaginal dissection 136f

G

Gasless laparoscopy 143
Glycine toxicity 36
Graft
    augmentation 136f
    replacement 136f

Graspers 105f
Gyncological endoscopy and minimal access surgery 143
Gynecare 159f

H

Heterotopic pregnancy 68
Hydrodissection 136, 136f
Hypothermia 147
Hysteroscopic
    anatomy of uterus 112
    lateral metroplasty 30f
    myomectomy 30
    surgery 144
        for intrauterine septum 143
    tubal cannulation 27, 118, 118f
Hysteroscopy 28f-30f, 112f
    endometrial ablation and resection 143f
    instruments 21
    uterine cornua 113f

I

Increased endometrial vascularity on hysteroscopy 98f
Indications of laparoscopic hysterectomy 78
Inferior epigastric artery 149f
Infertility 59
    treatment and ART 58
Injection
    needle 17, 17f
    of dilute vasopressin in fibroid 151f
Instrument cart 6
Instrumentation for hysteroscopy 115
Interstitial pregnancy 64
Intracorporeal
    ligation of inferior epigastric vessel 149f
    slip knot 101f
    technique 100
Intramyometrial cyst containing chocolate color fluid 98f
Intrauterine
    adhesions 28, 28f, 120f
    and cornual pregnancy 69f
    septum 26
Introduction of Veress needle and trocars 47
Inverted triangle shape of uterine cavity 113f
Ipsilateral suturing 107
Irrigation with fluid warmer 7f

K

Knee operated scrub sink 5f
Knot pusher 18

L

Laparoscope 13f
Laparoscopic
    adenomyomectomy 96
    adhesiolysis 143
    assisted vaginal
        hysterectomy 143, 156
    colposuspension 143
    hysterectomy 143
    instrument trolley 43f
    management of
        ectopic pregnancy 143
        ovarian cysts 143
        tubal pregnancy 64
        tubo-ovarian mass 143
    microsurgical tubal anastomosis 143
    myomectomy 143
    removal of broken myoma screw 153f
    retrieval bags 20
    round ligament plication 33
    sacrocervicopexy 92f
    salpingostomy and fimbrioplasty 143
    sterilization 143, 144
    supracervical hysterectomy 143
    surgery 143f
        for pelvic pain 143
    tissue approximation 143
    treatment of
        advanced endometriosis 143
        ovarian endometriomas 143
    uterine nerve ablation 143
Laparoscopy 31f, 33f, 60, 143, 144
    benign cystic teratomas 31f
    during pregnancy 143
    endometrioma 32f
    instruments 13
    team 6f
Large foot step 8f
Laryngeal mask airways 40f
Last part of tape in bladder 132f
Lateral peritoneal dissection 92f
Left
    ovarian ectopic pregnancy 67f
    salpingolysis 73f
    tubal ectopic 61f

Index

Leiomyomas and endometrial polyps 120
Levator ani muscle plication repair 93
Light cable 11
Linear salpingostomy 61
  technique 61f
Location of standard port placement 49
Lysis of intrauterine adhesions 120

M

Maintenance of pneumoperitoneum 39
Management of
  abdominal pregnancy 68
  ectopic pregnancy 26
  tubal ectopic pregnancy 60
Maryland grasper 16
Menstrual loss 100
Metallic reusable veress needle 13f
Metroplasty 118
Mild endometriosis 71
Mini-sling 160f
Monopolar
  cylindrical electrode for resectoscope 22f
  loops 122f
  puncture needle 16, 17f
Morcellated
  fibroid 20f
  pieces of uterus 87f
Morcellator 20, 20f, 159
Multiparameter monitor with display 47f
Multiseptate ovarian tumor 33
Myoma screw 18, 80

N

Needle
  holders 18, 105f
  insertion 106
  removal 108

O

Obturator foramen 130f
Operation
  table 6
  theater set-up 6, 43
    for safe gynecological endoscopy 3
Operative
  channel sheath 21
  hysteroscopy 117
  sheath 21f

Ovarian
  cyst 31, 31f
  cystectomy 144
  drilling 144
  ectopic pregnancy 66
  reconstruction 75f
    without suturing 76f
  tissue 74f
Ovariolysis assisted with third grasper 73f

P

Parking instruments big chamber without formalin 169f
Pelvis after conservative surgery 76f
Persistent ectopic pregnancy 62
Pneumo-omentum 148f
Pneumoperitoneum 39
Polycystic ovaries 143
Port placement 49f, 52, 105, 106f
Postabortion fetal bone 32f
Postadenomyomectomy cesarean section 102f
Postanesthesia care unit 5, 6f
Posterior vaginal wall repair 93
Posthysterectomy bleeding controlled by bipolar 152f
Posthysterectomy adhesions 33f
Postmenopausal bleeding 32
Postoperative care 94, 165
Pregnancy
  in rudimentary horn 64
  rates 100
Preoperative adenoma mapping 99
Preparation of endometrium 117
Presacral space dissection 92f
Primary trocars and cannula 14
Principles of laparoscopic hemostasis 143
Promonto fixation 92f
Proximal tubal occlusion 27
Puncture needle 17f

Q

Qadar's technique 88

R

Radical surgical treatment 63
Removal of
  ectopic 61f
  intrauterine foreign bodies 118
  IUD 118

Resectoscope 115f
  sheath 22
    with obturator 22f
Retrieval system in minimal invasive surgery 143
Right
  Cooper's ligament stitch 128f
  paraurethral helical stitch 128f
  rudimentary horn pregnancy 66f
Robotic sacrocolpopexy 93
Role of
  laparoscopic ultrasonography 143
  laparoscopy in
    abdominal pain syndromes 143
    gynecological malignancy 143

S

Sacrocervicopexy 91, 91f
Sacrocolpopexy 92, 93f, 138
Sacrospinous anchor in place 137f
Safe
  anesthesia for gynecological endoscopic surgery 35
  management of female urinary incontinence 126
Salpingectomy 144
Salpingo-ovariolysis 72, 74f
Salpingotomy 61f
Scissors and grasper for operative channel 22f
Seamless corners 4f
Secondary trocar vessel injury 149f
Septal resection 29f
Septate uterus 29f
Severe endometriosis 71f
Sexual function 135
Silastic ring applicator 20
  with loader 20f
Simple gynec operation table 43f
Single
  chip camera 10
  port access surgery instruments 21
  site laparoscopy access system 156f
Sites of ectopic pregnancy 59
Skin excision 136
Space of Retzius
  bladder 128f
  dissected urethra 128f
Spatula 17

Spoon forceps 15
Static posture 7
Steps of supracervical
　hysterectomy 87f
Sterile store station 5f
Sterilization and disinfections in
　laparoscopy 143
Storage inside operation
　theater 5f
Strategies for laparoscopic
　diagnosis of malignancy 143
Strengthening of myoma scar 56
Stress urinary incontinence 127f,
　159
Subendometrial adenoma on
　hysteroscopy 98f
　USG 97
Submucous
　fibroid 30f
　myomas and polyps 26
Suction
　cannula 17
　irrigation equipment 7
Superficial endometrial
　implants 71f
Supracervical hysterectomy 87, 88
Surgical
　management 60
　team 6
　technique 90
　trauma 38
Suture material 108
Suturing tubal incision 61f

T

Targeted hysteroscopic
　biopsy 118, 118f
Technical complications with
　instruments 152
Technique of
　adenomyoma resection 99
　endosuturing 100

panoramic hysteroscopy 117
salpingectomy 63f
segmental resection 62
endosuturing 101f
Tenaculum forceps 15
Tension free trot 130f
Three chip camera 10, 10f
Total laparoscopic
　hysterectomy 156
Training and credentialing in
　endoscopic surgery 141
Transvaginal
　ultrasonography 59, 96
Treatment of
　cervical ectopic pregnancy 66
　endometriosis in infertility 26
　heterotopic pregnancy 68
　interstitial pregnancy 64
　ovarian ectopic pregnancy 67
Trendelenburg position 39
Trivedi's
　adjustable tape 131, 131f
　obturator tape 127
Trocar
　and cannula 14
　placement 90f
T-shaped uterus 29f
Tubal
　cannulation 26
　factor 27
Types of
　hysterectomy 87
　laparoscopes 13f

U

Umbilical trocar inside adherent
　bowel 148f
Umbilicus 25
Unruptured tubal pregnancy 26f
Ureteric injury 88
Urinary
　retention 93
　tract injury 93

Urodynamics study strip 127f
Uterine
　artery bleeding 149f
　fibroid 31f, 121f
　polyp 121f
　prolapse 91
　septal resection with scissors
　　119f
　septum 29f, 118
Uterosacral
　dissected with harmonic 81f
　ligament
　　suspension 91f
　　uterine suspension 91

V

Vagina 82f
Vaginal
　closure 137
　remodeling 137
　tube 19, 19f
　vault
　　prolapse 91
　　sutured with interrupted
　　　stitches 82f
　　vertical incision 129f
Vault prolapse 92f
Venous gas embolism 37
Veress needle 13, 53f
Versapoint-gynecare bipolar
　generator 116f
Vessel
　injury 149
　sealing device ligasure 156f
Video
　demonstrations 144
　hysteroscopy 117
　monitors 7, 11

W

Weakening of scar 56f